Essentials of Teaching and Learning
in Nursing Ethics

University of Ulster
K   ANSTOWN

Commissioning Editor: Susan Young
Development Editor: Catherine Jackson
Project Manager: Frances Affleck
Designer: Stewart Larking

Essentials of Teaching and Learning in Nursing Ethics

Perspectives and Methods

Anne J. Davis RN PhD DSc(Hon) FAAN

Professor Emerita, Professor of Nursing Ethics, University of California, San Francisco, USA;
Professor Emerita, Professor of Nursing Foundations, Nagano College of Nursing,
Komagane, Japan

Verena Tschudin RN PhD

Editor, Nursing Ethics; *Reader in Nursing Ethics, University of Surrey, Guildford, UK*

Louise de Raeve PhD RGN

Lecturer, School of Health Science, University of Wales, Swansea, UK

Forewords by

The late Margretta Madden Styles RN EdD FAAN

Consultant; Professor Emerita, University of California, San Francisco, USA; Past President, American Nurses Association; Past President, International Council of Nurses

Mo Im Kim RN PhD

Dean and Professor, Red Cross School of Nursing, Seoul, South Korea; Former Minister of Health, South Korea; Past President, International Council of Nurses

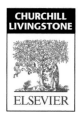

EDINBURGH LONDON NEW YORK OXFORD PHILADELPHIA ST LOUIS SYDNEY TORONTO 2006

CHURCHILL
LIVINGSTONE
ELSEVIER

First published 2006

ISBN 0 443 07480 1

British Library Cataloguing in Publication Data
A catalogue record for this book is available from the British Library

Library of Congress Cataloging in Publication Data
A catalog record for this book is available from the Library of Congress

Notice
Knowledge and best practice in this field are constantly changing. As new research and experience broaden our knowledge, changes in practice, treatment and drug therapy may become necessary or appropriate. Readers are advised to check the most current information provided (i) on procedures featured or (ii) by the manufacturer of each product to be administered, to verify the recommended dose or formula, the method and duration of administration, and contraindications. It is the responsibility of the practitioner, relying on their own experience and knowledge of the patient, to make diagnoses, to determine dosages and the best treatment for each individual patient, and to take all appropriate safety precautions. To the fullest extent of the law, neither the publisher nor the editors assumes any liability for any injury and/or damage.

The Publisher

your source for books, journals and multimedia in the health sciences

www.elsevierhealth.com

Working together to grow
libraries in developing countries

www.elsevier.com | www.bookaid.org | www.sabre.org

ELSEVIER   BOOK AID International   Sabre Foundation

The Publisher's policy is to use **paper manufactured from sustainable forests**

Printed in China

Contents

Biographies of contributors

Eli Haugen Bunch

In 1982 I received my doctorate from the University of California, San Francisco (UCSF) and returned to Norway as a research consultant with the Norwegian Nurses' Association. In this role I helped to develop and maintain the financing of the Center for Medical Ethics in Oslo that awards doctorates in medical ethics to health science students. Later, at the Institute of Nursing Science, University of Oslo, I taught healthcare ethics and research ethics courses. Now I am also engaged in the UCSF International HIV/AIDS Nursing Research Network and collecting data. I lecture widely in the Nordic countries on grounded theory as a research method.

Anne J. Davis

During 34 years at the University of California, San Francisco, I taught nursing ethics, served as a member of the Clinical Ethics Committee and the Research Ethics Committee, developed the Ethics Committee at a local hospice, chaired the California Nurses Association and the American Nurses Association Ethics Committees and worked with graduate students on research. I have visited 120 countries, working in the Middle East, Europe, Africa, India, and China. For six years I taught nursing in Japan. My research interests are end-of-life ethics and international nursing ethics. My honours include an honorary doctorate from Emory University and the first ANA Human Rights Award.

Louise de Raeve

In the early 1970s I began general nursing training, having first completed a philosophy degree.

It seemed an odd combination then but with the growth of healthcare ethics, I studied the subject and then took a teaching post in 1991 as the Macmillan Lecturer in Nursing Ethics, University of Wales, Swansea. More recently, my focus changed and I currently help run an MSc in Advanced Clinical Practice and teach clinical supervision skills. My belief in the value of supervision for nurses stems from my earlier experiences in a therapeutic community. I am also training as a psychoanalytic psychotherapist and hope to qualify in 2006.

Leyla Dinç

I graduated from nursing college in 1986 and worked as a clinical nurse at a university hospital for five years. In 1993 I received my Masters degree and in 1998 my doctorate in nursing. Since 1991 I have been on the faculty of Hacettepe University School of Nursing, Ankara, where I teach Nursing History and Ethics and with colleagues, Fundamentals of Nursing. I am a member of several national nursing organizations and serve as member of the Editorial Board on the journal *Nursing Ethics*. My major research focus is nursing ethics and teaching ethics to nursing students.

Theresa Drought

I recently joined the nursing faculty at the University of Virginia after seven years as co-director of the Northern California Kaiser Permanente Ethics Department. In California, I helped to establish a state nursing association, a regional collaborative group addressing ethical issues in long-term care, and a state-wide organization dealing with issues at the end of life. I have served as bioethics consultant to the California Medical Association, chair of the state's nursing association's ethics committee, and member of the American Nurses Association task force that produced the Code of Ethics for Nurses, 2001. My research focuses on medical decision-making and the discourse around the end of life.

Steven Edwards

I am a professor in the Centre for Philosophy, Humanities and Law in Healthcare, University of Wales, Swansea. I have authored books on philosophy of mind, relativism, nursing ethics, philosophy of nursing, and most recently, philosophy of disablement. In addition, I have published numerous articles in scholarly journals and with Joan Liaschenko, I am founding co-editor of the journal *Nursing Philosophy*.

Marsha Fowler

At present I am Professor of Ethics and Spirituality at Azusa Pacific University, California. I have taught ethics and served as an ethics consultant for the past 30 years. I am past chair of the California and the American Nurses Association ethics committees and was a member of the task force for the revision of the ANA Code of Ethics 1993–2001. For ten years I served as consultant on nursing education to the Ministry of Health, Republic of Russia. I am a recipient of the American Nurses Association's Honorary Human Rights Award. I am an ordained minister in the Presbyterian Church and I am a wood-worker, making furniture.

Ann Gallagher

I have a long-standing interest in, and concern with, the promotion of professional ethics in health care. I trained as a general nurse in Ireland and came to England to pursue mental health nursing training. Studies in philosophy and applied ethics followed and I became increasingly interested in ethics education in health care. My research includes empirical work relating to dignity in health care and theoretical work in relation to virtue ethics, human rights, and the teaching of ethics. Recent research interests include information giving in mental health and professional mis-

conduct. At the time of writing I worked at the Open University, England, overseeing a work-based, distance-learning curriculum. I am currently Senior Research follow at Kingston University, UK.

Nelly Garzón

After graduation from nursing school in Colombia, I received my BSN and MSN degrees in the USA. At the Faculty of Nursing, National University, Colombia I was Director of Postgraduate Education. Later I was Director, Planning Office of Human Resources, Ministry of Health and then Director, Academic Development, Ministry of Education. I studied bioethics at the Kennedy Institute, USA and the National Center of Bioethics, Bogotá. I have been active in the Colombian Nursing Association and served as President of the National Tribunal of Nursing Ethics. I served on the ICN Board of Directors and was ICN President 1985–1989. For the last 15 years I have taught nursing ethics and bioethics.

Chris Gastmans

As Associate Professor of Healthcare Ethics at the Catholic University of Leuven, Belgium, I teach and conduct research in the field of nursing ethics, care ethics, end-of-life ethics and empirical ethics. I chair several ethics committees in hospitals in Flanders. I am involved in national and European research projects on codes of ethics in nursing, suicide in elderly people, the involvement of nurses in euthanasia, and institutional ethics policies on euthanasia. In 2002, I was elected secretary-general of the European Association of Centers for Medical Ethics (EACME).

Maria Gasull

I began my professional career as a midwife and worked in delivery rooms for 11 years in Barcelona. In 1980 I became interested in nursing ethics and began to develop and teach ethics programmes at the University Nursing School of Sant Pau (Universitat Autonoma Barcelona) and still do. I have been a member of the Hospital Ethics Committee and the Advisory Committee on Bioethics for the Autonomous Catalan Government. At present, I am a member of the Deontological Commission of the Catalan Royal

College of Nursing and am working on national research concerning living wills for elderly people.

Miriam Hirschfeld

After receiving my doctorate from the University of California, San Francisco in 1978, I taught at Tel Aviv University and worked on a team to develop Chronic Care and Aging Programs for the Israeli General Federation of Labor Sick Fund. I worked at the World Health Organization, Geneva, in various positions including Chief Nurse Scientist and Director for home-based and long-term care from 1989 to 2002. My work has been recognized with several honours, including two honorary doctoral degrees. I have published widely, mostly on long-term care. At present I hold the position of Professor in the Department of Health Care Systems at Yezreel Valley College, Israel.

Emiko Konishi

For the past ten years I was a professor at Nagano College of Nursing where I chaired the Fundamentals of Nursing Department. I conducted research on ethical issues with Anne Davis when she taught there. I taught the graduate ethics course and was principal professor for graduate students' ethics research. As head of the International and Cross Cultural Nursing Research Center at the college, I chaired the Planning Committee and hosted the 2003 regional conference on Cross Cultural Nursing Research Collaboration in the Asia-Pacific region. My present position is Professor at Oita University of Nursing and Health Sciences, Japan.

Joan Liaschenko

As faculty in the Center for Bioethics and School of Nursing, University of Minnesota, I teach ethics to masters and doctoral nursing students and participate in ethics education in the medical and, occasionally, veterinary schools. My seven cats are particularly pleased about the latter. Feminist ethics seeks to dissolve hierarchies based on status and privilege and replace them by forms of social organization characterized by relationships of mutuality, respect, and friendship. In this book about teaching nursing ethics, it seems appropriate to say that, as a doctoral student at the University of California, San Francisco, I had, and still

have, just such a relationship with my mentor, Anne Davis.

Adamson Muula

I studied medicine at Flinders University, Australia and College of Medicine, Malawi, public health at Loma Linda University's Kenya programme, and palliative medicine in Uganda. My research interests include communicable diseases, medical ethics, health rights and human health resources. I served on the Malawi Medical Council Board, as Steering Committee member, Regional Network for Equity in Health, and as Director of the World Association of Medical Editors and founding member, Forum for African Medical Editors. Now I am Associate Editor of the *Malawi Medical Journal*. I practise medicine part time and am technical advisor to the Malawi National Assembly's Health and Population Committee.

John Paley

After a career as a jobbing researcher – doing it, teaching it, supervising it, managing it – I became a philosopher again – I already had a degree in philosophy. I still supervise empirical research and I am the director of Stirling University's clinical doctorate programme, which is the best course I have ever been associated with. I have also worked in publishing and have written a ton of open learning materials. In real life, I play bass in an old codgers' rock band, write weird comedy dramas and am obsessed with designer games (Die Siedler von Catan, not Monopoly). My current research interest is clinical cognition.

Samantha Pang

As Professor at Hong Kong Polytechnic University I teach, conduct research, and publish in the areas of nursing ethics, caring ethics, and decision-making of patients with advanced chronic disease. My nursing practice has been primarily focused on older adults with advanced chronic illnesses. I obtained my doctorate from the University of Hong Kong in 1999 and in 2002 received one of the first Fulbright Hong Kong Scholars awards to study cross-cultural differences in end-of-life decisions in the USA. As an editorial board member of *Nursing Ethics* and the International Center for Nursing Ethics, University of Surrey,

I am actively involved in studies of nursing ethics internationally.

Elizabeth Peter

I am an Associate Professor, Faculty of Nursing and member of the Joint Center for Bioethics, University of Toronto, Canada. I consider myself to be a highly fortunate individual in that I have been able to pursue two of my academic passions – nursing and philosophy – simultaneously. Both my undergraduate and graduate students challenge me to keep the theory of nursing and healthcare ethics relevant to practice and policy. I have learned as much from them as they have from me. I write widely in the field of nursing ethics and address ethical issues in home and community care.

Elizabeth Rozsos

Since 1992 I have taught nursing ethics at Semmelweis University Department of Nursing and Health Education Pedagogy, Budapest, Hungary. I led the Ethics Committee of the Hungarian Nursing Society from 1993 to 1998 and was a Consultant Editor of the journal *Nursing Ethics*. In Budapest I was the first hospital patient advocate. I served as member of the Ethics Committee for Clinical Pharmacology, Ministry of Welfare, and president of the Ethics Board for the Hungarian Association of Health Professionals. I published my first book for nurses in 1995, and a second in 2000, entitled *Knowing about nursing ethics*.

Nili Tabak

I am currently head of the Nursing Department and the Ethics Unit in the School of Professional Health at Tel Aviv University, Israel. I have a doctorate in nursing and an LL.B. in law. My main research interests are in psychogeriatrics, law and ethics. I attended law school at the same time as one of my sons was a student there.

Verena Tschudin

I became interested in ethics as a consequence of having trained as a counsellor in the late 1970s. Both disciplines continue to inspire me. Through the journal *Nursing Ethics*, which I have edited since its beginning, the international aspects of nursing and ethics have become increasingly relevant and also fascinating. Perhaps the best job I now have is looking for and helping to select the people for the yearly Human Rights and Nursing Awards given by the International Centre for Nursing Ethics (ICNE) at the University of Surrey, UK, which I now direct.

Foreword by Margretta Madden Styles

You hold in your hands an ideal resource for teaching, learning, and practising nursing ethics. The editors have called on colleagues around the globe to contribute chapters covering the field from the theoretical to the practical, from the retrospective to the prospective, from universalism to relativity/relativism. At your fingertips are segments on the history of nursing ethics and contemporary theories. The book concludes with an extensive section on the substance and methodology of teaching ethics from a broad international perspective, authored by experts from countries from most regions of the world. Food for thought about the future directions and dilemmas of ethics for nurses is put before readers in the final chapter.

Why is it important that such an informative, comprehensive, and provocative volume be available for teachers and nurses today? Teaching nursing ethics is rapidly expanding in dimension and shifting in emphasis. The subject appears more explicitly than previously on the curriculum of nursing schools, in the US as well as in other nations. Ethical issues will become even more complex in the decades ahead because of technology (or lack of it in poor countries) and advances in scientific knowledge, e.g. stem cell research and its spin-offs, an ageing population, cost and distribution of health care, and the global shortage of nurses.

With nurses increasingly playing a central role within the healthcare system, you will face more ethical dilemmas and be held more accountable for the environments you create and the decisions you make. There is a need to concentrate on preparing nurses for a 'true partnership' role in health care. Among other competencies, nurses require ethical knowledge and sensitivity to operate successfully within the larger policy and political arenas.

Because of these dramatic developments, it is likely that some faculties assigned to teach ethics have not been formally prepared to undertake such a critical responsibility. The section on teaching proposes explicit content, directions, and exercises for their use, with appropriate adaptation to accommodate differences in values and cultures and institutional environments.

This is an ethics book for a world of nurses for every step along the way, as they – you – progress from students, to practitioners/clinicians, to teachers.

The late Margretta Madden Styles, RN, EdD
Professor Emerita, University of California, San Francisco
Past President, American Nurses Association
Past President, International Council of Nurses
1930–2005

Foreword by Mo Im Kim

It is a great pleasure and an honour to write a fore-word for this important book. This is a very timely publication because ethical issues in nursing need to be critically analysed in the light of professional values, norms and virtues. They form the core of our professional responsibilities, and the need and desire to expand our boundaries depends on them.

This book is also interesting and helpful for an international audience because it raises questions about cultures that are different and distinct from those traditionally known.

I know that this book will help nurse educators and students who are advocating for ethical nursing practice and I wish it the success it deserves.

Mo Im Kim, RN, PhD
Dean and Professor, Red Cross School of Nursing,
Seoul, South Korea; Former Minister of Health, South
Korea; Past President, International Council of Nurses

Chapter 1

Editors' introduction

Anne J. Davis, Verena Tschudin, Louise de Raeve

This book is for teachers of healthcare ethics as well as for students in health professional schools. We hope that other people and professionals will also read and benefit from these pages. We, the editors, hope this focus on teaching ethics will further develop the field of nursing ethics by assisting people who teach and who practise in clinical settings. In these pages, contributing authors from numerous countries focus on various topics, but essentially this book is divided into four parts.

The first part provides a general background focusing on the history of nursing ethics, the social ethics of the nursing profession, and the sources of religious moral authority.

Part 2 presents four ethical theories or approaches: principle-based ethics, virtue ethics, caring ethics and feminist ethics. After an introduction to these ways of thinking about ethics, each theory or approach is critiqued and comments are made about teaching from this perspective. Each theory has limitations that may point to the need for a multifaceted approach in teaching ethics.

Sometimes the question of which ethics theory to use when teaching becomes one of seeing the situation as either–or, with a teacher using only one of these theories or approaches and not considering any of the others. We invite readers to think about going beyond that stance and to teach in a more inclusive manner. Theories give us lenses through which to see our world. They are especially helpful when we are dealing with more abstract ideas. It might be useful and informative to use all four theories presented here to discuss the same ethical problem. A given theory establishes our focus of concern, our language of dialogue and the outcome of our discourse.

Virtue ethics was for many years the only way that nurses thought of ethics. Questions about the characteristics of a 'morally good' nurse abounded. Florence Nightingale wrote of virtue ethics when she was trying to establish nursing as work for morally decent women. The dominant ethical theory in much of western medicine at present is principle-based ethics. It tends to be the one used in discussions of ethical problems whether in the clinical arena, in clinical ethics committees, or in research ethics committees. For this reason alone, it seems a good idea that nurses understand something of this ethical theory if they want to participate in these discussions. Some nurses say that to find the ethical voice of nursing, we need something other than principle-based ethics and have turned to caring ethics or feminist ethics. This means that they see some or perhaps many of nursing's ethical problems as different from medical ethical issues.

Much of the literature in healthcare ethics, often referred to as bioethics, deals with such questions as organ transplant, stem cell research, genetics and other high-technology developments. While these are all vitally important and need our attention, they may not be the most pressing ethical concerns for most nurses and doctors in their practice. What could be called the 'ethics of everyday practice' may require more attention than it has received.

It is important that readers realize that these four theories were developed in the West, with its specific history, influences, values and world view. Whether and to what extent they can be exported to non-western cultures is an open question. This statement raises the issue of whether we have universal ethics or whether our ethics is always embedded in specific cultural values. Do western and non-western cultures hold the same values and attempt to live by the same ethics? Not everyone agrees on this question, and for that reason readers of this book need to think carefully about this book's content and their own culture.

Just because something is done in a culture does not always make it an ethically right action; what people do is not always the same as what they ought to do. For example, in the nineteenth century AD (common era, CE) farmers in the southern USA owned slaves – people brought from Africa against their will. Slavery had become a tradition in the southern USA because the farms were large and the technology did not exist to do the farm work and therefore many hands were needed. Yet enslaving people was wrong then and is wrong now, although instances of slavery are regularly reported in newspapers today. A usual and traditional situation or action may be considered the norm, but that does not make it ethically right. In the case of American slavery, there was a terrible civil war with great loss of life to solve this ethical problem. And now, although the attitude of racism is still present in the USA, there is no slavery in this sense; laws can change people's status but not necessarily people's attitudes.

Slavery in the USA is just one example of socially embedded notions of right and wrong. This example serves to raise larger questions as to whether there are some actions that are right or wrong in every culture at a given time in history. The issue of universalism and relativism will arise in other parts of the book. It may well be that there are universals, but it is important here that people in non-Western cultures do not adopt ideas developed in the West without question. We see this as one problem in international nursing, although this may be changing. Ideas have moved mostly from the West, and especially from the USA and the UK, to other parts of the world, where they have been taken up and used sometimes without much thought as to their fit. In addition, nurses in the West, and especially those who speak English, have taken their ideas abroad, sometimes without thinking much about cultural differences.

One could say that fields of study can have new ideas that are treated like fads. Certain ideas catch on and many people in a field, such as nursing, begin to think this way and use this language. During our careers, we have seen several such new ideas that have been used, overused and even abused at times. We think ethics is an important aspect of professional life but we do not want these ideas to become fads. It is most important to be informed about new professional ideas and to think them through in a critical way. Dialogue and disagreement are also called for to advance nursing knowledge. Ethics can elicit passion because it has to do with values and we need to feel strongly about what matters to us, but we also need to remember that there may be different and convincing views that also need to be heard and respected. Although this is perhaps one of the most difficult aspects of ethics, it is also one of the most challenging and stimulating. How we balance the general value of tolerance for cultural differences with the questioning or condemning of cultural practices differing from one's own remains a central issue in discussions of human rights and international ethics, with ramifications for health-care and nursing ethics (Davis 2003).

The four theories presented here have all been critiqued, revealing both their strengths and weaknesses. We see a possible paradox in critiquing these four theories, which needs to be kept in mind as you read them. Two of these theories have a long history in the Western philosophical tradition. These earlier critiques assist the present authors to do their work and add to the weight of their own comments. As both virtue ethics and principle-based ethics were developed centuries (in the case of virtue) and decades (in the case of principle-based) ago, there has been time for ample critique and counter-response to these critiques. A genuine dialogue has occurred that has helped to refine these theories further and has also bared their weaknesses. The other two theories – caring ethics and feminist ethics – are fairly new, and although they have also been critiqued, there has been limited time for both critique and countercritique. One might therefore say that although theories are always evolving, the more recent ones have not benefited from an extended dialogue. If one agrees with this assessment, then we can say that the traditional theories are vulnerable because they have this history, while the more recent theories are vulnerable because they do not have this history.

The third part in this book begins with a chapter on the teaching of ethics drawn from a research project and this is followed by selected ethical problems presented from different countries: Columbia, Japan, Israel, Turkey, Norway, Hungary, Malawi and Spain.

The final part opens with a chapter focused on the future, which discusses the major demographic shifts in both developed and developing countries and what this means for healthcare systems, nursing, and our ethical responses. The editors have the last word with a summing up and the final raising of questions for your consideration. Now we want to explain why we think this book is timely.

WHY WE EDITED THIS BOOK

Over the last several decades, nursing ethics has taken a more central role in the profession's activities. The International Council of Nurses (ICN) has promoted ethics through its publications, by developing a session devoted specifically to ethics and by listing ethics as one of the topics for presentations at each quadrennial congress. National nursing associations in many countries have also focused on ethics in various ways that meet the needs of their members. In the academic world, nurse educators teach and conduct research about ethical issues. Clinical and administrative nurses participate in clinical ethics and research ethics discussions and people who influence policy have become more aware of potential ethical problems, such as the allocation of healthcare resources, which includes nurses.

The chapters on history and on social ethics show that these concerns about ethics and ethical dilemmas are not new, but have been central to nursing for many years. However, recently there seems to have been more focus on ethical issues not only in nursing, but in the health sciences generally. This focus is not limited to this field but has spread to other fields of endeavour such as industry, business, governments, and so on.

It has been suggested that an increased attention to ethics occurs at times when people feel confused about what are right and wrong thinking and actions. Whether this is true we cannot say, but it is apparent that in many places nurses practise in an ever more complex world of health care than was the case some years ago. For example, one of us graduated from nursing school in 1955 – 50 years ago. At this time we did not define death as brain death, could not transplant organs, had no reproductive technology, knowledge of genetics had made only limited impact in health care and antibiotics were fairly new. In addition there were no nurse practitioners with graduate degrees, many fewer nursing schools were in colleges and universities, and nursing students constituted most of the clinical hospital staff in many hospitals.

Some things in these 50 years have not changed much. Poor people still fare less well and die earlier than those who are better off economically, even in developed countries. Poor countries still have high infant mortality rates along with high maternal death rates. Infectious diseases are still rampant, HIV/AIDS has been added to that list and tuberculosis is on the increase. Many people, including some in healthcare ethics, are enamored with medical technology as the great benefit in extending life but give scant attention to public health measures. However, some believe that such advances as clean water and a sound sewage system have done more to keep people healthy and extend life than medical technology. Clearly we need both.

In some places in the world, neither adequate medical technology nor sound public health measures exist. Poverty is now recognized as a major factor in health status and life expectancy. The fact remains that many poor countries have limited healthcare services and even fewer public health measures. Some of us find it strange that this great disparity exists in a world that considers itself civilized; while some of us live among plenty, others die prematurely, often of preventable diseases, and do not have the most basic taken-for-granted necessities of life. Such a reality for so many raises many ethical questions and not only for health professionals and patients.

These questions encompass all aspects of life. We know that the ability to read, especially for women, has an impact on the health of a family. We know that population growth can have negative consequences for both families and entire countries. There is an age-old question that is in need of pondering: am I my brother's and sister's keeper, and who are my brother and sister? While we think that all of us have an ethical responsibility to ask and try to answer this question with some action, we do not believe that nurses have any special responsibility beyond what they can realistically undertake. Yet, what can nurses realistically undertake? Each nurse will need to answer this question for herself or himself. Many nurses engage in activities for the common good beyond their usual work and we need to know more about these activities.

The International Centre for Nursing Ethics (ICNE) at the University of Surrey, UK, has periodic one-day conferences where nurses who have made significant contributions to nursing and human rights are honoured and presented with the Human Rights and Nursing Award. At a preconference to the 2001 ICN Quadrennial Congress in Copenhagen, the ICNE sponsored the conference, *Human Rights and Nursing* when it presented the awards for the first time. The first people to receive them were Karla Schefter, from Germany, who organized and has administered a hospital in Afghanistan since 1989; Christine Schmitz, also from Germany, who had worked with Médecins Sans Frontières (MSF; in English, 'doctors without borders') for many years in numerous war-torn areas; and Glenda Wildschut, from South Africa, the only nurse commissioner on the Truth and Reconciliation Commission, who has worked in many places after conflicts, including Rwanda.

In 2003, the ICNE conference topic was *Responsibility and Vulnerability: A Global Perspective* and it honoured Cathy Crowe, a 'street nurse' working with homeless people in Toronto, Canada, and Mpho Sebanyoni-Motlehasedi from South Africa who has established a hospice for people suffering from HIV/AIDS that serves more than 80 communities.

The people given the awards in 2005 during the conference *Cultural and Historical Perspectives on Nursing Ethics: Listening to Each Other*, were Sister Grace Kodiyan, from India, who works with the poorest of poor people in north India, establishing health care, education, and social participation especially among women; and Fidelis Mudimu, from Zimbabwe's

Amani Trust which cares for people who are victims of organized violent crime.

These nurses were publicly recognized and given an award for exceptional service to humanity. It is important that we recognize and honour those of us in nursing who do outstanding humanitarian work. One could argue that all competent, ethical nurses engage in humanitarian work during their daily practice and those whom ICNE recognized were only special examples of this fact.

SOME GENERAL THOUGHTS ON TEACHING ETHICS

Little in life and teaching is value free and ethics is full of values. This raises questions about how to teach the subject to students. What do teachers do with their own values? This question assumes that all teachers have awareness of their values and this might not be the case. Perhaps most of us have experienced becoming aware of a value only when facing a specific situation of ethical choice. Or we have had our ethical position challenged by reality. For example, one of us had supported with reasonable arguments the idea of physician-assisted suicide but this was in the abstract. While caring for a terminally ill friend, this friend asked that she be killed. Now this abstraction became a reality and the firmly held position in the abstract came into question. It is much easier to deal with these profoundly difficult issues in the abstract, although even that is not always easy, than to be faced with the reality of a particular person in a particular situation.

We believe that there is an important difference between education and indoctrination. In some situations the latter may be necessary, such as in the military. Indoctrination in this case is for the common good and is meant to save lives, including the life of the one who is indoctrinated. When, if ever, is indoctrination an ethical good for most students? Should nursing students be indoctrinated? What is the difference between professional socialization and indoctrination?

We believe that education in ethics means that teachers place before health professional students different ways of thinking about ethical problems and help them learn to reason, using these ways with specific ethical cases. Not every problem is an ethical issue when there are conflicting claims involved. What flavour ice cream I should eat is not an ethical issue but whether I should eat ice cream or not might be an ethical issue, especially if I have diabetes.

In our opinion, these are some fundamental questions and concerns that teachers of ethics need to reflect on before, during and after they teach ethics. There is an irony that always occurs with knowledge. While conceptual knowledge gives us ways to think about our world, it also limits our ways of seeing and experiencing that world. This is also true with ethics knowledge. While one may not be able to change this, one needs to be acutely aware of it.

WHO SHOULD READ THIS BOOK

This book was written for teachers of healthcare ethics and their students. However, we sincerely hope that many other readers may find it useful. Like all books, it has limitations but we believe that it is a good addition to and advancement of the ethics literature and to our knowledge of ethics. In the spirit of colleagueship, we invite readers to send us their reactions about the contents of this book.

Reference

Davis AJ 2003 International nursing ethics: context and concerns. In: Tschudin V (ed) Approaches to ethics: nursing beyond boundaries. Butterworth-Heinmann, London, p 97

PART 1

Introduction and background

PART CONTENTS

Chapter 2

Introduction to history, social ethics and religion in clinical ethics

Verena Tschudin

Periodically, nursing is marked by grand ideas: the nursing process, nursing theories, advanced practice. Ethics also came like a wave, sweeping through the curriculum and leaving some nurses baffled as to why the fuss. They had been 'doing' ethics all along and could not understand why they suddenly needed to learn a new and different language.

The following three chapters show not only that nursing has a long history in ethics, but that ethics itself has a long history. Marsha Fowler is qualified in many disciplines, including nursing and theological ethics, both of which she teaches; she is an ordained minister in the Presbyterian Church, holds a Karate black belt, does excellent woodwork, is a marvellous cook, and grows exotic fruit. Some of these talents are evident in these chapters by her truly encyclopaedic knowledge of the subjects covered.

Ethics has always been concerned with how power is used, who has it and why. Religions have tried to regulate power and social structures have aimed at developing, keeping and ordering the powers needed to guide any society. The perceived lack of power within nursing as a whole has been the subject of many studies worldwide. Was it the combination of Victorian society with its understanding of the role of women, religion and military backgrounds that led nursing to the place it occupies today? It must not be forgotten that nursing is far older than medicine. Even physicians were able to do little else than give nursing care to the sick for most of western history. Anyone visiting the islands of Rhodes and Malta in the Mediterranean will see there some imposing palaces from as far back as the eleventh century (Common era), built by the Knights Hospitallers of St John, 'a community of monks set up to nurse Christians who fell ill while on pilgrimage to the Holy Land' (Aquilina Ross 1991). Indeed, the term 'hospice' stems from that era and was essentially a place where pilgrims could rest and be nursed to health and strength again. These tasks were not carried out by women; on the contrary, the Hospitallers were noblemen and 'nobility was an essential qualification for knighthood'. While the records of history tell stories of noble people caring for brave people, probably the less well-off were cared for at home and by women. However, the nurses at St Thomas' Hospital in London, where Florence Nightingale established the now recognized form of training, were known in the UK as 'the ladies' until the 1960s. Some languages use the word 'sister' for any nurse, regardless of any religious component to the role. Nursing has a long history, and the gendered use of power has evolved with many twists and turns. Today's concerns with professional autonomy are only one of these turns.

The history of any family or institution is important for moving forward. Ethics can be understood only if some basic concepts are known and understood, as will be shown in the later theory chapters. The social dimensions of nursing are crucial if the profession is to advance in the areas that will be outlined in the last chapter. It is important, therefore, to understand present situations in order to make sense of the past and the future. Ethics often happens at the boundaries of the accepted and the not-yet acceptable, at the fuzzy edges and in the grey zones. When these grey zones are taken seriously and are reflected on, then ethics will not simply be yet one more thing to learn, but it will be the exciting tool for the future and that which brings colour into the grey areas between absolute right and absolute wrong.

These zones are often the areas where religion either has in the past played or is now playing a major role. Religions have always intended to guide their adherents to the right or the best decisions for the good of individuals and society. As traditional practices lose their hold, people are looking for new ways of making sense of the new kinds of dilemmas they face, most of them concerning the beginning or end of life. New religious practices are shaping life, but it is often less the formal religion that matters, as a need to express a spirituality that encompasses the whole of life. Rituals tied to power structures have become suspect and nurses, patients and clients alike search for the best ways of expressing their needs. Hence the ethical imperative to tell a story and the need to listen to the story and the person telling it. It is as if each person has a need to tell their own story starting with 'In the beginning . . .'. The history, the lived experience, and the transcendent combine in how a person is enabled to tell her or his story. Ethics is about how such stories are heard and acted on.

Reference

Aquilina Ross G 1991 Malta. APA Publications, Hong Kong

Chapter **3**

Ethics in nursing: an historical perspective

Marsha Fowler and Verena Tschudin

A persistent interest in ethics has been demonstrated in modern nursing since the 1870s. In that time, nursing has amassed an extraordinary body of moral literature, has suffused its curricula with ethics content, and has developed codes of ethics to guide practice. This moral energy has not been limited to the USA and Europe, although this chapter will principally address the history of nursing's ethics in these regions.

THE MORAL LITERATURE: USA

The rather ample body of moral literature in nursing begins in the 1800s with a focus on an ethics of virtue within the multiple relationships formed in nursing practice. Frequent mention is made as well of 'etiquette'; this should be understood as a part of the larger virtue ethics that governed the moral thinking of the profession. The shift away from a virtue and relationally based ethics is even slower than that same shift in general society by about 10 or 15 years. This lag reflects the social situation of nursing, and to some extent women, in the USA in its self-contained, hospital-based, all-female, semi-sequestered, tightly regulated education and living arrangements. The shift toward a more duty-based ethics is gradual and the relational categories are actually never lost, although they become more covert, as can be seen in the overview of the literature that follows (Fowler 1984).

The first 'true' nursing journal', *The Trained Nurse and Hospital Review*, was initiated in 1888. Within a year the journal published a six-part series on ethics in nursing, the first extant articles on ethics in the nursing literature

(H.C.C. 1889). The series divided the duties of nurses into 'seven classes' of relationship and dealt with them sequentially in the articles. For decades to come, nursing would address ethics in this relationally based fashion; overtly in the 1950s and then more subtly in succeeding years. These included the nurse-to-physician, nurse-to-nurse, nurse-to-patient, nurse-to-self relationships, and so on. In succeeding years, as nursing came to assert itself, the nurse-to-physician relationship became the nurse-to-other-health-professionals relationship, and physicians were no longer mentioned.

In 1900, the *American Journal of Nursing* (AJN), the official journal of the American Nurses' Association (ANA), began publication. In July of that year an article entitled 'Ethics in Nursing', by Isabel McIsaac, was published (McIsaac 1900). This was the first AJN article that focused directly on ethics, although Isabel Robb preceded McIsaac when she addressed ethics in her article 'Hospital Economics', which was published in January (Robb 1900a). This article, however, simply incorporated a section on ethics and was not entirely devoted to the topic. Thereafter, the AJN consistently included articles devoted in whole or in part to topics in ethics. From 1900 (e.g. Robb 1900b) until the early 1980s, when the field of bioethics began to flourish, there were approximately 450 such articles. Between 1926 and 1928, and 1931 and 1934, the AJN included a feature column entitled 'Ethical Problems', which tackled mostly clinical–ethical concerns solicited from the readership. Some of these columns tackled 'bedside' ethical issues but others answered non-clinical questions such as when nurses may wear their cape in public. The AJN also published the ANA's 'Code for Nurses' and its successive revisions, beginning with 'A Suggested Code' in August 1926 and 'A Tentative Code' in September 1940, neither of which was formally adopted by the Association (ANA 1926, 1940, Fowler 1984).

From 1900 to mid-1965, when the field of bioethics began to develop more fully, approximately 65 books on ethics in nursing were published. Many of these books were nurse-authored, others were written by Roman Catholic priests or social workers. The citations for these works are given in Appendix 1. In the 1960s, the ANA published a position paper that began the movement of nursing schools away from hospital-based programmes and into institutions of higher education. Although this move enabled the profession to come into its own, it also resulted in a significant loss. When the hospital schools were closed, their libraries, archives, collections and other materials of historical importance were disbursed and in many instances lost. There are some books on ethics in nursing, published in the 1800s and alluded to in the later literature that have not, to date, been recovered. As nursing matured, it took control of its moral literature (as it did its clinical literature) and works on nursing ethics by non-nurse authors became rare. By the 1980s, with the notable exception of philosopher Andrew Jameton's fine work, and a few nurse–spouse teams, works on ethics and nursing are the exclusive domain of nurse authors (Fowler 1984, Jameton 1984).

One unusual work should be noted: Sister Rose Helene Vaughn's 'dissertation' (Master's thesis, Catholic University of America) entitled 'The

Actual Incidence of Moral Problems in Nursing: A Preliminary Study in Empirical Ethics'. To date, this is the first identified and extant work of ethics research in nursing. In this thesis, nurse Vaughn culled 2265 ethical incidents from 288 diaries kept by 95 nurses for the study. She then categorized the incidents into 33 categories. The clinical–moral problem with the greatest frequency is that of co-operation between nurses and physicians. Interestingly, she placed a number of incidents that today would be labelled 'sexual harassment' in a category called 'lust' (Fowler 1984, Vaughn 1935).

THE ETHICS CURRICULUM IN AMERICA

These books formed the bedrock of ethics education in nursing schools, curricular standards for which were established by varying agencies. In some instances, individual States established standards for ethics education in nursing, incorporating them (sometimes including specific lecture content) in regulatory law. By 1916, the Board of Registration of Nurses in California required all schools of nursing to include a course in ethics in five of six 'half years' of a 3-year programme. The only subject matter requirement that equalled ethics in volume is what would be called medical–surgical nursing today. The curricular requirements included clinically based ethical concerns, but extended to social–ethical concerns as well, including such issues as 'housing reform' and 'the spirit of youth and the city streets'. Issues that ultimately derive from poverty received considerable attention (Bureau of Registration of Nurses (BRN) California State Board of Health 1916, Fowler 1984).

In 1917, the National League for Nursing Education (NLNE) also established curricular requirements for ethics in nursing education within its 'Standard Curriculum for Schools of Nursing'. The standard called for 10 hours of ethics instruction in the second year, a number of hours co-equal to that of other major topics. The basic lectures were to include content on ethical theory, personal ethics, professional ethics, clinically applied ethics, and social ethics (Fowler 1984, NLNE 1917).

Although not a part of an ethics curriculum, the Nightingale Pledge, written by Lystra Gretter (1893) of the Farrand (later Harper–Farrand) Training School of Nursing in Detroit, Michigan, was often administered to graduating classes at their commencement. When it was administered to the combined Detroit area schools' graduation during the years 1939–1945, the Pledge fell into the public domain and appeared in such odd commercial places as Hollywood movie advertisements. In an attempt to reclaim and protect the Pledge, Gretter modified it in 1935 and copyrighted it. This move, however, came too late and the original Pledge became the prevailing version (see Appendix 2). With regard to the revision of the Pledge, an autograph note by Gretter states the following: 'Commensurate with the broader activities of the Farrand Training School of Nurses the Florence Nightingale Pledge has been revised to include service to the community within its scope. [signed] Lystra E. Gretter' (Fowler 1984, Gretter 1935).

Reflecting the wider society, nursing ethics in the USA embraced an ethics of virtue over an ethics of duty. The notion was that if the nurse is a person of virtue and a morally good will, she (sometimes he) will do what is right. The shift to an ethics of duty did not take place until nursing moved out of hospital schools of nursing and into colleges and universities. The nursing moral literature, both indirectly and directly, reflected the emergence of women as more fully recognized participants in the professions and in society, as well as the emergence of nursing as a scientific profession struggling for public recognition as such.

THE DEVELOPMENT OF AN AMERICAN CODE OF ETHICS

In 1922 the Advisory Committee on Ethical Standards of the NLNE formally proposed the formulation of a code of ethics for nurses. A code of ethics is a means to specify for the profession and its members, as well as for the public, the moral expectations of its practitioners. At a joint meeting of the boards of the NLNE and ANA (see Chapter 4), the president of the ANA requested that the task be undertaken under the aegis of the ANA, to which the NLNE agreed. In January of 1926 the ANA Committee on Ethics had published in the AJN 'A Suggested Code'; it was never formally adopted. This code retained the relational structure that had first appeared in *The Trained Nurse*. It was written in rhetorically effusive narrative that was quite dated even for its time. The most important contribution that this unadopted code made was its specification of the central moral motif of nursing: the ideal of service. It was followed by 'A Tentative Code', published in 1940. This code also employed the relational format of *The Trained Nurse* articles. Reflective of the social location of nursing, this code contained considerable material that is not appropriate to a code of ethics, such as a defence of nursing as a profession. This Tentative Code was also not adopted. Throughout the 1940s and into the 1950s, nursing in the USA retained a sense of a 'call' (vocation), even as a religious vocation. Thereafter, as nursing professionalized, the public expression of nursing as a calling or vocation (*vocare*, to call) waned (Fowler 1984).

In 1950, a Code for Professional Nurses was presented to the ANA House of Delegates. It was unanimously adopted and became the first official code of ethics for the nursing profession. The 1950 code contained a brief preamble and 17 enumerated provisions. Although it was not made explicit in the provisions, they retained the relationally based format of the articles published in 1888 in *The Trained Nurse*. In 1956 a minor change related to nurses and advertising was made to the Code. Nursing was still seeking to legitimate its claim to being 'a profession' and, as a consequence, adopted some of the supposedly ethical constraints of the 'classical professions' of law and medicine, specifically that professionals do not advertise. In reality, the prohibition against advertising in law and medicine, although made pristine for the public, strengthened attempts in the nineteenth century to prevent 'fee wars' among physicians and attorneys, thereby securing a level of income thought befitting of a physician or lawyer.

The first major revision to the Code came in 1960. In the preceding decade, nursing had moved towards a heightened sense of the importance of its contribution to patient care, and hence an increased sense of co-participation in patient care and a decreased sense of subordination to physicians. The next revision came in 1968. This trajectory suggests that a code of ethics begins to feel dated about 8 years after its adoption. By 10 years, it is less serviceable. This requires, then, that codes of ethics be revised approximately every 8 to 10 years so that they retain a fit with the current state of practice. It is less the precepts that are embodied in a code than their application that needs revision. The 1968 revision reduced the number of provisions from 17 to 10. This particular Code was important in that it provided the basis for the provisions of the 1976 and 1985 Codes. For 28 years, the provisions of the Code remained the same, although 'interpretive statements' published with the codes changed. In this period of time the ANA Committee on Ethics could revise the interpretive statements but any change in the actual provisions of the Code had to be voted on by the House of Delegates. By 2001, when the latest Code was adopted, both the provisions and the interpretive statements had to be approved by the House of Delegates.

The 1968 Code is the last to retain a provision on the personal ethics of the nurse. For the next 33 years there would be no reference to the personal ethics of the nurse. In the Code of 2001, however, it is recognized that persons really do not have two distinct and separate spheres of ethics; a person is one person. In 1968, the Code became duty based and moved away from the virtue-based moral tradition of nursing that had prevailed until then.

In 1976, interpretive statements were published for the first time with the Code itself. For previous codes, interpretation was incorporated in articles on the code published in the AJN. The Code of 1976 retained the provisions of the 1968 Code, as did the successor Code of 1985. The 1976 Code's interpretive statements were more assertive and activistic in nature, reflecting the changes that had taken place in the profession as nursing became science oriented and medicine became technology oriented. A variety of civil rights concerns entered in, as did an increased awareness of medical paternalism. Patients were accorded more autonomy in the 1976 Code, perhaps aggressively so. In accordance with the prevailing influence of the field of bioethics, this Code also reflected the heightened bioethical sensibilities and specialization of its framers. It was thus more 'technically ethical' than previous revisions and reflected much of the then standard bioethical vocabulary (Fowler 1984).

By the time the 1985 Code was released 'ethical principlism' held sway in the field of bioethics and heavily influenced the language and content of the interpretive statements of this Code. Much of the more legal and less ethical language of previous codes was omitted. At this time, unwanted and unwarranted technology at the end of life was receiving considerable public as well as professional attention, and was accordingly so represented in the 1985 Code. This Code also reflected an increased awareness of various forms of social prejudice, of problems relating to access to care, of a right to health care for all (not only citizens), of the rise of nursing research, theory and standards, and of the expanded role of the nurse. By 1996, however, this excellent work had become dated and no longer reflected the social and clinical context of nursing nor the development of the field of ethics in nursing. In 1996, the ANA formed a task force to explore the need for a new code. The task force recommended not only a revision of the interpretive statements but a full revision of the provisions of the Code itself, which had not been revised since 1968 (Fowler 2000).

In late 1996, a committee of ten people was appointed and charged with the task of revising both the provisions and the interpretive statements of the code. Because of changes in the organizational structure of the ANA, it was now necessary for the committee to have the House of Delegates approve both the code and its interpretive statements. The process took 7 years before it came to final overwhelming approval by the House in 2001.

The Code of Ethics of 2001 is a dramatically different code. It expands its focus beyond clinical roles alone to all nursing roles. For the first time, it incorporates a provision solely devoted to the duties-to-self of the nurse. It also now includes a provision regarding the moral responsibilities of the profession as a whole through its professional and practice associations. In addition, this Code moves to incorporate other approaches to ethics, apart from ethical principlism (Fowler 2001).

These codes of ethics, adopted and unadopted, are important documents not simply because they provide moral guidance for nurses, but also because they reflect the changes in the profession over the past 75 years and nursing's moral reflection on these changes.

THE UK AND WESTERN EUROPEAN CONTRIBUTION

The influence of Florence Nightingale on nursing cannot be underestimated. Nightingale was a deeply religious woman, trained by nuns in Germany, and her main experience of nursing was in a military setting. Thus religion, religious practice and military concepts formed the background to Nightingale's understanding of nursing. She had the attention of influential people and because she bestowed 'her *imprimatur* upon secular vocational nursing she gave it standing in Victorian Britain and throughout the world' (Smith 1982 p 155).

Europe today consists of nearly 50 countries 'encompassing a vast diversity of values, languages, cultures, races and religions' (Tadd 1998 p 1). Many of these countries have in turn influenced cultures and practices in other parts of the world through their missionary and trading activities, notably Britain, Spain, Portugal and the Netherlands.

Ethics was not a subject specifically taught in nursing schools in the early parts of the twentieth century in Europe. The Nightingale Pledge (see Appendix 2), although known, was not as widely used as in the USA. Throughout Europe, many nursing schools were originally directed by deaconesses: religious sisters whose sense of mission was to serve others.

Their rise in the number of nurses coincided significantly with the establishment of nursing as a profession. Hence it can be argued that in Europe nursing was for a longer time span within the ambit of 'vocation' and therefore the ethos of religious thinking and arguing than in the USA. Nightingale herself bitterly opposed registration and the underlying concept of professionalization because of her belief that nursing was a vocation; she saw registration 'almost a sacrilege to this ideal' (Bradshaw 1994 p 136).

A short overview of practices in some European countries will testify to the diversity of the continent and its approach to ethics within nursing.

In the UK, a significant text was *Ethics for Nurses* (Way 1962), which was originally published as a series of articles in *Nursing Times*, and reprinted for the last time in 1971. Today it reads like a text from a different world. Almost on the last page is the heading 'Respect for the Doctor'. This starts:

> *Ward routine has a certain pattern to encourage respect for the doctor; he is always accompanied by the sister, the ward is quiet, he is never contradicted; and by various means he is shown to be a person of pre-eminent skill and wisdom.* (Way 1962 p 22)

The entire text is in the style of 'what nurses always do' and 'what nurses never do'. The (then) UK regulatory body, the United Kingdom Central Council (UKCC) issued the first Code of Professional Conduct for Nurses, Midwives and Health Visitors (Based on Ethical Concepts) in 1983 (UKCC 1983). This was considered an important document, with nursing leading the way among healthcare professionals. A significant component of that Code was in fact the first clause:

> *[In fulfilment of professional responsibility and in the exercise of professional accountability the nurse, midwife or health visitor shall:] 1. Comply with the law of any country, state, province or territory in which she works, and have due regard to custom and practice.*

A second edition of the Code was issued only 16 months later with a remarkably changed text (UKCC 1984).

In 2002 the UKCC ceased to exist, and in its place came the Nursing and Midwifery Council (NMC), whose first act was to issue a new version of the Code, based on eight values that are now shared by all the main UK health professional regulatory bodies (NMC 2002). It is noteworthy that this is a code of professional practice, based heavily on duties, rather than being a 'code of ethics' where the moral sensitivities and principles form the basis.

In the Nordic countries (Denmark, Finland, Greenland, Norway, Sweden) ethics is still largely taught by clergy in nursing schools. It is to be noted that nurses in these countries are also the most active in publishing on ethics in journals, largely in English.

In some other European countries, notably Switzerland (Shaha 2004) and Italy (Sala & Manara 1999), nursing struggles even now to be accepted as a fully independent profession, rather than being considered supplementary to the medical profession.

A Decree of the President of the Italian Republic (No 225/1974) was published in 1974 to replace an earlier Royal Decree of 2 May 1940 'concerning nurses' assignments'. This so-called *Mansionario* was a type of job description in which the duties of nurses were precisely described. It was called an 'instrument', but often it was not at the service of the professional, rather the professional seemed to serve the *Mansionario*; that is, despite their freedom and autonomy in professional behaviour, nurses had to respect the instructions in the *Mansionario*, without the possibility of discussing them. The *Mansionario* was replaced in 1994 by the so-called *Profilo professionale*. The *Profilo* places emphasis on the autonomy of professionals, and speaks of technical, scientific and relational competencies all having equal importance (Sala & Manara 1999).

Alongside this document is the Deontological Code of 1999, which is an updated version of the 1977 Code. Sala & Manara (1999) consider this new code to reflect the growing development of nursing as a science and to be expressive of a growing self-consciousness in the profession, particularly concerning ethical issues. While this is welcome, they also express that the teaching of ethics has to be improved. However good and useful a code is, it cannot 'provide moral sensibility and the faculty to act ethically' (Sala & Manara 1999 p 461).

The Swiss Nurses Association published a document in 1990 under the title 'Ethical Principles for Nursing' (SBK/ASI 1990). This describes the responsibilities of nurses towards patients and clients, themselves and the profession, colleagues, and society and the environment. It also contains the ICN Code of Ethics of 1973 and the UN Declaration of Human Rights. This document was reissued and updated in 2003 but it does not represent a code as such, and only considers four principles of bioethics as guiding the ethics of nursing.

The law concerning the regulation of health care in Switzerland is in a state of change, and with it the place of the nursing profession. Under civil law, nurses cannot be held directly responsible for their actions, but they can be held indirectly responsible. Discussions are underway among the profession and in parliament, 'to recognise nursing interventions as the visible expression and particular characteristic of the nursing profession' (Shaha 2004).

Switzerland is not part of the European Union, and is not expected to be a member state for the time being; nevertheless, many European directives have been taken on board by the Swiss people, and tertiary education for nurses is one of these. However, in 2004, only one school of nursing offered tertiary nurse education at basic level.

Belgian nurses have until now rejected the formulation and use of a national code of ethics for nurses. One possible explanation for this is that 'nursing practice in Belgium is already strongly influenced by legal regulations in which ethical values and norms are implied. . . . Professional ethics is acknowledged as an important aspect of nursing practice and education in professional documents, including advisory documents for the nursing profession and professional and nursing ethics textbooks' (Verpeet et al 2003 p 655).

This diversity of practice and cultural norms maintains a certain national character, but with the European Union growing in size and the labour force able to move between EU countries without restrictions, a growing problem is the safety and professional work of nurses who might not be familiar with their new country's cultural practices.

ETHICS EDUCATION

For the various reasons outlined, ethics education in Europe has also been diverse and less dependent on American literature. Ethics was for the first time a specific item in the curriculum of nurse education when the 'Project 2000' programme was introduced in the UK in the early 1980s. This programme has been replaced by 'Fitness for Practice' and ethics does not figure any longer as a discrete subject but is taught across the curriculum. However, many tutors and lecturers who have to teach ethics, or be versed in the subject when teaching social subjects, do not themselves have a background in ethics. Thus it can be argued that many nurses know about ethics and certain theories and principles, but do not know how to apply them in ethical analysis, or indeed how to think ethically about what a nurse is to be or to do.

THE IMPACT OF THE JOURNAL *NURSING ETHICS*

The journal *Nursing Ethics* has made a significant contribution to ethics internationally. It is a UK publication and, since its beginning in 1994, has not had a competitor within nursing. This means that its readers and contributors are virtually the entire population of nurses worldwide interested in the subject.

Early contributions to the journal were concerned with issues such as feeding severely demented patients (Norberg et al 1994), confidentiality and personal integrity (Edgar 1994, Ngwena & Chadwick 1994) and patient advocacy at the end of life (Love 1995). Contributions came mainly from the UK, Scandinavia and the USA. By 2004 and 2005 many contributions came from Turkey and Korea, but on not dissimilar topics (Kim et al 2004, Özkara et al 2004). This highlights a gap in knowledge transmission. In science it seems to take 10–15 years for ideas to impact generally, and something similar may be happening here. These early articles address what have come to be the settled topics in clinical ethics that were of great controversy only 10 years ago. They addressed testing the use of four ethical principles by student nurses, how far patients should have autonomy, and what informed consent might mean.

Increasingly, articles have been of a more reflective and subtle type, challenging the status quo of healthcare systems in which the authors work. They also tend more to be written in the first person, showing a readiness by the authors to own their perspectives. It seems pertinent therefore to mix the various stages of consciousness and exploration of ethics in one journal, not only providing an international overview at a glance, but enabling individuals and professional groups to gain and develop their ethical awareness and practice in appropriate ways that might not otherwise have been so transparent. There is a sense in which the 'butterfly effect' – a butterfly flapping its wings in Tokyo affecting the weather in London – is true also in nursing and ethics, where the action of one nurse in a remote part of the world will affect that of another nurse in another part, and vice versa. This is particularly true in ethics.

If space would permit, this discussion could be deeply enriched by a history of ethics in nursing in Canada, Mexico, Colombia and throughout Latin America, as well as in Japan, Korea, Australia, New Zealand, Russia and throughout the world. Everywhere there is organized nursing, there is both a present concern for ethics and an enduring history of ethical discourse. Perhaps the larger task is both to amass and analyse a comprehensive worldwide history of nursing's ethics, but more importantly to bring together nurses from around the world to shape the future of nursing ethics education, research and scholarship.

CONCLUSION

The development of nursing's ethical literature and the teaching of ethics in nursing have proceeded differently in different nations. However, in all instances the sociopolitical location of nursing has influenced both the process and content of its development. When and where nursing is less autonomous, it is reflected in its ethics. When and where nursing is emerging as a profession, seeking public recognition of its science and professionalism with the attendant allocation of social resources to support research and education, it is reflected in its ethics. When and where nursing is well established as a profession and a science with a distinctive body of knowledge that contributes to regional, national and global health, it is reflected in its ethics. Where nursing is a female-dominant endeavour, the sociopolitical location of women in the particular society is also reflected in its ethics. Ethics in nursing has never been an algebraic calculus; it has always reflected nursing's residence within and concern for its service and the society it serves.

APPENDIX 1: EARLY BOOKS ON ETHICS IN NURSING

The following list is taken from Fowler 1984 *Ethics and nursing, 1893–1984: the ideal of service, the reality of history.* Los Angeles: University of Southern California. The books are listed in order of publication.

Robb, Isabel Adams Hampton 1900 Nursing ethics: for hospital and private use. New York, EC Koeckert. 273 pages. Reprinted without revision in 1911, 1916, 1920.

Lounsberry, Harriet Camp 1912 Making good on private duty: practical hints to graduate nurses. Philadelphia, JB Lippincott.

Aikens, Charlotte 1916 Studies in ethics for nurses. Philadelphia, WB Saunders.

Parsons, Sara 1916. Nursing problems and obligations. Boston, Whitcomb and Barrows. 149 pages. Reprinted 1919, 1922.

Stoney, Emily & Catlin, Lucy 1917 Practical points in nursing for nurses in private practice. Philadelphia, WB Saunders.

Spalding, Henry 1920 Talks to nurses: the ethics of nursing. New York, Benziger Brothers. 128 pages.

Murphy, Richard 1923 The Catholic nurse: her spirit and her duties. Milwaukee, WI, Bruce. 147 pages.

Brogan, James 1924 Ethical principles for the character of a nurse. Milwaukee, WI: Bruce. 128 pages.

Talley, Charlotte 1925 Ethics: a textbook for nurses. New York, Putnam's. 140 pages. 2nd edition 1928.

Garesche, Edward 1926 A vade mecum for nurses and social workers. Milwaukee, WI, Bruce.

Talley, Charlotte 1927 Lesson plans in ethics for nurses. New York, Putnam's.

Garesche, Edward 1928 Couriers of mercy: friendly talks to nurses. Milwaukee, WI, Bruce.

Edgell, Beatrice 1929 Ethical problems: an introduction to ethics for hospital nurses and social workers. London: Methuen and Company.

Garesche, Edward 1929 Ethics and the art of conduct for nurses. Philadelphia, WB Saunders. 341 pages. Also 1944, 358 pages.

Russell, Frederick 1929 Ethics in general and special. Emmitsburg, MD: Sisters of Charity. 74 pages.

Gladwin, Mary 1930 Ethics: talks to nurses. Philadelphia: FA Davis. 2nd edition 1937, 365 pages. 3rd edition 1938, 281 pages.

Jamieson, Elizabeth & Sewell, Elizabeth 1931 Ethics notebook for nurses. Philadelphia, JB Lippincott. 22 pages. Also 1933, 1935, 1940, 1944.

Harrison, Gene 1932 Ethics in nursing. St Louis, MO, CV Mosby. 163 pages.

Gabriel, Sr John 1932 Professional problems: a textbook for nurses. Philadelphia, WB Saunders. 158 pages.

Goodrich, Annie 1932 The social and ethical significance of nursing: a series of addresses. New York, Macmillan. 401 pages.

Moore, Dom Thomas Verner 1935 Principles of ethics. Philadelphia, JB Lippincott. Also 1937, 1939, 1943.

Vaughn, Sr Rose Helene 1935 The actual incidence of moral problems in nursing: a preliminary study in empirical ethics. Washington, DC, Catholic University Press. 123 pages.

Dietz, Lena Dixon 1935 Professional problems in nursing. Philadelphia, FA Davis.

Evarts, Arrah 1935 Ethics of nursing. Minneapolis, MN, Burgess. 40 pages.

Rothweiler, Ella 1938 Davis' cumulative continued study units on ethics. Philadelphia, FA Davis. 51 pages.

Spaulding, Eugenia 1939 Professional adjustments in nursing, being professional adjustments II. Philadelphia, JB Lippincott. 436 pages.

Dietz, Lena Dixon 1940 Professional adjustments I. Philadelphia, FA Davis. 226 pages.

Goodall, Phyllis 1942 Ethics: the inner realities. Philadelphia, FA Davis. Also 1943, 239 pages.

Harrison, Helen 1942 Professional adjustments [no place or publisher given].

Hansen, Helen 1942. Professional relationships of the nurse. Philadelphia, WB Saunders. 382 pages.

Densford, Katherine & Everett, Millard 1946 Ethics for modern nurses: professional adjustments, I. Philadelphia, WB Saunders. 260 pages.

Price, Alice 1946. Professional adjustments, I [no place or publisher given].

McFadden, Charles 1946 Medical ethics. Philadelphia, FA Davis. 356 pages. Also 1949, 438 pages.

McAllister, Joseph 1947 Ethics with special application to the medical and nursing professions. Philadelphia, WB Saunders. Also 1955.

Gounley, Martin 1949 Digest of ethics for nurses. Paterson: St Anthony Guild. 82 pages.

Pearce, Evelyn 1953 The nurse and the patient: an ethical consideration of human relations. London: Faber and Faber. 184 pages.

Hayes, Edward et al 1956 Moral handbook of nursing: a compendium of principles, spiritual aids, and concise answers regarding Catholic personnel, patients and problems. New York, Macmillan. 180 pages.

Godin, Edgar & O'Hanley, J 1957 Hospital ethics: a commentary on the code of Catholic hospitals. Bathurst, New Brunswick, Canada, Hotel Dieu Hospital.

Way, Hillary 1962 Ethics for nurses. London: Macmillan. 24 pages.

Plachata, Sr Mary Miranda 1963 Spiritualize your nursing [no place or publisher given].

Pelley, Thelma 1964 Nursing: its history, trends, philosophy, ethics and ethos. Philadelphia, WB Saunders. 238 pages.

Hayes, Edward, Hayes, Paul & Kelly, Dorothy 1964 Moral principles of nursing. New York, Macmillan. 257 pages.

Additional early references for which insufficient data were available to trace the work:

Landes 1955.

National League for Nursing 1957.

Storey 1958.

Southard 1959.

APPENDIX 2: THE NIGHTINGALE PLEDGE

From Fowler 1984 *Ethics and nursing, 1893–1984: the ideal of service, the reality of history* (full publication details appear in the Reference list).

NIGHTINGALE PLEDGE, 1893

I solemnly pledge myself before God and in the presence of this assembly, to pass my life in purity and to practise my profession faithfully. I will abstain from whatever is deleterious and mischievous, and will not take or knowingly administer any harmful drug. I will do all in my power to maintain and elevate the standard of my profession, and will hold in confidence all personal matters committed to my keeping, and all family affairs coming to my knowledge in the practice of my calling. With loyalty will I endeavour to aid the physician in his work, and devote myself to the welfare of those committed to my care.

NIGHTINGALE PLEDGE, 1935 RECENSION

I solemnly pledge myself before God and in the presence of this assembly to pass my life in purity and to practise my profession faithfully. I will abstain from whatever is deleterious and mischievous, and will not take or knowingly administer any harmful drug. I will do all in my power to maintain and elevate the standard of my profession, and will hold in confidence all personal matters committed to my keeping, and all family affairs coming to my knowledge in the practice of my calling. With loyalty will I endeavour to aid the physician in his work, and as a 'missioner of health' I will dedicate myself to devoted service to human welfare.

References

American Nurses' Association (ANA) 1926 A suggested code. American Journal of Nursing 26(8):599–601.

American Nurses' Association (ANA) 1940 A tentative code. American Journal of Nursing 40(9):977–980.

American Nurses' Association (ANA) 1950 The code for professional nurses. ANA, Kansas City, MO.

American Nurses' Association (ANA) 1956 The code for professional nurses. ANA, Kansas City, MO.

American Nurses' Association (ANA) 1960 The code for professional nurses. ANA, Kansas City, MO.

American Nurses' Association (ANA) 1968 The code for nurses. ANA, Kansas City, MO.

American Nurses' Association (ANA) 1976 The code for nurses with interpretive statements. ANA, Kansas City, MO.

American Nurses' Association (ANA) 1985 The code for nurses with interpretive statements. ANA, Kansas City, MO.

American Nurse's Association (ANA) 2001 The code of ethics for nurses with interpretive statements. ANA, Washington, DC.

Bradshaw A 1994 Lighting the lamp; the spiritual dimension of nursing care. Scutari Press, London.

Bureau of Registration of Nurses (BRN) California State Board of Health 1916 Schools of nursing requirements and curriculum. State Printing Office, Sacramento, CA.

Deloughery GL 1998 History of the nursing profession. In: Deloughery GL (ed) Issues and trends in nursing. Mosby, St Louis, MO, p 1–52.

Edgar A 1994 Confidentiality and personal integrity. Nursing Ethics 1(2):86–95.

Fowler MD 1984 Ethics and nursing, 1893–1984: the ideal of service, the reality of history. University of Southern California, Los Angeles.

Fowler M, Daly, B 2000 Task Force for the revision of the Code for Nurses "The Need for change," American Journal of Nursing 100(7):69–72.

Fowler M, Benner P 2001 Current controversies: the new Code of Ethics for Nurses. American Journal of Critical Care Nursing December:434–437.

Gretter L 1893 The Nightingale pledge. Harper Training School of Nursing, Detroit, MI.

Gretter L 1935 The Nightingale pledge. Revised edn. Harper–Farrand Training School of Nursing, Detroit, MI.

H.C.C. [author identified by initials only] May 1889 Ethics in nursing: talks of a superintendent with her graduating class. Trained Nurse and Hospital Review 2(5):179–183.

H.C.C. July 1889 Ethics in nursing: a nurse's duty to herself: talks of a superintendent with her graduating class. Trained Nurse and Hospital Review 3(1):1–5.

H.C.C. August 1889 Ethics in nursing: a nurse's duty to herself: talks of a superintendent with her graduating class. Trained Nurse and Hospital Review 3(2):40–43.

H.C.C. September 1889 Ethics in nursing: talks of a superintendent with her graduating class: the doctor. Trained Nurse and Hospital Review 3(3):81–85.

H.C.C. October 1889 Ethics in nursing: talks of a superintendent with her graduating class: duties of a nurse to her patient's family, friends, and servants. Trained Nurse and Hospital Review 3(4):121–124.

H.C.C. November 1889 Ethics in nursing: talks of a superintendent with her graduating class: a nurse's duties to her own friends. Trained Nurse and Hospital Review 3(5):121–124.

H.C.C. December 1889 Ethics in nursing: Talks of a superintendent with her graduating class: a nurse's duty to her own hospital or school and to her fellow nurses. Trained Nurse and Hospital Review 3(6):199–201.

Jameton A 1984 Nursing practice: the ethical issues. Prentice Hall, Englewood Cliffs, NJ.

Kim Y-S, Park J-W, Son Y-J, Han S-S 2004 A longitudinal study on the development of moral judgement in Korean nursing students. Nursing Ethics 11:254–256.

Love MB 1995 Patient advocacy at the end of life. Nursing Ethics 2:3–9.

McIsaac I 1900 Ethics in nursing. American Journal of Nursing 1(7):483–488.

National League for Nursing Education (NLNE) 1917 Standard curriculum for schools of nursing. NLNE, New York.

Ngwena C, Chadwick R 1994 Confidentiality and nursing practice: ethics and law. Nursing Ethics 1:136–150.

Norberg A et al 1994 Ethical reasoning concerning the feeding of severely demented patients: an international perspective. Nursing Ethics 1:3–13.

Nursing and Midwifery Council (NMC) 2002 Code of professional conduct. NMC, London.

Özkara E, Civaner M, Oglak S, Mayda AS 2004 Euthanasia education for health professionals in Turkey: students change their opinions. Nursing Ethics 11(3):290–298.

Robb IAH 1900a Hospital economics. American Journal of Nursing 1:29–33.

Robb IAH 1900b Nursing ethics: for hospital and private use. EC Koeckert, New York.

Sala R, Manara D 1999 The regulation of autonomy in nursing: the Italian situation. Nursing Ethics 6(5):451–467.

SBK/ASI 1990 Ethische Grundsätze für die Pflege Schweizer Berufsverband der Krankenschwestern und Krankenpfleger. (SBK/ASI) 1990 Ethische grumidsäge für die pflege. SBK/ASI, Berne.

Shaha M 2004 Country profile: Switzerland. Nursing Ethics 11(4): 418–424.

Smith F 1982 Florence Nightingale; reputation and power. Croom Helm, London.

Tadd W 1998 Setting the scene. In: Tadd W (ed) Ethical issues in nursing and midwifery practice; perspectives from Europe. Macmillan, Basingstoke, UK, p 1–9.

United Kingdom Central Council (UKCC) 1983 Code of professional conduct for nurses, midwives and health visitors (based on ethical concepts). UKCC, London.

United Kingdom Central Council (UKCC) 1984 Code of professional conduct for the nurse, midwife and health visitor, 2nd edn. UKCC, London.

Vaughn RH 1935 The actual incidence of moral problems in nursing: a preliminary study in empirical ethics. Catholic University Press, Washington, DC.

Verpeet E, Meulenbergs T, Gastmans C 2003 Professional values and norms for nurses in Belgium. Nursing Ethics 10(6):654–665.

Way, Hillary 1962 Ethics for nurses. Macmillan, London.

Chapter **4**

Social ethics, the profession and society

Marsha Fowler

Nursing's ethics in the USA has never been focused solely on clinical ethical issues. It has, from the beginning, always been intimately concerned with the shape of society and its affect on health and illness. Hence, American nursing's ethics has always been in good measure a social ethics. This is reflected in early nursing ethics curricula as well as in the role of nursing associations, as recently articulated in the 2001 revision of the Code of Ethics for Nurses of the American Nurses' Association (ANA). The social ethics of a profession is most often, although not exclusively, exercised through its professional associations, that is, through collectives of nurses rather than by individual nurses. The question to be asked is: what is the moral role and responsibility of a professional nursing association (or any social structure) that seeks to be a socially transforming professional association? The answer is: the moral role and responsibility of the professional association is to preserve, develop and assert the meaning and value structures of the nursing profession, that is, to exercise the social ethics of the profession in society.

The meaning and value structures are those aspects of social–professional life that embody the ideals, values and ethics of a professional group; in this context those of nursing. Meaning and value structures are juxtaposed against power structures: the social structures that embody power in any of its forms, for example, politics, economics, prestige and authority. To establish the claim that the role of a professional association is to safeguard and vouchsafe the profession's meaning and value structures, it is necessary to examine the interplay of profession, ethics and society. More specifically, this means to examine the social role of professions, the structure and function of professional associations, and the role of social ethics.

THE SOCIAL ROLE OF PROFESSIONS

The social role of a profession is to prepare practitioners with the knowledge and skill necessary for the exercise of that profession's practice. This would seem a simple task, and yet there is much that is hidden here. For instance, the public must be able to trust the profession and believe that all its members will possess a particular level and quality of knowledge and skill, that is, a particular expertise. The public must be able to trust that the members of the profession are persons of a morally good will, that is, that they have a genuine desire to help those who come to them, and will do so with integrity. In the case of nursing, this means with compassion. The public must be able to trust that the members of a given profession will be characterized by a particular set of moral virtues and ethical guidelines that they exercise even when unobserved. In order for this social trust (sometimes called a social contract) to exist, the profession's members must be 'schooled' in both the knowledge and techniques of its practice. This is the task of the profession's educators. However, this is not enough. When the formal and basic education ends, the professionals must find an affiliation that will motivate them to continue to learn throughout life, to practise the craft with virtue, to seek to enhance the knowledge base of the profession itself and to observe the moral guidelines of the profession. This is the task of the professional association. Thus, both education and professional associations are essential to the moral life and excellence of a profession. It is therefore necessary to look more closely at professional associations and their functions.

THE STRUCTURE OF PROFESSIONAL ASSOCIATIONS

Any social structure is itself comprised of two substructures, whether it is a governmental bureau, a business, a school, a professional association, a polyclinic, a local church or even a club. The first substructure is the 'power structure' and the second is the 'meaning and value structure'.

Power structures are those aspects of an institution, agency or group that allow it to 'get things done' or to bring about changes according to its desires or values. In governments, power structures are asserted through such means as legislation or regulation. A business might exert its power structure through the use of social trust in a particular product or service, or its name recognition. Around the world, everyone recognizes the names McDonald's, Pizza Hut and Coca Cola. Even if the quality of their products is questionable in terms of actual nutritive value, these businesses can assert power through their name recognition and association with youth worldwide and through the consumer knowledge that the quality of the product will be consistent. It is a power to cultivate new consumers and maintain old ones, especially within a particular age range. A school, university or academy exerts power through its prestige. This is related to the public perception of the quality of its instruction, the quality of the faculty, the faculty's scholarly and research productivity, the renown of its graduates, the difficulty of acceptance for admission, and so on. A local religious institution might demonstrate its power structure when its leader is known for great wisdom, learning, and piety such that inquirers, or troubled souls, persons in crisis, or spiritual journeyers, seek that person out. A profession asserts its power structure, as one example, when it is able to affect legislation and regulation for the advance of the profession's practice by sharing its expertise and recommendations with those who make law. Another example might be found in instances wherein the professional association takes measures that enhance the public's understanding of the profession or improve the image of the profession in the public mind. Professions most often assert their power structures through the vehicle of a professional association.

THE ROLE OF THE PROFESSIONAL NURSING ASSOCIATION

As professional associations are social structures that thus possess two chief substructures, their role is to assert both of those substructures in balance with each other. The professional nursing associations must assert their power structures to accomplish many tasks, including:

- Assuring the essential quality of practice of their members
- Fostering appropriate legislation and regulation regarding professional practice
- Collaborating with educators in establishing standards of education
- Assisting in the development of standards of practice expected of all practitioners
- Identifying expert practice
- Positively influencing and enhancing the public image of the profession and its practice

Collectively, the tasks of the power structure of the professional associations are thus to bring about social change within the profession, in society and in the minds of the public. The role of professional associations in relation to the meaning and value structures of a profession is to preserve, to develop and to assert the meaning, values and ethics of the profession. This is done by establishing moral standards for practice, as in promulgating and maintaining a code of ethics for the profession. It is also done by cultivating specific virtues within its members through motivation and modelling of virtues. For instance, creating an expectation of lifelong professional learning or modelling caring and compassion toward nurses themselves and providing a 'home' for the expression of their needs and concerns. It is also done by moral reflection on the goals of the association itself.

Within professions and their organizations, power can be used for good or for ill. Power itself is value neutral; it is the use of power that determines its moral praiseworthiness or blameworthiness. There are therefore two views of the goodness of professions. Some have seen professions as affiliative moral communities that serve to reinforce ethics and ideals in a society where other affiliative ties have been loosened. Others have taken a sharply critical view of professions, seeing them as elitist oligarchies concerned with maintaining and enlarging their own monopolistic powers at the expense of those who would use their services. Thus, some have seen professions as the innocent Red Riding Hood and others as the predatory Big Bad Wolf (many other fairy or folk tales can also make a suitable analogy). The truth is to be found in both of these views, and in neither of these views.

Emile Durkheim (1933) developed a more optimistic view of professions and a less optimistic view of society. He saw the evolution of society as a move towards general disintegration wherein social and relational ties, and hence moral ties, became looser and morally less binding. This does indeed characterize the USA, although readers will need to understand their own context to make comparisons. Durkheim saw increased mobility, urbanization and the nuclear family as factors contributing to the devolution of society. Professions provided an altruistic moral community that formed new moral ties for those otherwise left adrift by the loosening of their moral moorings. In this happy view, professions are seen as self-policing, where individuals and the group itself are directed by the coercive force of moral suasion and restrained by moral penalty. These would avert individual or collective attempts at pursuit of a wholesale egocentric ethics at the expense of clients, the profession, or society. Neither professionals nor a professional association could then become a runaway train of abuse, greed or manipulation. It is, however, an unhappy fact that in the USA Durkheim's view flies in the face of evidence of political power brokering, contemptible failures at self-policing and a paucity of altruism coupled with gross professional excesses (Durkheim 1933). One has only to read the daily news to see such failures powerfully evident among the classical professions of law and medicine, as well as among many other professional groups.

The second and much more cynical view of professions essentially sees them as predators laying in wait to seize on a social need to turn it to their own pecuniary advantage in such a way that their own social power and prestige would be enhanced. Here, professions are specialized and monopolistic power elites that serve their own ends of social dominance, further power, privilege, exclusive authority, suppression of competition and a secured position through the exploitation of a social need rooted in a profound human need (e.g. health, hunger, pain). In this community, ethics serves to keep its members in line. It is a grim reality that professions in the USA sometimes resemble this portrait (caricature, even) better than Durkheim's (Durkheim 1933, Geison 1983, Hatch 1988, Veatch 1972). Nonetheless, this view, too, fails to accord with actuality. While in any instant we can see professional abuses, such as state health-insurance fraud, police brutality and insider trading in the stock market, we can also find examples of profound selflessness for the benefit of individuals and society. Some names that come to mind are Marie Curie, the nurse Clara Maas and Catholic priest Damien of Hawaii; we can see both Little Red and Big Bad Wolf.

Of these two views, the first errs on the side of giving too much weight to meaning and value structures and the second on the side of giving too much weight to power structures. The truth of professions and their professional associations, in terms of their moral mandate, is to achieve a balance between power structures and meaning and value structures.

Meaning and value structures must stand in a reciprocal relationship with power structures; associations must be balanced in their concern. Structures of social power include all the various forms of power: authority, position, money, prestige and so on. Power structures have the capacity to 'implement', that is, the power to act towards the realization of the community's values, meaning and goals. Meaning and value structures of which ethics is a part, set boundaries, such as what constitutes legitimate means or ends. They inform and critique power structures and reshape power structures according to the community's values and meaning.

Within any organization it is possible for the power structure to overwhelm meaning and value structures and to engage in run-away self-interest. It is also possible, although less often the case, that the meaning and value structure immobilizes the power structures. The socially transforming professional nursing association must therefore seek a balance in which power structures are informed by meaning and value structures; it must empower and live out those values in the real world. The meaning and value structures critique power structures and reshape them according to the value of the community. Although it is rarely the case that meaning and value structures render power structures impotent, it is the case that power structures can leave the meaning and value structures behind in the dust of demise. In the view set forth here, power structures and meaning and value structures (including ethics) must be maintained in dynamic and social equilibrium with one another. To realize this tension, the professional nursing associations act within and outside the larger social power structures to transform them, but do so by embracing, implementing, and proclaiming their own professional meaning and central values. This is accomplished through the professional associations' exercise of what is formally understood as 'social ethics', which will be examined below. First, however, this abstraction might be helped by a concrete example.

ETHICS, SOCIETY AND PROFESSIONAL ASSOCIATIONS IN NURSING

Of necessity, I take as an example one from my own nation, that of the American Nurses' Association. As always, readers will need to modify what I say according to their own context.

The oldest professional general association in nursing in the USA was created in 1896 at the meeting of the Association of Superintendents of Training Schools of Nursing. It was named the Associated Alumnae of Training Schools of the United States and Canada. It eventually became the National League for Nursing Education, and then the National League for Nursing; the latter became the American Nurses' Association (ANA). In its articles of incorporation, the ANA set forth the objectives of the Association as follows:

> *The object of the Association shall be: to establish and maintain a code of ethics, to the end that the standard of nursing education be elevated; the usefulness, honor, and interests of the nursing profession be promoted; public opinion in regard to duties, responsibilities, and requirements of nurses be enlightened; emulation and concert of action in the profession be stimulated; professional loyalty be fostered, and friendly intercourse between nurses be facilitated.* (Convention of training school alumnae delegates 1896)

The first object was the creation and maintenance of a code of ethics for nurses; in 1950, the first Code for Nurses was formally adopted by the ANA House of Delegates. The Code is periodically updated, most recently in 2001 (see Chapter 3). The ANA is recognized nationally and internationally as the spokes-organization for nursing in the USA, and as the basis for the US membership in the International Council of Nurses (ICN) based in Geneva, Switzerland.

Various collateral nursing organizations arose over the years, for instance for public health nurses, for African–American nurses and others. With increased specialization of nursing after the 1960s, there has been a proliferation of nursing specialty organizations, such as the:

- American Association of Critical Care Nurses
- Perinatal Nursing Association
- Association of Operating Room Nurses
- Health Ministries Association
- Emergency Nurses Association, and so on

Such organizations are of two types: practice associations and professional associations. Nursing 'practice associations' remain practice focused, with some outward concern for legislation affecting patients in their specialty. Their chief concern is for continuing education of the members, for the constant improvement of practice through clinical innovation, research and knowledge development. The ANA, however, is a 'professional association', which is to say that its direct interest in bedside practice is low and that the advance of nursing as a profession per se is its major concern. This is a task of the power structure of an association. (Note that the objects of the Association, as set forth in the articles of incorporation, do not include the provision of continuing education for clinical practice.) Thus, the ANA will become involved in power-structure issues of regulation of nursing schools and curriculum, of the economic and general welfare of the nurse, legislation for funding of nursing traineeships or research, and establishing national standardized testing for nursing registration. In short, the ANA is concerned with the political, economic, educational, ethical and other large non-clinical aspects of nursing. It has also been the task of the ANA to develop and maintain the Code of Ethics for Nurses. This is a task of the meaning and value structure of the association.

Specialty associations, such as those noted above, bring specialist concerns and experience to the generalist perspectives of the ANA. They often prepare standards for clinical practice and seek collaboration with the ANA for the adoption of these standards by the ANA. The same kind of collaboration between professional and practice associations ought to hold true for ethics statements. Nursing associations often undergo a process of development and evolve from a practice association into a professional association that retains a practice emphasis.

The first several years in the life of a professional organization are spent in establishing the organization by cultivating a constituency that becomes a membership and financial or resource base, by defining the primary interests and activities of the group, and by establishing various aspects of the organization, such as structure, authority and communication. As an organization solidifies and matures, it generally enlarges its original scope of involvement, reaching beyond those activities that consumed its first energies. On the whole, practice-based associations are involved initially in continuing education of the membership for clinical practice, but eventually move into the area of establishing standards for education and practice, and later into the policy arena in areas that affect their target patient population or nurses within their specialty. They move from practice to professional association functions and from self- or patient-focused concerns to include more social concerns. As standards for practice are developed, initial standards attend to focal clinical concerns such as medications, treatment interventions, nursing process, and so forth. It is generally the case that later in the development of practice and education standards, concern for the ethics of clinical practice surface, initially taking the form of recommendations for moral content in education and moral standards for practice, but ultimately taking the formal form of a code of ethics. Eventually, however, the goal is that of 'social transformation' in accordance with the moral values of the profession. This requires the exercise of social ethics by the professional associations.

SOCIAL ETHICS

Social ethics can be defined as dealing with 'issues of social order – the good, right, and ought in the organization of human communities and the shaping of social policies. Hence the subject matter of social ethics is moral rightness and goodness in the shaping of human society' (Winter 1966). There are three major functions of social ethics, all of which fall within the legitimate and essential purview of the professional association: reform of the profession, epidictic discourse and social reform (Fowler 1989).

Reform of the profession, the first function of social ethics, ensures that the profession itself keeps its own house in order. It contends for change within the professional community itself, seeking to move the profession towards an envisioned ideal, to bring the 'ought' into conformity with the reality of the profession's development, practice and efforts. This is the critical, self-reflective and self-evaluative aspect of social ethics. 'Epidictic discourse', the second function of social ethics, is that form of communication that takes place within the group, seeking to reaffirm and reinforce the values that the community itself embraces. It 'sets out to increase the intensity of adherence to certain values, which might not be contested when considered on their own but may nevertheless not prevail against other values that might come into conflict with them' (Perlman & Obrechts-Tyteca 1969). Epidictic discourse reinforces the group's values, to and for the group, to strengthen the values that are held in common by the group and the speaker 'making use of dispositions already present in the audience' (Perlman & Obrechts-Tyteca 1969). Epidictic discourse galvanizes the group to employ the values cherished by the group to bring about the reform of the profession that the first function of social ethics would seek. It also provokes the group to enter into the third function of social ethics, that of speaking the values of the group into society at large to help bring about social change that is congruent with the group's values (Fowler 1989).

THE FUNCTIONS OF SOCIAL ETHICS

Any professional association that seeks to develop its social ethics must first look to itself to see whether the association is consistent with its expressed values. An example from the USA might help. If an association rejects prejudice in clinical practice on the basis of a patient's personal attributes or the nature of his or her illness, it must also examine itself to ascertain that the association does not permit those same forms of prejudicial discrimination in any of the aspects of the association's life, such as membership practices, advance within the association leadership, committee membership, awards or scholarships and so forth. The association ought to keep its own house in order in line with the ethical values it claims to affirm.

Epidictic discourse develops over time as the profession's ethical tradition grows and develops. The moments in the profession's history that brought about a moral unity and an advance of practice, the profession, the welfare of the nurse, or the welfare of society must be recorded and retained for the collective memory of the profession. In addition, concerted attention must be paid to the function of epidictic discourse and its value in bringing about a cherished unity.

The third function of social ethics, to speak the values of the group (nursing) into society must be developed with specific attention paid to education and legislation. It must be noted that this function of social ethics occurs later in the development of an association than do the other two. It is generally the case that a group attempts to secure conformity to its ethical norms by its own membership first. Only later, as strength of membership and perspective grow, does the group move into the arena of the critique of society and effecting social change.

As the ANA revised its Code of Ethics for Nurses, it added to the 2001 revision a provision on the moral role of professional associations. This reads: 'The profession of nursing, as represented by associations and their members, is responsible for articulating nursing values, for maintaining the integrity of the profession and its practice and for shaping social policy' (ANA 2001). This is a groundbreaking addition in that it is the first instance of any such statement appearing in an American nursing code of ethics. Its interpretive statements do, in fact, encompass the three functions of social ethics.

The role of a professional association in relation to ethics is to preserve, develop, and assert the meaning and value structures of the profession. This is not a simple task; it involves several concerns:

- Attention to the analysis of the profession
- The power structures of society, the profession and the professional association ethics
- The current situation of society relative to nursing
- The meaning and value structures of nursing
- The need for ethical reform within nursing and its association
- The ways in which epidictic discourse should be employed to increase group adherence to its values
- The ways in which a profession and professional association can effect change in society according to the ethics of the profession

This is no mean task. It is, however, one that can move a professional association in a direction that will balance meaning and value structures over against power structures in a way that protects, preserves and develops the association's values to the end of serving patients, society, and the individual nurse. The foremost task in this direction is the development, maintenance, and promulgation of a code of ethics for all nurses.

References

American Nurses' Association (ANA) 2001 Code of ethics for nurses with interpretive statements. ANA, Washington, DC, p 24.

Convention of training school alumnae delegates and representatives from the American Society of Superintendents of Training Schools for Nurses 1896 Proceedings of the Convention, 2–4 November 1896. Harrisburg Publishing Company, Harrisburg, PA.

Durkheim E 1933 The division of labor in society (trans. G. Simpson). Macmillan, New York.

Fowler MDM 1989 Nursing and social ethics. In Chaska NA (ed) The nursing profession: turning points. CV Mosby, St Louis, p 24–30.

Geison GL (ed) 1983 Professions and professional ideologies in America. University of North Carolina, Chapel Hill, NC.

Hatch NO 1988 The professions in American history. Notre Dame University Press, Notre Dame, IN.

Perlman Ch, Olbrechts-Tyteca L 1969 The new rhetoric: a treatise on argumentation. Notre Dame University Press, Notre Dame, IN.

Veatch R 1972 Models for ethical medicine in a revolutionary age. The Hastings Centre Report 2:5–7.

Winter G 1966 Elements for a social ethics. Macmillan, New York, p 215.

Further reading

Bixler GK, Bixler RW 1959 The professional status of nursing. American Journal of Nursing 59:1142–1146.

Frankena W 1972 Ethics. Prentice Hall, Englewood Cliffs, NJ.

Johnston T 1972 Professions and power. Macmillan Education, London.

Knowles JH 1977 Doing better and feeling worse: health in the United States. WW Norton, New York.

Kultgen J 1988 Professions and professionalism. University of Pennsylvania, Philadelphia.

Sleicher MN 1981 Nursing is not a profession. American Journal of Nursing 81:186–192.

Stackhouse M 1973 Ethics: social and christian. Andover Newton Quarterly 13:173–191.

Styles M 1982 On nursing: toward a new endowment. CV Mosby, St Louis.

Troeltsch E 1925 Historiography. In: Hastings J (ed) Encyclopedia of religion and ethics, vol 6. T & T Clark, Edinburgh.

Chapter 5

Religious and clinical ethics

Marsha Fowler

Religious moral discourse extends approximately 6000 years from oral tradition to approximately 3000 years of written reflection. In this light, any brief essay on religious ethics will have to restrict its focus severely. Perhaps the most expedient approach is to ask about the practical aspects of religio-moral authority and its incorporation into ethics in nursing practice. Thus, the question that this chapter will address is 'What are the sources of religious–ethical authority that give rise to moral norms and how might they inform clinical nursing practice?' Here, moral norms are understood to be the criteria by which we judge what we ought to be or do as moral beings. Four broad categories of religious–ethical authority that may serve as sources of moral norms will be examined: religious writings, religious tradition, reason and experience. Although some religions may emphasize one source over another, all four together comprise the basis for religious–ethical decision making.

Although the present discussion is narrowly limited to sources of authority in religious ethics and their incorporation in the exercise of nursing ethics, the world around us is aflame with religiously coloured strife. These desperate situations are actually more than strictly religious and combine power, politics, oppression and culture. These overshadow the aspects of religion that foster human flourishing and sustain human community. An understanding of religious authority and ethics serves not only to inform our understanding of ethical decisions by nurses or their patients but also to inform our understanding of the world.

SACRED WRITINGS AS A SOURCE OF RELIGIO-ETHICAL AUTHORITY

Religious writings span a wide range of authority within any given religious tradition. They range from sacred to devotional writings. The faith community in which they arise regard as sacred or canonical writings those that have prior, or the most vigorous, or perhaps absolute, authority. Canonical writings are seen as having their ultimate origin in God, the divine, or the transcendent, and are customarily regarded as having binding authority because of their transcendent origin. This is not to deny that they have been written by human hands but these writings are seen to be somehow uniquely inspired in their recording. The writings vary in how they are viewed: as having been dictated by the divine, as divinely inspired through the vehicle of human expression, or as reflecting divinity in having been set down by a singular individual who has reached a transcendent state of spiritual progress.

Examples of canonical writings, or scriptures, include the:

- Torah
- Tanakh
- Bible
- Qur'an
- Mahabharata
- Tipitaka
- Mahayana Sutras
- Tao De Ching

Tanakh is an acrostic for Torah (law), Neviim (prophets) and Ketuvim (writings), the three categories of works that are combined into the Jewish Bible. The Tanakh forms the basis for the first portion of the Christian Bible, commonly referred to by Christians as the Old Testament. The second of the two portions of the Christian Bible is the New Testament. Both the Tanakh and the Christian Bible are the work of multiple writers and redactors, inspired by God in their recording of the sacred writings.

The Qur'an precisely records the words of God revealed by the angel Gabriel to the prophet Muhammad and contains the sacred writings of Islam. The Qur'an is recorded as the word of God through a single individual.

The Hindu sacred scriptures fall into two categories: the Shruti (that which is heard), which includes the Vedas and Upanishads, and Smriti (that which is remembered), which includes the post-Vedic Hindu Mahabharata and the Ramayana. The authority of the Shruti is given greater weight. The Bhagavad Gita, widely known in the non-Hindu world and considered to be sacred text by almost all Hindus, combines elements of both Shruti and Smriti.

The Tipitaka is the scripture of Buddhism. Theravada Buddhists regard the Tipitaka as the complete teachings of the Buddha while Mahayana Buddhists regard the Tipitaka and the Mahayana Sutras together as sacred scripture.

Other sacred writings include the Guru Granth Sahib (Sikhism), the Tao De Ching (Taoism), the Avesta of Zarathustra (Zoroastrianism) and others too numerous to list. Some religions, such as Shintoism, have no written scriptures. Many of the scriptures listed here began as oral tradition, passed down verbatim for centuries before being recorded, so that the life of the sacred scriptures is often considerably longer than its life in written form. In cultures where the primary mode of transmission is through oral tradition, that transmission should not be regarded as less accurate than contemporary written transmission.

These sacred writings comprise some of the primary texts for the followers of their respective religions. As such, they are read and followed as the basis for the tradition's world view, as authoritative guides to the religious life and its practices, and as a source of moral authority and teachings. They are regarded as authoritative, trustworthy, and binding in matters of faith, including the moral life.

The development of the field of textual studies (lower criticism), as well as the rise during the nineteenth century of modern higher critical methods of study of ancient texts, have served to advance the modern understanding of sacred scriptures. Today, sacred scriptures are understood by scholars to be works of faith, not works of science, geography or history, and as being shaped by the language, culture, literary genre, setting-in-life (*Sitz im Leben*) and redactional purposes (the theological purposes of the editor) of the work. These studies make it clear that in a plain and simple reading of sacred texts today, particularly ancient texts, there is very little that is plain and simple about them. A brief discussion is necessary here because a poor or uninformed interpretation of sacred texts is most frequently when followers of a religion go awry.

There are three fundamental sequential phases of interpretation of sacred scriptures: exegesis, interpretation (together referred to as hermeneutics) and application. Exegesis is the process of examining a text to uncover how the text's first readers would have understood its meaning. Interpretation involves discerning how we are to understand the text today in the light of what it meant to the first readers. Application addresses the question of how we should live in the light of this interpretation. Understanding of the texts customarily requires some study to accompany the reading if one is to see how, for instance, the literary genres/subgenres serve to limit possible exegetical interpretations of the text. Works such as commentaries can be used to shed considerable hermeneutic light on passages of scriptures, from which the members of the faith community can move towards application in daily life.

Many religious traditions also have written works such as devotional or instructive writings that are revered, although not regarded as canonical. They are seen as authoritative and reliable, but are subordinate to sacred scriptures. In most instances these works serve as general guides or further explication for the life of faith. Persons within a given faith community will draw on the sacred writings as well as these other religious works for guidance in the moral life. Yet the question remains: how are moral norms drawn from sacred writings?

There are several approaches to the derivation of ethical precepts from scriptures. One way is to view sacred writings as books of rules that are concrete, material norms. This is perhaps the least satisfactory means of deriving moral norms, and is methodologically unsound on at least three grounds. First, it is a precritical approach to sacred writings that generally ignores the necessity for exegesis. It wrests portions of scripture from their broader context that specifies the nature of the communal context in which these norms are operative. It neglects the interpretive boundaries that are set by such things as literary genres and original setting-in-life, applying them to contexts that do not bear the same hallmarks. Second, it grants normative stature to particular portions of sacred writings without testing those portions against the whole of the corpus. Third, this approach is often a means of proof texting a pre-existing disposition not actually based on faith. Rather, it is a disposition in search of a justification, thereby using sacred writings in such a way as to make them mean what the reader wishes them to mean rather than what they actually mean, or bootlegging meaning into a passage. This approach to the derivation of moral norms from sacred writings can prove dangerous when such interpretation deviates from the tradition's dominant interpretation(s). It must be noted that some persons reject the use of sacred scriptures as sources of moral authority altogether, on the grounds that their antiquity makes them dated and therefore unusable and inapplicable to life today. This dismissive approach is flawed in the same way in that it, too, treats sacred writings like a cookbook.

Religious scriptures do contain concrete, material prescriptions and proscriptions for moral behaviour, but such specifications customarily give way to the authority of more formal norms. For instance, concrete norms against misrepresentation in the marketplace would give way to formal norms enjoining us to treat one another as we ourselves would wish to be treated. At the level of formal norms, there is considerable concurrence among world religions. For instance, many religions have a similar norm about the way in which we are to treat others, often called 'the golden rule'. Rabbi Hillel has stated it as:

> *What is hateful to you, do not do to your neighbor: that is the whole Torah; all the rest of it is commentary; go and learn.* (Talmud, Shabbat 31a)

A similar formal norm is found in many other religions, for example:

> Hinduism: *'One should not behave towards others in a way that is disagreeable to oneself. This is the essence of morality. All other activities are due to selfish desire.'* (Mahabharata, Anusasana Parva 113.8)
> Islam: *'Not one of you is a believer until he loves for his brother what he loves for himself.'* (Forty Hadith of an-Nawawi 13)

While religions do not collapse into the same moral norms, there is some agreement in the moral norms that religious persons will use. Indeed, these norms may bring about similar applications and similar conclusions such that the religious world view resident behind them is imperceptible in moral discourse. Similar norms may also produce divergent interpretations even within one tradition (e.g. the 'sanctity of life' as encompassing animal as well as human life). In some instances the divergence relates to a difference in interpretation of a fact, rather than the value itself. Formal principles such as these require reflection in order to be applied.

Setting aside less adequate means of deriving moral norms from scripture, at least three different general approaches emerge. Sacred scriptures may be seen as divinely revealed moral law that should govern the actions of the faithful; as a glimpse of the nature of the divine or transcendent from which one derives moral norms according to the attributes, character, or nature of the transcendent; or as providing a moral context and vision for the life of faith from which themes such as destiny, oneness, salvation inform and guide moral deliberation and choice (Gula 1982 p 33). Within these three basic approaches, formal moral norms are given concrete specification for particular settings by means of reflection that employs reason, tradition and experience and sacred writings themselves to give further specification in any given situation.

RELIGIOUS TRADITION AS A SOURCE OF RELIGIO-ETHICAL AUTHORITY

Religions are by nature lived out in the context of a community of faith. The extent to which ordinary followers are at liberty to interpret the tradition and its sacred writings varies widely within as well as among religions; sometimes that task is reserved for the tradition's leaders or scholars.

Religions, as religious cultures, often become embedded in the wider civil culture to the extent that the religion and the culture may merge at points. In many instances, religion and culture can be difficult to disentangle. Aspects of the civil culture may even become de fide, or essential tenets of the faith even when they have no actual basis in the faith (Niebuhr 1951). For example, specific forms of national political organization, such as 'democracy', may be seen as an approved and essential expression of the faith rightly understood, when, in fact, it is not. The culture of a religion, rather than its beliefs, may govern many aspects of non-moral behaviour, including how one reacts with joy or sorrow, success or disappointment, forgiveness or anger. At times, beliefs may actually be at odds with religious culture. Examples are when the beliefs condemn homosexual behaviour but not the condition of homosexuality and yet the culture rejects homosexuals per se. Or when equality between the sexes is affirmed and adultery is roundly condemned by the faith but winked at when men are caught, while women are damned for the same offence. This is rather more complex than simple hypocrisy: it is a religio-cultural response that takes a veneer of religious belief; it *may* entail a degree of cognitive dissonance and yet not actually be hypocrisy.

Our concern here is with the more formal aspects of a religious tradition wherein the official statements, beliefs, rules and customs are handed down to the faithful. This would include formal authoritative pronouncements regarding religious ethics, moral issues and moral expectations of followers. Today, the internet can be a rich source of religious bioethical perspectives. A search of the terms 'Islam' AND 'end-of-life' returns more than 1 630 000 results; many of these are clearly articulated, formal statements by widely respected Moslem scholars. In addition, the internet also provides access to official religious sites. For instance, there are websites for the Chief Rabbi of the Commonwealth (British), the Vatican, the Church of Scotland, His Holiness the fourteenth Dalai Lama of Tibet, the Sikh Network and the Golden Temple Kar Seva, His Holiness Patriarch Alexy II of Moscow and all Russia, the Pagan Federation, The British Druid Order and so on. Through the internet it is now possible to obtain official statements on a wide range of faith-based questions and concerns, including bioethical issues of interest to nurses, for virtually all world religions. A number of religious traditions have scholarly journals available online as well.

In the realm of nursing and bioethics, religious traditions usually have an understanding of what constitutes health, beliefs about disease, mental illness, suffering, death and dying, health care and medical treatment. They often formally address issues related to end-of-life care, withdrawal of treatment, reproduction, access to health care, healthcare delivery systems, cloning and all current bioethical issues. The statements that are produced are position statements for the tradition itself and serve as guidance for individual believers. When a tradition issues such statements, there is an expectation that adherents of the tradition follow this guidance. Depending on the gravity of the issue being treated and its implications for the faith, some traditions allow a degree of latitude among believers based on conscience.

A religious tradition may also have a body of teachings on health-related personal ethics that are also considered to be authoritative of its followers. For instance, faithful members of the tradition may be taught that an obedient lifestyle that fully embraces the tradition may lead to freedom from disease or suffering. Where disease or suffering exists, it represents a life not fully lived in the faith. A number of religious traditions view personal health maintenance as a part of one's religious obligation. The particular ends of the religion (e.g. salvation, mukti, nirvana, paradise, the beatific vision, or oneness with the universe) also inform how one is to live life in relation to our corporeal existence. Moreover, there may be specific religious practices, such as fasting or vegetarianism, that some traditions encourage that can have health implications. The degree to which an individual nurse or patient is influenced by the official teachings and statements of a tradition is dependent on several factors. These include its cultural aspects, its vision of human life and its ends; its views of health, illness, mental health, death, dying and suffering; and its moral perspectives and guidance. They are based on many factors, such as the degree of devotion or adherence of the believer, the level of religious integration, limitations on the exercise of disagreement or conscience, the individual level of self-reflection, and the personal religious support structures of the individual.

REASON AS A SOURCE OF RELIGIO-ETHICAL AUTHORITY

Religions in general give a systematic account of reality, usually referred to as a world view. Within that world view there are claims about knowledge (epistemology) and its acquisition, claims about the nature of humanity (ontology) and its ends, and claims about the way in which the life of faith should be lived (ethics and aesthetics). It is by way of reason that the individual believer will evaluate the claims of the religion for coherence, consistency, comprehensiveness, congruity or compatibility with facts known of the material world, explanatory power, and sense-making potential. This is a critical rationalism applied to faith for the purposes of evaluation and of deepening an understanding of the faith (Peterson et al 2003). Although related, this is different from the reasoned, critical reflection necessary to elucidate the truths, precepts or formal guidelines of the faith that might be brought to bear on ethical decision making and action. For instance, a religion may contain a basic rule in its sacred writings 'do not kill'. Searching the context of the rule in sacred scripture leads one to believe that it refers to killing humans and not animals or plants or, more broadly, not something like the environment. Yet, even with this clarification, the norm against killing cannot be applied as it stands, for we still do not know what is meant by killing. A search of commentaries is of some assistance in that it clarifies that do not kill means do not murder, but it still does not take us far enough. Is withdrawal of treatment murder? Are abortion, euthanasia or suicide? What types of killing constitute murder? The difficulty with a formal rule is that it is without content yet requires that reason be used in order to specify how it should be applied. How then might reason be used within religious ethics in exploring and employing moral norms? Two fundamental methods of moral reasoning may be broadly sketched.

The first method is essentially deductive. It begins with abstract and universal formal principles drawn from reason or sacred writings, or the tradition. These principles are seen as timeless and free from historical or cultural conditioning. As such they can be applied rationally with rigour, clarity, coherence and consistency, independent of the context. Although not entirely formulaic, this approach shares with formulas a certain conceptual precision and a degree of objectivity or impartiality. Reasoned evaluation and application thus show a degree of orderliness and stability and provide for a historical continuity by moving from formal to concrete material norms applicable by all people everywhere and across time. On the other hand, life is not generally known for its neatness. The deductive approach fails to take account of the complexity and imprecision of the human situation, the social construction of reality, the fluidity of human freedom or the uniqueness of particular moral contexts.

A second general method of moral reasoning takes greater account of the messiness of life by beginning inductively with experience and particularity, rather than logic and universality. It is empirical in nature and draws intentionally on the social sciences in its reflection. Norms are more malleable in this approach and, unlike the deductive approach, it risks relativity at its farther end. As examples within the ethical literature of nursing, the deductive approach is more closely associated with what has been called ethical principlism, and the inductive approach that starts with experience is familiarly seen in various approaches to feminist ethics in the nursing literature. Both approaches are a part of religious moral reasoning.

These two basic approaches to religious ethics ought not to be cast in an either/or standoff. The deductive approach does indeed allow for rigour and precision, for the exploration of nuance, dispassionate discussion, resistance to relativization, and consistency and evenhandedness in application. These are strong reasons to retain a deductive approach. The inductive approach pays close attention to the experience of the moral community and its members as a valid source of moral knowledge and judgement, and to the complexity of moral dilemmas. Other aspects to consider are the non-universal aspects of those dilemmas, and the fact that our reason is suffused with elements drawn from culture, tradition and the historical context. For these strong reasons, an inductive approach should be retained. Although the inductive method has gained the ascendancy in religious and secular western circles, both the deductive and inductive methods should be used, bringing their respective strengths to moral reflection, discourse and decision making.

RELIGIOUS EXPERIENCE AS A SOURCE OF RELIGIO–ETHICAL AUTHORITY

Religious experience is an encounter with a transcendent reality and is understood by the person as an experience of a supernatural presence or being, or a sense of an ineffable reality. Such experiences tend to be intimate, intensely real, awe-filled, perhaps overwhelming or frightening, and as having a depth of mystery. These experiences may produce religious moral insight. To speak of religious experience is, in the end, to address the issue of what is customarily called the inner or interior life, or spirituality.

Religious spirituality can serve as an interpretive lens that is important for a discussion of experience as a source of religio-ethical authority. For some persons, however, religious experience is less a part of their moral evaluation or outlook. Much of what has been said here is true only of persons who have determined intentionally to live their faith as an intimate part of daily life, i.e. they have chosen to live seeing through the lens of their religious world view and to act in a manner congruent with it. Those who affiliate more loosely with a faith tradition or embrace it only nominally or culturally will probably not demonstrate as full an attempt to draw on its resources.

A second issue relating to the use of sources of religious ethical authority has to do with what might be called the spiritual maturity. The various theories of spiritual development share some basic understandings. Spirituality is generally seen as a life journey, a process of development and maturation. In general, greater spiritual maturity demonstrates:

- Intentionality
- Critical reflection and reasoning
- Coherence of basic beliefs
- A higher level of integration
- Familiarity with the tradition, history, literature, and practices
- Involvement with the religious community
- Personal practices of piety
- A commitment to spiritual growth

Such persons see the world through the lens of their religious world view. Persons with less well developed spiritual lives tend to compartmentalize their faith to a greater degree and it has less influence on daily life.

In general, religious traditions and their communities would seem to retain an overt emphasis on virtues to a greater degree than does the larger secular society. These could include such virtues as peaceableness, equanimity, kindness, generosity, love, goodwill, awareness, carefulness, wisdom and so forth. Moral agency, then, would be rooted in the spiritual character of the person as much as in specific religio-moral duties.

Religious experience may also be felt as an encounter with the divine, the numinous or the absolute that is in and of itself religiously and morally authoritative, and a source of moral knowledge. Here the importance of a community of faith as a community of reference cannot be overstressed as it may serve as a source of correction. The People's Temple, the Order of the Solar Temple, the Branch Davidians and Heaven's Gate, are examples of groups with privatized religious experience and interpretation, and without a larger community of reference and thereby without a source of correction. These religious groups demonstrate the lethal triad of isolation, complete subjection to a charismatic leader and anger (Gilmartin 1996). They tend to be regarded as 'cults' because they stand in tension to society and other religious groups. Whether for religious experience or for interpretation of sacred writings, a larger community of faith that serves as a community of reference also serves as the guardrails at the edge of the cliff.

That community of reference should not, however, be a box that holds timeless truths in a time warp. Where this is the case, spiritual exemplars and heroes are less likely to emerge. Such persons can be forces for social change. Religious experience may lead a believer to critique the community itself, or to step out and take risks so that the world might be changed for the better. There are many examples of this, but Walter Rauschenbusch, Reinhold Niebuhr and the Pastor's Emergency League immediately spring to mind. Rauschenbusch sought to restate Christian doctrine in terms of a greater social ethical consciousness. His particular concern was for the poor and the industrial workers in America's industrial revolution. Reinhold Niebuhr was an ardent social activist concerned for the welfare of factory workers. He later wrote vigorously about and against the self-deceptions of nations. At great peril, a group called the Pastor's Emergency League organized in Nazi Germany as an alliance of German Pastors to resist Hitler's usurpation and co-optation of the Protestant church as a tool for the propagation of Nazism (Scholder 1989). In these three examples we see a profound and public moral critique of their own societies, based on their understanding of sacred writings and tradition, reason and religious experience. For all three, deeply held religious ethics and distress at the sociopolitical situation came together in the form of social criticism and social activism, that is, social ethics. Examples of such 'faithful persons' are too numerous to name but we must not continue without mentioning Archbishop Desmond Tutu, Archbishop Romero and Tenzin Gyatso, the fourteenth Dalai Lama.

In particular, the experience within a community helps to nurture that faculty called conscience and helps to imbue a sense of duty. It can foster virtues such as humility in the face of moral complexity, and grace or forgiveness for error that springs from human limitation. It can help to sort out the official position that must be expressed in daily life. Experience, personally and within the community, can also help to navigate those few instances in which religious and secular ethics come into conflict in nursing practice.

RELIGIOUS ETHICS AND NURSING ETHICS

Those sources of religious ethical authority that have been discussed – sacred writings, tradition, reason, and experience – are also the same sources of moral authority found within nursing. Although not precisely sacred, the codes of ethics for nurses formulated by nursing associations in many nations, or by the International Council of Nurses (ICN), serve as authoritative moral standards governing practice. The issue-based position statements produced by those nursing associations and documents that extend the codes of ethics comprise the subordinate standards. Nurses may also draw from the tradition of service and more recently of caring as a source of moral norms. Reason is also a source of moral knowledge in nursing; the debate over an ethics of caring is an example. The clinical experiences of those human tragedies that we call moral dilemmas serve as sources of moral norms as well.

The question remains, however: what about those instances in which religious ethics may come into conflict with professional ethics? Competing values are not new to nursing, particularly in an economically constrained environment where cost competes with care, and quantity competes with quality. Competing duties are also not new to nurses, for example, where doing good for the patient also inflicts harm, or where keeping a confidence may harm someone else. There are occasions where religious values or duties might conflict with professional values or duties. Basic values, such as human dignity and well-being, tend not to find conflict with religious values. More often, when they occur, the conflicts are situated in conflicts of duty. For instance, the nursing ethical literature deals extensively with distributive justice, while many religious traditions emphasize compensatory justice, and with it a particular duty to care for underserved, marginalized, disadvantaged and vulnerable persons. In some religious traditions, refusal or withdrawal of end-of-life treatment may be prohibited, placing nurses who are assigned as caregivers in a morally difficult position. In conflicts such as these, the nurse must weigh the religious values and duties over against those of the profession or the setting, and choose between them.

However, such conflicts are relatively infrequent; more often, religious ethics affirms and sometimes expands professional ethics. Where conflict occurs, the degree to which nurses (or patients) embrace a religious tradition, as well as their point of spiritual development, will in part determine the scope and depth of their reliance on that religion's moral norms in facing moral dilemmas in health care. If their level of commitment is less than moderate, it is the case that other values may overwhelm their religio-ethical values and claim priority. It is more frequently the case, however, that the religiously based ethics of the nurse will produce moral responses, decisions and actions that are not dissimilar to those of other practitioners. A mature and reflective religious world view that underpins and grounds a nurse's moral position may in fact remain transparent to colleagues and not cause conflict, while yet enriching the moral discourse.

References

Gilmartin K 1996 The lethal triad: understanding the nature of isolated extremist groups. Federal Bureau of Investigation (FBI) Law Enforcement Bulletin, September. FBI, Washington, DC.

Gula R 1982 What are they saying about moral norms? Paulist Press, New York.

Niebuhr HR 1951 Christ and culture. Harper Torchbooks, New York.

Peterson M, Hasker W, Reichengach B, Basinger D 2003 Reason and religious belief. Oxford University Press, Oxford.

Scholder K 1989 A requiem for Hitler (trans. J Bowden). Trinity Press International, Philadelphia.

Further reading

Bellah R 1992 The good society. Vintage Books/Knopf Publishing Group, New York.

Carter S 1993 The culture of disbelief. Basic Books, New York.

Desai PN 1989 Health and medicine in the Hindu tradition. Crossroad, New York.

Feldman D 1986 Health and medicine in the Jewish tradition. Crossroad, New York.

Harakas S 1989 Health and medicine in the Eastern Orthodox tradition. Crossroad, New York.

Holifield EB 1989 Health and medicine in the Methodist tradition. Crossroad, New York.

Hultkranz A 1997 Shamanic healing and ritual drama: health and medicine in the native North American religious traditions. Crossroad, New York.

Leech K 1985 Experiencing God: theology as spirituality. Harper & Row, New York.

McCormick R 1984 Health and medicine in the Catholic tradition. Crossroad, New York.

Marty M 1983 Health and medicine in the Lutheran tradition. Crossroad, New York.

Marty M, Vaux K 1982 Health/medicine and the faith traditions: an inquiry into religion and medicine. Fortress, Philadelphia.

Niebuhr HR 1932 Moral man and immoral society, vols 1, 2. Simon and Schuster, New York.

Numbers R, Amundsen, D 1986 Caring and curing: health and medicine in the western religious traditions. Macmillan, New York.

Presbyterian Church (PC USA) 1989 How and why the church makes a social policy witness. PC (USA), Louisville, KY.

Rahman F 1997 Health and medicine in the Islamic tradition. Crossroad, New York.

Rauschenbusch W 1997 A theology for the social gospel. Westminster/John Knox, Philadelphia.

Smith D Health and medicine in the Anglican tradition. Crossroad, New York.

Snyder G, Marty M, Wind J 1995 Health and medicine in the Anabaptist tradition. Crossroad, New York.

Sullivan LE 1997 Healing and restoring: health and medicine in the world's religious traditions. Crossroad, New York.

Sweet L 1994 Health and medicine in the evangelical tradition. Crossroad, New York.

Thiselton A 1980 The two horizons: new testament hermeneutics and philosophical description. Grand Rapids, MI, Eerdmans.

Vaux K 1984 Health and medicine in the reformed tradition. Crossroad, New York.

PART 2

Theories of ethics

PART CONTENTS

Chapter 6

Introduction to the theory chapters

Louise de Raeve

The chapters in this part of the book are varied and fascinating. They are split into four sections in which one moral theory is presented in the opening chapter, followed by a chapter where the theory is critiqued and a chapter that explores what it might mean to teach ethics from such a theoretical perspective. The authors of the critique chapters have not been asked to comment specifically on the chapter preceding theirs, therefore chapters can be viewed in a standalone sense. As editors, however, we would recommend reading each theoretical section in the order in which they appear in the book, i.e. presentation, followed by critique, followed by application to nursing (with a specific focus on teaching). The sections themselves have also been given a specific order, commencing with the principle-based approach. We believe this is the most widely known theoretical perspective in healthcare ethics and even though the virtue approach has a longer history, its re-emergence in healthcare ethics seems to have been in response to perceived inadequacies with the principle-based approach. Caring ethics is a more recent candidate but it has strong links with virtue theory, certainly in the form presented in this book. Feminist ethics, the last of the four theories, is the most historically recent and while also rejecting the principle-based approach, it shares with caring ethics a similar definition of what it is to be a person and the importance of context and narrative when thinking about moral issues.

In the introduction to this book we suggested that a moral theory establishes 'our focus of concern, our language of dialogue and the outcome of our discourse'. Moral theories share an attempt to provide a 'reasoned response to practical questions such as 'How should we live?' or 'What should we do?', asked of matters ranging from the public and political to the intimate and domestic' (O'Neill 1991). In the case of health care, these questions are more specific, for example:

- How should we treat patients?
- How should we prioritise care in contexts of multiple need and inadequate resources?
- How should we teach nurses what it means to be a good nurse or a kind and competent nurse and how can we help them to achieve this?

Moral theories aim at helping with these deliberations by systematizing and clarifying what is at stake and each has attempted to provide a universal account of morality. In view of this, it is not unreasonable to hope that they would provide answers, or at least give us more certainty that the outcome of our deliberations would be the right answer. This, however, seems to be a forlorn hope because no moral theory is without criticism; while individuals may prefer one or another, none can claim final authority. Indeed it may be the case that moral discourse, by its highly evaluative nature, is an area of enquiry for which there could never be a universal theory or anything amounting to 'moral answers'.

If this is the case, it does not prevent the insights of these different moral theories being of great value but it may then be a question of comparing and contrasting them and taking from them what seems most useful. This 'pick and mix' approach might lead one to talk of moral perspectives, rather than theories. However, it may not be so simple to do this, because a 'pick and mix' approach might ignore the fact that many moral theories are set up in opposition to each other. Their language and concepts are different and the way in which, for example, they give respective weight to reason or emotion, or particular states of affairs versus general situations, may be so different as to be contradictory. With this in mind, we introduce the respective chapters below and invite you to read them carefully but also critically.

Steven Edwards begins his chapter by examining the principle-based approach and from this emerges what he calls a 'modest' and 'immodest' proposal. He concludes that both approaches are defensible but suggests that the latter approach, which gives supremacy to the principle of autonomy, needs to be suffused with care. Samantha Pang, in her critique, introduces an interesting cross-cultural dimension by comparing what a nurse might decide in the USA as opposed to Hong Kong. After a logical analysis of these two cases, she concludes that the principle-based approach is inadequate to capture what is morally at stake in nurse–patient relationships. The generality of the principles ignores the intimacy of this relationship. Theresa Drought argues that the principle-based approach is not a 'template for action' and her framework makes this clear with its 'other concerns' section. However, she suggests that this approach to moral decision making is a useful tool.

This section is followed by three chapters that examine virtue theory. Inherent in this inquiry is the question of whether or not virtue theory is in fact a theory, or an anti-theory. In its theoretical form, it has a long history from the Greek philosopher, Aristotle, to the present day. The focus of the virtues is not on general principles to guide action but on character and, specifically for nursing, on those qualities of character that would describe the good nurse. Louise de Raeve concludes that the virtues might be enhanced within nursing by the provision of good role models, by the study of medical humanities and by participation in clinical supervision.

Chris Gastmans gives a thorough description of what might be meant by 'care' and 'caring ethics'. He links this firmly to the virtue tradition, making caring ethics an aspect of virtue ethics but not equivalent to it.

He sees it as a 'stance from which we can theorize ethically' rather than it being a 'full blown ethical theory'. He stresses the importance of relationship, narrative and interpretation and also comments that because care is a virtue, 'emotion and reason are intrinsically bonded together' in this approach. John Paley follows with a hard-hitting critique of the care-based approach. He presents a strong version and a weak version of this and demolishes them with equal intellectual force, concluding that care within ethics would only have adequate meaning if it was incorporated into a deontological or utilitarian system of thought. This conclusion is not so dissimilar from that of Steven Edwards in the first chapter, although it is reached for quite different reasons. What I think John Paley perhaps ignores is that, whether nurses wish it or not, the dependency of patients tends to give rise to them becoming attached to their nurses (or to them fighting against this). Ethics cannot ignore these aspects of the nurse–patient relationship, for nurses need help to think about the best way to respond, in the interests of patient care and recovery. Anne Davis and Marsha Fowler complete this section with an overview of some very useful literature on the topic and helpful questions to invite students to consider.

Joan Liaschenko and Elizabeth Peter present feminist ethics. With its interest in power and oppression, it is a kind of reforming ethics but with links to the care-based approach. The expressive collaborative model advocated by Walker (1998) is promoted and this acknowledges that 'morality is fundamentally interpersonal and negotiated'. Persons are viewed as largely restricted in their autonomy by their relationships. In the critique, Elizabeth Peter considers the accusation of 'relativism' that could be levelled against this approach and she refers to a 'hard' and 'soft' version of this. In response, she suggests that moral pluralism is a better description of feminist ethics than moral relativism. In these two chapters, general rules and principles of morality are rejected. Nevertheless, there seems to be an implicit commitment to an underlying principle of justice, which I would argue is necessary to give meaning to language like 'oppression'. In my reading of the chapter, I cannot quite work out where Elizabeth Peter stands on this. Both authors write the final chapter in this section concerning the teaching of feminist ethics. Ideas such as 'moral ethnography' and 'geography of responsibility' are explained via the use of a very interesting case example. It is claimed that 'feminist ethics is not a subject matter but a way of doing ethics' and in this, it has something in common with the chapter exploring the teaching of virtue ethics.

In reading these chapters, you may be surprised to discover that three authors (Samantha Pang, Theresa Drought and Chris Gastmans) use clinical examples concerning patients where there is an issue of whether or not to continue feeding. We did not ask them to use a common example; perhaps this indicates that the issue is particularly troubling for nurses, at least in the countries from which these authors come. It might even have broader meaning, for it could be that our professional commitment and motivation makes the issue of food and feeding a particularly painful one for us. The word 'nurse' comes from the old French word *nourice*, which derives from the Latin *nutricia*. In Latin *nutrive* meant 'to nourish', so *nutricia*, the nurse, is 'the nourisher' (Collins English Dictionary 1986).

References

Collins English Dictionary 1986 Second edition. Collins, London.

O'Neill O 1991 Introducing ethics: some current positions. Bulletin of Medical Ethics November:18–21.

Walker M 1998 Moral understandings: a feminist study in ethics. Routledge, New York.

Chapter 7

A principle–based approach to nursing ethics

Steven Edwards

This chapter presents a sympathetic account of a principle-based approach to nursing ethics. Two versions are used and defended: modest and immodest versions.[1] The value of this approach in either version is proposed for both nursing ethics education and practice.

TWO CONDITIONS A THEORY OF NURSING ETHICS MUST MEET

Two of the main conditions of adequacy for any credible approach to nursing ethics are:

- The approach must recognize the complex nature of moral judgement
- Any such approach must be compatible with the requirements of professional practice

MORAL JUDGEMENT

One common response to questions about the nature of moral judgement is to point to the many disagreements that exist about moral matters. For

---

[1] The 'modest' form of the principle-based approach, as I am using that term here, signifies a way of applying the approach merely as an aid to moral decision making. This is in contrast with the 'immodest' form of the approach, in which one particular moral principle is held to 'trump' or outweigh all others.

example, within western cultures there is disagreement concerning the moral defensibility of abortion, capital punishment, use of animals for medical research, distribution of healthcare resources, the extent of foreign aid that should be given, etc. These are simply some present-day disagreements; they are multiplied many-fold when considering disagreements across cultures and historical periods.

It is also common to contrast this apparent state of disarray in moral judgements with other types of judgement. Although there is disagreement within and across cultures regarding moral matters, no such disagreements appear to be present in arithmetic. Two people might disagree about the morality of capital punishment but they will agree that $2 + 2 = 4$. Similarly, two people may disagree about whether assisted conception services should be provided by the National Health Service (NHS) in the UK, but they are hardly likely to dispute that New York is west of London.

If there is a dispute concerning a simple empirical matter, such as a dispute between two people concerning how many chairs there are in this room, this can easily be resolved by simply counting the number of chairs in the room. In a case of this kind there is agreement on what counts as a chair and on how to count the chairs: on what counts as one chair and what counts as two. Finally, there is agreement on which outcome will resolve the dispute.

By contrast, in a moral dispute, such as that concerning the moral defensibility of abortion, there may be disagreement over the very subject of the debate. For one party, the termination of the life of a fetus may be equivalent to the killing of an adult human being. For the other, the fetus has no such moral status and the moral significance of its death does not remotely compare with the significance of the death of an adult human being. There is debate about what counts as morally right and wrong action. The two parties in the dispute plainly disagree about this.

There is agreement about what counts as a chair and there may be agreement about what counts as a fetus, but there is disagreement over the *moral status* of the fetus. There seems no equivalent of this in the chair dispute.

In the chair dispute, each party accepts the procedure for resolving the dispute, but this seems not to be so in the abortion dispute. Although both parties may agree on the empirical 'facts', e.g., that this is a fetus of 10 weeks' development, there remains disagreement about what it is 'right' to do.

Both parties can *see* the chairs and thus verify the count to see who is correct, but there seems to be no equivalent empirical tribunal to 'see' the rightness or wrongness of abortion. One can see chairs, desks, human beings and so on, but not moral rightness or wrongness, it seems. Two parties can agree about all the empirical facts relevant to a disagreement, yet still disagree about what is morally right or wrong. For example, two people might agree that renal dialysis is withheld from patients over the age of 65, but one person may say that this is morally indefensible while the other maintains it is morally correct.

These characteristics of moral judgement need to be borne in mind in any approach to nursing ethics.

PROFESSIONAL PRACTICE

The second constraint stems from the requirements of professional nursing practice. An approach to nursing ethics that obliges a nurse not to consider the interests of all the patients for which he or she has clinical responsibility would plainly violate the requirements of professional practice. Similarly, an approach that obliges a nurse to exhaust herself or himself, thus neglecting obligations to his or her own family, would also breach such requirements. Any credible approach to ethics must respect the standards of professional practice.

A PRINCIPLE-BASED APPROACH TO NURSING ETHICS

The best-known statement of the principle-based approach to healthcare ethics is detailed in Tom Beauchamp and James Childress' book *Principles of Biomedical Ethics* first published in 1978 and now in its fifth edition (2001). In this approach, four levels of thinking about moral matters are identified (1994 p 15), each of which involves a greater degree of generality:

- Level one: particular moral judgements
- Level two: moral rules
- Level three: moral principles
- Level four: theories

Level 1 concerns particular moral judgements, such as decisions to tell a patient the truth or to withhold it.

At *level 2*, Beauchamp and Childress posit four moral rules central to the relationships between healthcare professionals and patients (2001 p 283). These are as follows. First, *the veracity rule*. This is a rule that refers to obligations to be truthful to patients and to cultivate their understanding of relevant considerations (2001 p 284). Second, *the privacy rule*. This concerns obligations to respect people's privacy in a range of senses. These include an informational sense, a sense relating to people's 'personal space' and also to privacy in decision making: not to encroach upon people inappropriately (2001 p 295). The third rule is about *confidentiality*. Breaches of confidentiality are defined thus:

> An infringement of a person's confidentiality occurs only if the person (or institution) to whom the information was disclosed in confidence fails to protect that information or deliberately discloses it to someone without first-party consent. (Beauchamp & Childress 2001 p 304)

Thus, although related to obligations to respect privacy, obligations to respect confidentiality are more specific. They apply only when a person has divulged information in confidence and this has been passed on to other parties without the consent of the person concerned, or the information is not kept secure. Fourth, *the fidelity rule* concerns obligations 'to act in good faith, to keep vows and promises, fulfil agreements, maintain relationships, and discharge fiduciary responsibilities. . .' (2001 p 312). As Beauchamp and Childress conceive of such obligations, they stem from recognition that the relationship between patients and healthcare professionals is not morally equivalent to that between consumers and service providers. In the latter, relationships are contractual in nature: one party contracts the services of another party. Such a contractual relationship is not morally appropriate in health care, mainly due to the vulnerability of patients. The example that Beauchamp and Childress give as a breach of fidelity is that of 'abandonment' (2001 p 313).

This can be explained with an example from nursing: a nurse walks down a ward to care for patient A. On the way, patient B asks for help from the nurse. The request does not concern any urgent health issue requiring an immediate response (perhaps the patient is asking to be made more comfortable). The nurse says 'I'll be back in one moment. I promise I won't forget.' The nurse then cares for patient A, taking a little longer than expected. The nurse finishes the procedure 5 minutes before the end of her shift. She recalls the promise made to B but decides to get ready to finish her shift and go home, without seeing patient B. She does not know if B was attended to by any other colleague. The nurse's act would count as a breach of fidelity. (It may be a *justified* breach perhaps, if the nurse has another more urgent commitment.)

Two comments need to be made here: (1) This concerns the relationship between judgements and rules. Particular judgements are instances of moral rules. For example, a level 1 judgement to tell a person the truth is an instance of a level 2 rule of veracity (or a rule to the effect that one ought to be truthful). (2) Rules provide moral justification for judgements. Hence a judgement to tell a person the truth may be justified by reference to the veracity rule.

Level 3 of Beauchamp and Childress's framework is the level at which the principles feature, of which they posit four:

1. THE PRINCIPLE OF RESPECT FOR AUTONOMY

The first principle they discuss is respect for autonomy. They stress this does not mean that this is the weightiest or most important moral principle (Beauchamp & Childress 2001 p 57). The principle of respect for autonomy includes obligations to 'acknowledge a person's right to hold views, to make choices, and to take actions based on personal values and beliefs' (2001 p 63). Also, it requires more than non-interference in others' personal affairs. It includes obligations to build up or maintain others' capacities for autonomous choice. This moral principle involves more than simply acknowledging that people are entitled to their opinions and to act on these. It involves, in some circumstances, enhancing a person's capacity to make autonomous choices. One means of doing so is by providing relevant information to someone. In the nursing context this may mean information relating to a patient's health condition, such as information regarding side effects of medication or adverse consequences of surgical interventions. Respecting autonomy also entails respecting a person's choices 'so long as their thoughts and actions do not seriously harm other persons' (2001 p 64).

2. THE PRINCIPLE OF NON-MALEFICENCE

The second moral principle Beauchamp and Childress describe is that of non-maleficence (2001 p 113). On the face of it, the principle can seem simple to define. It concerns obligations not to harm others. However, what counts as harm might not always be easy to determine. This raises the question of who is best placed to judge what counts as harm: the patient, the nurse, or some other party. A patient who refuses life-saving blood products on religious grounds may consider the blood products more harmful than mortal death if receipt of the blood product leads to 'eternal damnation'.

3. THE PRINCIPLE OF BENEFICENCE

The principle of beneficence points to obligations to act in ways that promote the well-being of others. As Beauchamp and Childress say, '[the moral] principle of beneficence refers to a moral obligation to act for the benefit of others' (2001 p 166). As with the previous principle, in practice it can be problematic to determine just what will benefit another person. Other people's opinions about this may be at odds with one's own. Nonetheless, this principle obliges nurses to act in ways that benefit others.

4. THE PRINCIPLE OF JUSTICE

The fourth is the principle of justice. This is an extremely complex concept but, simply put, the principle of justice concerns obligations to treat others fairly. This may entail giving others what they are entitled to, what they deserve, what they need or what they have a right to. Beauchamp and Childress identify a formal principle of justice according to which 'Equals must be treated equally, and unequals must be treated unequally' (2001 p 227). Justice in the distributive sense, i.e. involving the distribution of a benefit (or a burden), can be shown by an example from nursing. The nurse in the example above considers how her care should be distributed; should she go to patient A or B? The principle of justice obliges her to 'treat equals equally and unequals unequally'. Since patient A is in greater need than patient B, she goes to care for patient A, thus fulfilling obligations of justice. In this example, the determination of what counts as being equal focuses on need. Another example would be that of a nurse who is asked by a patient about the side effects of medication. The nurse gives the information. If the nurse is then asked the same question by a patient with the same condition and in the same state of health as the first patient, the nurse is obliged to give the same information to the second patient, unless some relevant moral difference between the two patients can be identified, such as the second patient's inability to make decisions for himself, e.g. due to severe dementia.

Rules are specifications of principles, that is, principles are more general than rules but can be recognized in rules. For instance, the moral rule of veracity is a specification of the principle of respect for autonomy. Part of the obligation to respect autonomy is to be truthful, and thus to foster autonomy. Principles can also serve as justifications for rules: A nurse may justify telling a patient the truth (veracity) by appealing to the principle of respect for autonomy. A similar story can be given of the relationship between other principles and rules.

In *Level 4*, moral theory is considered. There are a number of moral theories, such as utilitarianism, deontology, virtue ethics, communitarianism and so on (Beauchamp & Childress 2001 p 384–408). It is not necessary here to spell these out in detail (see Singer 1991). Each moral theory identifies something of great importance in morality. They fail primarily because they try to 'compress' all moral thinking into the one dimension that happens to be the focus of the theory, thus providing a distorted view of morality. Utilitarians emphasize the maximization of good consequences but are forced to ride roughshod over individual rights. Deontologists, in emphasizing the importance of motive and of absolute duties, neglect to consider the importance of consequences. In spite of this, all moral theories have a key place for the kinds of moral values represented in the four moral principles. Both utilitarians and deontologists see the importance of respecting autonomy (Kant 1785/1948, Mill 1863/1962) and other key values, such as avoiding unjustified harms, promoting well-being and acting fairly.

Given this, and in the light of the poor prospects for a solid foundation for the moral sphere, Beauchamp and Childress recommend a 'coherentist' model of moral judgement (2001 p 397–401). In this model there is no ultimate foundation for moral judgements. Rather, in making judgements one considers the kinds of values represented in moral rules, principles and theories. One should try to systematize these by avoiding contradictions and by acknowledging commonsense morality as a constraining factor. Thus if a judgement, motivated by a theory or principle, conflicts seriously with commonsense morality, one would revisit the reasoning that led to the judgement and consider revising it.

An example will help. Some theorists have defended the view in nursing ethics that the principle of respect for autonomy is the weightiest moral principle. It is so vitally important that it should be respected even if respecting it will lead to terrible consequences, even if respecting it leads to moral judgements that appear to conflict radically with commonsense morality. Suppose a person expresses an intention to end his own life without any apparent reason: he has no health or financial problems, but this person simply decides that life is not worth living. The 'autonomy-weighted' principle-based position allows that such a desire must be respected. Many people find this counterintuitive. Could a credible approach to moral problems in nursing imply such a view?

Another example might be an elderly and frail patient with severe mobility problems who needs pressure area care. However, the patient refuses this. Even when the consequences of this refusal are spelt out to the patient, she still refuses. The 'autonomy-weighted' approach implies that the patient's wishes should simply be respected in spite of the inevitable deterioration in the patient's health that such a refusal will lead to.

Beauchamp and Childress' 'coherentist' approach permits one to revisit the train of reasoning that led to a position in which it is considered morally justified to respect such wishes expressed by people, be they suicidal or frail and in need of pressure area care. They recruit the term 'reflective equilibrium' for this process: 'The goal of reflective equilibrium is to match, prune and adjust considered judgements in order to render them coherent with the premises of our most general moral commitments' (2001 p 398). To arrive at the 'considered judgement' that the frail patient's wishes should be respected, one should also have considered other principles and other values before having arrived at a final conclusion. The other principles involved are beneficence, non-maleficence and justice, in addition to the values gained from moral rules and theories, such as fidelity from the level of rules, and at least duties and consequences from the level of theories.

PRINCIPLE-BASED ETHICS AND NURSING EDUCATION

I have been involved in the teaching of nursing ethics for several years and over that time I have learned that Beauchamp and Childress' approach contains something of great value and of considerable use in such teaching.

I found that novice nurses were often unaware of the moral dimension of nursing practice. They were unable to articulate coherently any misgivings they had about specific instances of nursing practice in which they had been involved. Using Beauchamp and Childress helped me with both these problems. As all decisions by nurses impact on the well-being of patients, it is plain that nursing (and all healthcare work) has a deeply ingrained moral dimension. This had largely gone unnoticed previously, and certainly most curricula for nurses in the UK did not include any mandatory ethics component until 1991. Merely emphasizing Beauchamp and Childress' principles as *moral* principles promoting well-being, being fair, etc. as *moral* values helped to show the moral dimension of nursing practice.

I also found that the principles provided a means of structuring the thoughts of the nurses I taught when they were faced with moral problems in their practice. In applying the four principles to their experiences it became clear that, for example, decisions to withhold information from patients typically involved conflicts between the principles of respect for autonomy and those of beneficence or non-maleficence. The principle of autonomy points to obligations to provide information but beneficence or non-maleficence can be deployed to argue that information should not be provided, e.g. if doing so will cause distress to a patient. Nurses who were until then unable to articulate their sources of moral concern, exploited the vocabulary of the principle-based approach to do so.

Indeed, many moral problems faced by nurses in their practice are analysable in terms of the four principles. The theories highlight different ways of thinking about moral matters, such as the importance of consequences and of duties, and so do the moral rules.

It is tempting to suggest that Beauchamp and Childress' framework simply provides a kind of checklist of considerations to aid moral decision making. It is possible to recognize that a decision with a moral dimension has to be made and then simply consider the decision from the perspective of the moral rules, principles and theories. Would such decisions involve violations of autonomy, justice, confidentiality, etc?

This can in fact be a helpful process. It does not provide nurses with answers to moral problems, but it can help their moral deliberations by signalling the relevant moral dimensions of their decisions. I describe this way of using the principle-based approach as a *modest* approach because it does not attempt to produce moral decisions; rather, it structures moral thinking and fosters moral sensitivity. This *modest* use of the principle-based approach can be usefully contrasted with what can be termed an *immodest* use of the approach.

AN IMMODEST USE OF THE PRINCIPLES

The principle-based approach set out by Beauchamp and Childress intentionally refrains from claiming that the principle of respect for autonomy is the weightiest principle (1994 p 105; 2001 p 57). However, as many moral problems in nursing involve conflicts between the principle of respect for autonomy on one hand and those of beneficence or non-maleficence on the other, some authors have articulated a position that does involve giving greatest weight to respect for autonomy (Benjamin & Curtis 1986, Edwards 1996). Hence, in a conflict between this principle and others, respect for autonomy always wins out and is always accorded the greatest weight. For obvious reasons this can be known as the 'autonomy-weighted' principle-based approach. The fairly cautious *modest* principle-based approach set out by Beauchamp and Childress has therefore become something much more ambitious and even crude, by subsequent commentators.

In this cruder or *immodest* version, when there is a clash, the principle of respect for autonomy is given greatest weight. It is worth indicating that this position can be supported by good arguments. For example, the following considerations all seem to lend support to the view that autonomy is of singular importance:

First, the importance of autonomy in our lives is reflected in the law. For example, the most serious crimes possible to commit are murder, assault and theft. They are so serious because they involve violations of personal autonomy. Murder involves the thwarting of a lifetime of autonomous choices. Assault violates a person's autonomous choices concerning who should have access to his or her body. Theft negates the owner's autonomous choices concerning what to do with her or his possessions. Conversely, punishments seek to curtail the offender's autonomy of action by imprisonment, fine, or enforced community service (or at the most extreme the death penalty).

In English law, people are allowed to refuse life-saving treatment, providing that their refusals are informed and competent (Mason & McCall Smith 1994). Some laws seem to overrule the autonomous wishes of people, such as legislation requiring car users to secure themselves with seat belts, or motorcycle riders to wear helmets. Nonetheless, the weight attached to the importance of autonomy in the legal context is evident from the fact that one can refuse life-saving treatment (other legal systems may weigh things differently).

These brief considerations suggest that there are good reasons to give the principle of respect for autonomy more weight than the principles of non-maleficence and beneficence. A general consensus exists according to which people can decide for themselves whether they wish to act in ways that promote their own well-being or, equally, to pursue activities that involve high risks of harm. Such activities include heavy smoking and drinking, not exercising, mountain climbing, boxing, and numerous other risky pursuits. A general position is reflected in ordinary common-sense morality according to which respect for autonomy is the most weighty moral principle.

The 'autonomy-weighted' principle-based position clearly cannot apply to non-competent people. In relation to moral problems arising from care of very young children or seriously intellectually disabled people, the role of autonomy appears negligible. In moral problems arising from care of these groups of people, obligations of beneficence, non-maleficence and justice require balancing. Also in situations where there are limited resources it will not be possible to meet all autonomous requests for resources. Hence, autonomy is constrained by the principle of justice and the 'autonomy-weighted' position cannot apply.

CRITICISMS

Principle-based approaches to nursing ethics, whether modest or immodest have come in for considerable criticism; some are here set out and responded to.

The first criticism is that it can sound an extremely callous approach to ethics. One can think again of the person who expresses an intention to end his own life without any apparent reason: he has no health or financial problems, he simply decides that life is not worth living. The autonomy-weighted principle-based position seems to allow that such a desire must be respected.

The principle-based approach here seems unproblematically to accept that the suicidal person should be allowed to get on with it. Surely, a plausible position in morality would find such a verdict strongly counterintuitive. The suicide example leads to related criticisms.

Second, the approach seems to suppose that patients unequivocally know what they want. A colleague described a situation in which, as a public health doctor, he was called to visit an elderly, frail man. The man had some serious health and mobility problems; he could barely move from his armchair. It was put to this man that he should go into hospital or sheltered accommodation but he refused. Did his choice reflect an appreciation of the alternatives available, i.e. go into hospital, perhaps temporarily, or stay and probably die at home? Was the man's conception of what would happen to him in hospital or in the sheltered accommodation an accurate one? Eventually the man was admitted to hospital against his wishes (although he did not resist and seemed to welcome having the decision made for him).

It seems reasonable to suggest that people do not always know what they want because they do not have a clear conception of the alternatives available to them. They may simply prefer to stick with the option that involves least short-term inconvenience in their view.

Third, and also related to the last two examples, is the criticism that the principle-based line is excessively 'first-person centred'. The primary focus in the suicide example is on the person: does he wish to end his own life or not? Commentators from other theoretical perspectives have pointed to the fact that in these analyses there is no mention of the people who are in some kind of relation with the person, such as his family, friends and colleagues. A criticism is therefore developed that the autonomy-weighted principle-based approach derives from a crude and inaccurate view of persons. According to the 'crude' view, persons are like 'atoms' identified without reference to other people; they are 'pure' individuals who simply choose what they prefer or seems best for them. The rival view stresses that persons are defined by their relations to others and that these relations have a moral dimension. For example, the fact that one is a son implies that one has or has had parents. This relationship is not simply a biological one. It has a moral dimension of obligations and concern built in to it, as do almost all other relationships.

This third criticism claims that the moral position in which respect for autonomy is given greatest weight stems from a view of persons that is seriously mistaken. According to the criticism, persons are not unique social 'atoms' but are constituted by their relations to others.

A fourth criticism is that the principle-based line omits care and emotion, which are crucial aspects of morality. Any theory that denies a role for care and emotion is open to objection. For example, care is central to morality in the sense of defining the scope of our moral obligations. We recognize obligations to those we care about. Emotion appears to be central in the sense that our identification of moral problems seems to derive from an emotional response to them; certain situations are identified as moral problems because they demand an emotional reaction from us.

This fourth criticism suggests that in focusing on the principles, other equally important elements of moral experience are obscured.

A DEFENCE: SAVING THE PRINCIPLES

I think plausible responses can be made to each of these four criticisms. I addressed the 'callousness' charge in an earlier work (Edwards 1996) as follows. Reconsider the example above of the frail, elderly patient who refused pressure area care, who would apparently be left to decay in horrible circumstances for the sake of respecting her autonomy. I suggest that the principle of autonomy should be applied in a way that is infused with care. Thus if a patient makes a decision that is plainly counter to her best interests, the patient should be engaged with and given the proper opportunity to explain the rationale behind her decision. She should be made aware of all the various options, differing types of pressure area care and so on. All this should be done sympathetically and in an appropriate context with privacy and time. Given all these opportunities, and if respecting the autonomy of the patient does not cause serious harm to others, then the patient's decision should be respected. Forcibly to manipulate the patient against her express and competent wishes seems the morally worse course of action. The hope is that the patient would change her mind. To impose physical manipulation on her seems hard to defend. Much could also be said about this situation concerning the autonomy of the nurses involved and the interpretation of the term 'harm'.

The second concern implies that patients do not know what they want, therefore it is difficult to respect their autonomy. As an initial response, it should be stressed that it is dangerous and morally dubious to presume that people do not mean what they say they mean (that they say 'no' and mean 'yes'). If there are good grounds to suppose a person is mentally competent, these wishes should be respected. In the example above, the elderly man seemed relieved to have the decision made for him. It could have turned out differently. He could have been outraged that his last days could not be spent in the place he loved most, his own home. Such cases indicate the importance of continuity of care and of relationships between patients and nurses. Continuity makes it more likely that subtle cues are picked up and that the patient's wants are respected.

The third criticism is more abstract than the previous two. This maintains that the principle-based view is wedded to a philosophically flawed conception of the person and that it erroneously conceives of persons as isolated atoms. This is a mistake, the critic argues. Persons are constituted by 'webs of relationships', by their social ties, and so on (see Edwards 2001, Taylor 1991). However, this is an ontological point, not a moral one. One can accept that persons are socially constituted but at the same time allow that their own views about what they want are of vital moral significance. The fact that I am socially constituted does not mean that my views should be disregarded or considered less important than others' views.

The final criticism is that the principle-based approach omits some essential aspects of moral experience, such as care and emotion. In response, it seems to me that moral responses to others are in fact prompted by moral sensitivity, which is inseparable from care. One is moved by the plight of others because one cares about them, even if they are strangers or animals. Seeing this as a moral problem stems from moral sensitivity to the plight of such persons. One is troubled by their situation because one cares about the individual. One is moved emotionally by their predicament. It seems that the principles need not obscure these central components of the moral life that are care and emotion.

I return to the two conditions of adequacy on any credible approach to ethics with which this chapter began. The principle-based approach (in either form) seems to me to meet the first condition. It recognizes the absence of a clear foundation for resolution of moral differences and offers an appropriate response. It is a response grounded in key aspects of commonsense morality, values such as respect for the views of others, the importance of self-determination, justice, etc. It also meets the second condition, that is, compatibility with professional nursing practice. Many codes of practice stress the centrality of values such as respecting patients' wishes, promoting their well-being, not harming them and treating them fairly.

CONCLUSION

After identifying two conditions of adequacy on any credible approach to nursing ethics, I set out the principle-based approach to nursing ethics as this is presented in Beauchamp and Childress' text. This was then applied in the context of ethics education in nursing. Following this, a so-called 'immodest' principle-based approach to nursing ethics was described and defended from criticism. Such an approach, I claimed, is capable of meeting the two conditions of adequacy with which this chapter began.

References

Beauchamp TL, Childress JF 1994 Principles of biomedical ethics, 4th edn. Oxford University Press, Oxford.

Beauchamp TL, Childress JF 2001 Principles of biomedical ethics, 5th edn. Oxford University Press, Oxford.

Benjamin M, Curtis J 1986 Ethics in nursing. Oxford University Press, Oxford.

Edwards SD 1996 Nursing ethics, a principle-based approach. Macmillan, Basingstoke, UK.

Edwards SD 2001 Philosophy of nursing, an introduction. Palgrave, Basingstoke, UK.

Kant I 1785 Groundwork of the metaphysic of morals. In: Paton HJ (trans.) 1948 The moral law. Hutchinson, London.

Mason JK, McCall Smith RA 1994 Law and medical ethics, 4th edn. Butterworth, London.

Mill JS 1863 Utilitarianism. In: Warnock M (ed) 1962 Utilitarianism. Fontana, London.

Singer P 1991 A companion to ethics. Oxford University Press, Oxford.

Taylor C 1991 Sources of the self. Cambridge University Press, Cambridge.

Further reading

Nozick R 1974 Anarchy, state and utopia. Blackwell, Oxford.

The National Commission for the Protection of Human Subjects of Bioemedical and Behaviural Research: the Belmont Report 1978 US Department of Health, Education and Welfare, Washington, DC.

Chapter **8**

The principle-based approach to nursing ethics: a critical analysis

Samantha Mei-che Pang

INTRODUCTION

This and the previous chapter analyse the way in which principle-based ethics can meet the two conditions of a credible approach to nursing ethics. While Chapter 7 provides a sympathetic account, this chapter will take a critical stance. First, I will examine the role of principle-based ethics in addressing the complex nature of moral judgement, and second I will examine whether the principle-based approach to moral reasoning is compatible with professional practice. The often-cited criticisms of principle-based ethics revolve around understanding Beauchamp and Childress' (2001) approach to bioethical principles and its application to resolving ethical quandaries in the clinical context. In Beauchamp and Childress' approach all bioethical principles are considered important, therefore no one principle trumps:

- How, then, within the system, can one resolve clashes between these principles?
- How, in any given complex context, would one know which principles were relevant without recourse to moral sensitivity, which would therefore seem to precede using any principle? This suggests

that principles are not the complete answer to moral questions in health care.

- Principle-based ethics emphasizes duties and this is essential, particularly when health care involves the care of strangers or caring for people one does not particularly like. However, an emphasis on duty alone would seem to go against the moral intuition that we often value actions carried out with right feelings, as distinct from mere duty, such as keeping promises and being hospitable to strangers in need.

- What is meant by 'right feeling' cannot be defined enough in general terms because its meaning belongs to specific contexts on specific occasions. What follows is an attempt to illustrate, with real-life examples within the clinical context, the issues raised in applying principle-based ethics for resolving difficult care situations.

CLINICAL DECISION-MAKING IN THE PRACTICE CONTEXT

To provide the best possible care for patients requires competent nursing judgements. With an emphasis on evidence-based practice in health care, many nurses believe that making clinical judgements depends on the level of scientific evidence that can be gathered. The higher the level of evidence available about a particular care phenomenon, the more certain we are how to improve the relevant care for patients. The example I will use is of pressure ulcer care. Low pressure ulcer incidence is usually viewed as an indication of quality nursing care (Pang & Wong 1998). Evidence-based pressure ulcer risk calculators have been developed since the 1960s and research efforts continue to identify which risk calculator can produce a higher predictive power for local application (Kwong et al 2005).

No one risk calculator possesses 100% accuracy, yet nurses can use these data to make decisions to start preventive measures for patients considered at high risk of pressure ulcers. However, pressure care cannot be adequate if only evidence-based data is used. Two cases from ethnographic case studies that I conducted with colleagues in the USA and Hong Kong during 2002–2004 are presented (Pang et al 2004, 2005). Both patients (Mr A and Mr B) suffered from advanced progressive Alzheimer's disease and lived in long-term care facilities for terminal care. Mr A lived in the USA and Mr B in Hong Kong, China. Making an advance directive or living will is rare in Hong Kong whereas in the USA it is common (Pang & Chung 2002). The Hong Kong Hospital Authority Clinical Ethics Committee (2002) has issued guidelines on forgoing life-sustaining treatment for terminally ill people but as patients with advanced dementia are not considered to die imminently, it is common practice to insert a feeding tube when they develop eating difficulties.

Case A   Mr A is 70 years old but when he was in his early 60s he drew up an advance directive to forgo artificial nutrition and hydration in end-of-life care, including tube feeding and intravenous therapy. He was not cognitively impaired then. On admission to hospital, his wife and the clinical staff affirmed this directive. Mr A could not recognize his wife and his ability to speak was largely impaired. He had sensitive skin that required special care. He could not control his bowel or bladder. He spent most of the day in a wheelchair because he could not move by himself. He did not eat well and had lost weight over the past weeks. One day he developed an ulcer on his ankle and reddened skin over several pressure areas. The ulcer became worse and two new ulcers developed despite the use of pressure-relieving measures. His wife worried about the deteriorating ulcers and the quality control nurse regularly reminded the ward staff of possible substandard care. After exhausting all the extrinsic pressure-relieving interventions, the clinical team eventually formed a clinical opinion that the ulcers would not be controlled unless the patient's nutritional status improved. The option was to provide nutritional supplement through a feeding tube.

Case B   Mr B, an 89-year-old man lived with his adult son until one day he fell and broke both hips. Once hospitalized, he was put on tube feeding and ordered conservative treatment for his fractured hips. He was transferred to a long-term care facility after his condition had stabilized. He could not recognize his loved ones but was responsive to them. He strongly rejected the feeding tube and made every attempt to pull it out after reinsertion. His arms were restrained but despite this he appeared very determined to get rid of the tube and tried every posture in bed to release himself from the constraints. Frequent reinsertion of the feeding tube traumatized his naso-oesophageal passage, his mobility was reduced, and friction and sheer force were increased. His adult son questioned whether it would be better to forgo tube feeding. The nurses worried that he would develop pressure ulcers soon.

In both cases, the nurses were drawn into difficult decisions over tube feeding so that the risks and burdens of pressure ulcers would be reduced. Mr A's nurse would have liked to place a feeding tube to correct the nutritional deficit; this might have reduced the risk of further skin breakdown. Mr B's nurse wanted to withdraw the tube because the patient resisted it, thus increasing the chance of pressure ulcer formation. Both decisions may go contrary to the customary practice of the two countries. Mr A's nurse had to overrule the patient's advance directive, whereas Mr B's nurse had to challenge the current practice. Apparently, simply applying the scientific formula of pressure ulcer risk calculation fails to provide an answer for the nurses to deal with these two difficult care situations. The question of tube feeding to improve pressure care for Mr A and Mr B takes us into the realm of moral argument. The term 'argument' here does not refer to an angry dispute but to a set of reasons being given to support or refute a conclusion as to the right action to take. What follows is an analysis of the argumentation process in principle-based ethics.

MORAL JUDGEMENT AND PRINCIPLED THINKING

To make a judgement about the moral worth of tube feeding patients, nurses who use the principle-based approach on which to argue need to ask the following questions:

- Which ethical rules and principles are at stake?
- Which duties emerge from these rules and principles?

The reasons given by principle-based thinkers to justify any course of action will be grounded in the ethical rules, principles and duties they recognize as necessary for their professional roles. Examples of ethical rules and principles that principle-based thinkers will seriously consider in making a judgement of the moral worth of an act are described in Chapter 7 and I will not repeat them here.

Even though we hold some bioethical principles as universal, these principles are interpreted and practised differently in different places (Pang et al 2003, Tao & Lai 2002). Fan (1997) contends that there are three reasons or levels for this:

- Are there differences in the crucial moral vocabulary and fundamental moral principles employed within two cultures?
- Are there differences in the meaning of a moral principle that appears to be accepted by any two cultures?
- Are there differences in ranking of moral principles or goods even if the same principles or goods are endorsed in both cultures?

Drawing on different ethical theories, people using the principle-based approach may have different attitudes to these principles and rules when applying them in practice. Some take principles as absolute, overarching and binding so that no compromise can be made. Some take principles as prima facie, that is, always binding unless a competing moral obligation overrides or outweighs it in a particular circumstance. More interesting is that people using the principle-based approach may have different combinations of the principles they take as absolute and those principles they take as prima facie. The following is an illustration of this by making reference to deontology and utilitarianism.

For a deontologist, the categorical imperative is the criterion for judging the acceptability of any rules that direct actions. In Kant's words, 'I ought never to act except in such a way that I can also will that my maxim become a universal law.' Simply put, I should not act in a particular way if I do not want people to act in such a way for all relevantly similar circumstances. This means that I should not tell a lie to a patient unless I can also accept as a moral right that other nurses would lie to me if I were the patient in any relevantly similar circumstances. Rules that can pass the categorical imperative test become binding, and thus will form the basis of morality for obligatory duties (Beauchamp & Childress 2001 p 350–351).

Utilitarian theory holds that actions are right or wrong according to the balance of good and bad consequences. The utility principle states that an action is right if it can produce the maximum balance of positive value over disvalue and a utilitarian will use this as the overarching principle in ethical justification. An act is obligatory if it produces the best overall result, judged from an impersonal perspective that gives equal weight to the interests of each affected party (Beauchamp & Childress 2001 p 340–341).

Both ethical positions raise issues of which duties or acts are to be defined as obligatory and hence are strong duties that everyone has to follow, and which duties or acts are moral ideals and thus are supererogatory, that is, beyond obligation (Beauchamp & Childress 2001 p 41–42). With this in mind I return to the two cases.

In both cases, the principles of respect for autonomy and beneficence are at stake. Both patients had severe cognitive impairment and therefore the issue is how to respect their autonomy when they cannot indicate their preference in words. Although Mr A had an advance directive, he made it a decade ago. People tend to change their mind about treatment options when their conditions change (Drought & Koenig 2002). How can the clinical team and his wife be certain that Mr A indeed prefers not to have any form of artificial nutrition in this particular situation? Even if patients can express their dislikes, as in the anti-tube behaviour of Mr B, nurses are not comfortable in taking his behaviour as an 'informed decision', because Mr B might not be competent to give informed consent. Paternalism is apparently justified in both cases because the principle of beneficence should be the overarching concern for justifying tube feeding Mr A and Mr B. Paternalism is considered justified for incompetent children in need of parental supervision. In health care, justified paternalism extends to incompetent patients in need of care similar to beneficent parental guidance (Beauchamp & Childress 2001 p 177). The principle of beneficence points to obligations to act so as to promote the well-being of others. What constitutes the well-being of Mr A and Mr B? Inevitably we are drawn into the sanctity-of-life and quality-of-life arguments for justifying whether or not to tube feed the patients and therefore whether prolonging life or promoting dignity should be taken as more important. Both cases present an ethical challenge to principlism, regardless of whether this is underpinned by a deontological or utilitarian justification. A justified course of action can pass either the categorical imperative test or the utility calculation.

The second question in a principle-based argument is how to justify the kinds of moral duties that nurses should abide by when responding to the clinical situations of Mr A and Mr B. In view of the dilemmas raised in the principles at stake, the possible scenarios will be:

Case A	Not to institute any artificial nutrition (obligatory duty), nurses are held accountable to respect Mr A's advance directive (respect for autonomy, upheld in the Patient Self-Determination Act). Or: To institute tube feeding as a corrective therapy (obligatory duty), given that the patient is not likely to die in a few days and his nutritional inadequacy may be reversible (beneficence).

Case B	To provide optimal comfort care to Mr B by withdrawing the tube (obligatory duty) because he does not like it (substituted judgement based on respect for autonomy), and the tube is a source of discomfort contributing negatively to his well-being (beneficence). Or: To continue tube feeding (obligatory duty) because to do otherwise will deprive Mr B of adequate nutrition, which may hasten his death (beneficence in terms of removing the possible harms on the patient's life).

Moral dilemmas arise when two or more moral values apply but support mutually inconsistent courses of action. In this regard, both cases exemplify typical moral dilemmas:

A deontologist will meet the dilemma by asking: 'In view of conflicting but equally strong duties, which course of action can produce the greatest balance of rightness over wrongness?'

A utilitarian will question: 'Which course of action can produce the best consequences in terms of, for example, happiness, pleasure and health for persons most affected?'

These analyses are examples, not exhaustive descriptions, of the chains of arguments structured by principled-based thinking. Issues such as how to enact 'respect for persons' and 'safeguarding the best interests of the patient' in these difficult care situations are opened to competing interpretations in different ethics traditions, such as caring ethics and virtue ethics.

ATTRIBUTES OF PRINCIPLE-BASED MORAL JUDGEMENT

In differentiating whether a person is acting morally or ethically, Beauchamp and Childress (2001) contend that a person can act *morally* by following a set of rules of right conduct. However, to act *ethically* the person must go through a formal reasoning process that ends in selecting one specific behaviour from alternatives. For principle-based thinkers, the task is to arrive at the best and right judgement that is logical, rational, systematic and defensible. The following will describe these four attributes.

The first attribute of principle-based moral judgement is logic. In answering the question 'what ought I do?' principle-based thinkers try to identify the maxims or fundamental principles of action that ought to be adopted, then move from principles to deductive reasoning and to concrete application in the actual situation. A classic example of deductive reasoning is the syllogistic argument, as follows:

> All men are mortal (major premise)
> Socrates is a man (minor premise)
> Therefore Socrates is mortal (conclusion)

The logic of this argument is that if we accept the major and minor premises as true, we have to accept the conclusion, because it is drawn from these premises. Applying this logic to make a moral argument, people using the principle-based approach will draw their conclusions from the premise(s) they uphold as ethical principles. For instance:

> A person's right to self-determination should be honoured at all times (major premise)
> Advance directives are a means to protect a person's right to self-determination when he or she cannot speak for himself or herself (minor premise)
> Therefore advance directive should be honoured at all times (conclusion)

Based on this argumentation, the principle-based position is not to tube feed Mr A. Another argument will go like this:

> Patients should have the right to refuse medical treatment (major premise)
> Tube feeding is a form of medical treatment (minor premise)
> Therefore patients have the right to refuse tube feeding (conclusion)

Based on this argumentation, principle-based thinking does not insist on tube feeding Mr B if Mr B's anti-tube behaviour is taken as a strong expression of his objection to be tube fed. This situation is problematic because Mr B is not considered competent. A surrogate decision is deemed necessary for a representation of Mr B's will.

The same premise will arrive at logically coherent conclusions, but conflicting conclusions will be drawn from competing premises. For instance:

> Provision of food and fluid is a form of basic nursing care and hence is an obligatory nursing duty (major premise)
> Tube feeding is a means of providing food and fluid to those who cannot eat and fail to maintain adequate nutrition (minor premise)
> Therefore tube feeding is a form of basic nursing care that nurses are obliged to provide when patients fail to maintain adequate nutrition (conclusion)

When applying principle-based thinking, holding these three arguments as equally valid means being drawn into an unresolved dilemma regarding whether or not to tube feed Mr A and Mr B.

The second attribute is rationality. Principle-based ethics is committed to a view that moral obligations derive only from reason and that God, human authorities, communities and preferences or desires of human agents are not involved. When good reasons support a moral judgement, those reasons are good for all relevantly similar circumstances. This position is far-reaching in formulating rules for ethical practice.

The two other attributes, to be systematic and defensible, are well demonstrated by the sympathetic account in Chapter 7.

In summary, in difficult care situations one cannot rely solely on scientific evidence to make clinical decisions. To arrive at a morally justified course of action in dealing with the issue at stake, nurses should be able to appreciate and discern the conflicting moral values at stake and at the same time have their own ethical stance examined.

The second concern raised at the beginning of this chapter was compatibility between moral theory and professional practice. The best test of compatibility of the principle-based approach to moral reasoning in professional practice is to see what actually happens in practice.

PRINCIPLE-BASED ETHICS AND PROFESSIONAL PRACTICE

Research on ethics in nursing began to flourish in the late 1970s, inquiring primarily into two areas of ethical concern in nursing: the approaches used by nurses in ethical decision making, and the ways in which ethical practice can be fostered in actual patient care. Evaluating the relevance of the principle-based approach in informing ethical nursing practice was a regular topic.

Pence (1987) suggested that nursing ethics entered a new beginning in the late 1970s, characterized by an increasing awareness of nurses' role in exercising professional judgement to safeguard patients' best interests, something that until then was monopolized by physicians. Although many would agree that nurses should participate in ethical decision making, concerns were raised about whether nurses were prepared for such a role. As Fromer wrote:

> The real tragedy with regard to ethical dilemmas in nursing practice is not that nurses do not recognize that such dilemmas exist, rather it is their lack of preparation to solve these dilemmas using ethical principles. (1982 p 20)

This is open to questioning. It is far from clear that any curriculum could provide such preparation. Research activities at the beginning of the 1980s primarily focused on assessing nurses' capability in principle-based thinking. One of the most often used theoretical frameworks is Kohlberg's theory of moral development. Of the three levels and six universal stages identified in the process of moral development, Kohlberg argued that the highest level of moral development is characterized by making moral judgement based on universal ethical principles. In his words:

Principles are universal principles of justice: the equality of human rights and respect for the dignity of human beings as individuals. These are not merely values that are recognized, but are also principles used to generate particular decisions. (1981 p 412)

Research on nurses' level of moral reasoning revealed that nurses were predominantly at the conventional level of moral reasoning. This level stresses obedience to authority and the need to maintain harmonious relationships with the institution's authority figures, even at the expense of patients' rights (Munhall 1980, Murphy 1981). Arising from this, it could be claimed that nurses need knowledge and understanding of ethical theories and principles for ethical practice.

Principle-based thinking requires nurses to scrutinize their own judgements, attitudes and actions in the light of their impact on the autonomy and values of others. From this perspective, ethical theories provide the structure and the tools of ethical analysis and decision making, while the principles form the content of thought and reflection. It was optimistically thought that if nurses were equipped with moral reasoning skills, everyday moral problems in clinical practice would then be ethically addressed. As Fowler suggests:

Ethical arguments help to relieve moral uncertainty by clarifying the questions and by illuminating the ethical features of the situation, thereby providing a measure of comfort. They help to clarify moral dilemmas by revealing general and specific obligations and values, and they help to reduce moral distress when they can be used for the formulation of institutional policies that support moral action. (1989 p 957)

The need to prepare nurses to reason morally is generally shared by nurse ethicists, but doubt is also raised whether ethical decision making within the clinical context follows the logic of the principle-based approach. Few political philosophers today accept Kohlberg's claim that concern for universal principles represents a 'higher morality' than concern for relationships, or deny that any decent moral theory will contain both elements. The difficult question is how to proceed in cases of conflict (Barry 1995).

Studies focusing on nurses' responsibilities in practice situations revealed that even though nurses were prepared with principle-based thinking, it was too optimistic to believe that ethical practice would be fostered. Swider et al (1985) examined the priorities reflected in the decisions made by senior nursing students when they encountered an ethical dilemma in their practice. They used quantitative measures to categorize the students' responses as patient-centred, physician-centred or bureaucratic-centred; the bureaucratic-centred responses were in the majority. These findings suggested that the nursing students were confused and unclear about their ethical responsibilities. They argued that the conflicting loyalties and responsibilities of nurses to physicians, hospital administration and patients had created problems for nurses. They could not arrive at sound and justifiable resolutions. Yarling and McElmurry (1986) believed that nurses needed to have autonomy in practice before they could act as free moral agents, that is, acting according to their own sense of moral integrity.

Holly (1989) conducted a survey to measure critical care nurses' perceptions of various types of support in relation to ethical issues. Environmental work support, social support and tangible support was given to nurses when their views were not in line with the institutional views in situations where they needed to make ethical decisions. Holly found that, in general, nurses did not feel free enough to engage in ethical decision making in hospital environments or to act in an advocacy role in such situations. She suggested that the essential elements for making ethical decisions were a supportive environment, open and clear lines of communication, including individual nurses' perspectives, and competence in ethical decision making.

Davis (1989) conducted a descriptive study focusing on nurses' ethical decision making in situations of informed consent. The findings suggested that institutional influences, such as patients' compliance with institutional and medical authority, institutional hierarchy and physicians' claims of authority were potent variables affecting the nurses' decisions. Davis recommended that collective strategies should be developed for conflict resolution in order to safeguard ethical practice.

Chambliss (1996) gathered data from field observations and interviews for 15 years for his research into nursing ethics within the hospital context. While affirming Davis' findings, he gave a detailed account of the issues nurses were dealing with in actual situations. Chambliss contended that nursing ethics did not speak in the language of bioethics. Rather:

> Nursing's moral core, its commitment to the welfare of the patient as a 'whole person', has been buried under medical directives and the financial and administrative imperatives of the modern medical centre. (1996 p 3)

With a belief that nursing's problems in particular reflect the organizational structures in which nurses work, Chambliss suggests that any serious discussion of ethics in nursing must deal with these realities.

Studies drawing on nurses' narratives of their moral experience in practice situations have flourished in recent years. Most of these studies emerge from a critique of the inadequacy of emphasizing principled thinking in resolving ethical issues in practice situations (Parker 1990, Søderberg & Norberg 1993, Viens 1995). These studies challenge the assumptions underlying this principle-based approach. As Beauchamp and Childress explain (2001 p 353), deontological constraints are essentially negative duties specifying what we cannot justifiably do to others; they do not specify any actions that we should perform for the sake of others. Although principled thinking can address issues related to the public sphere, it is ill equipped to explain the moral bases of the private sphere, such as friendship and relationships between family members. In particular, the impartial assumptions of the principle-based approach cannot account for the moral concerns of personal relationships. As nurses encounter patients in the patients' most vulnerable moments, sharing an intimacy found in few other human relationships, Chambliss (1996) doubts the relevance of principle-based ethics to help nurses resolve the dilemmas they encounter within the clinical context.

Pang (2003) conducted an ethnographic study to understand the nature of ethical issues encountered by nurses in China. She found that Chinese nurses conceptualize ethics in terms of six role relationships and eleven facets of nursing responsibilities. The six role relationships are nurses in relation to: society, the profession, practice, healthcare institutions, patients and patients' families. Responsibilities in relation to society comprise two facets of responsibilities: the doctrine of socialist humanism and healthcare access. Responsibilities in relation to practice comprise three facets: (1) the nurse's personal qualities, (2) the nurse's professional qualities and (3) attitude toward work. Three facets are identified in relation to the patient. These are: protectiveness, quality of care and treating the patient as an individual. The facet of responsibilities in relation to healthcare institutions is institutional rules and regulations; in relation to the profession it is respect for nurses; and in relation to the patient's family it is the holistic inclusion of family members. Within this web of relationships, Chinese nurses inevitably encounter ethically difficult situations characterized by conflicting values and competing role requirements. In making sense of the moral experience of nurses in China, we need to take this contextual complexity into serious account.

CONCLUSION

This chapter has shown that contextual understanding is crucial in making sense of the moral experience of nurses in practice situations. Following the procedures of principled ethical argumentation cannot guarantee morally appropriate responses in dealing with the difficult care situations nurses encounter in their day-to-day practice. From a care-based perspective, we find that principle-based thinkers fail to capture fully the moral essence of clinical encounters. As Beauchamp and Walter commented:

> *Whenever the feelings, concerns, and attitudes of others are the morally relevant matters, rules and principles are not as likely as human warmth and sensitivity to lead us to notice what should be done.* (1994 p 18)

We find this comment particularly relevant in responding to the question of 'what ought nurses do to be ethical' in the cases of Mr A and Mr B. The core issue goes beyond the justifications of the moral worth of tube feeding or not tube feeding. We think the major concern should be how to understand and relate to Mr A and Mr B as unique individuals in their stage of advanced dementia, and how to orchestrate individualized care for them in a sensitive and responsive way that can conform with the patients' values, beliefs and preferences and that can help sustain the relationship between the patients and their families.

Similar to advocates of evidence-based practice, principled ethicists hold a sense of optimism that systematic ethical argumentation based on rationality will help us arrive at a justified course of action in resolving ethically difficult situations with moral certainty. As shown in the above examples of possible chains of competing arguments in justifying tube feeding or not tube feeding, we are doubtful that principled thinking can help to provide such an answer. Engelhardt (1996) arrived at a similar conclusion after he examined the intellectual basis of moral arguments in the principle-based ethics tradition. He proposes that the fundamental basis for ethics discourse is procedural, with an aim to have 'peaceable agreement' among interested parties. Another approach to resolve competing views is through consensus building (Veatch 1998).

References

Barry B 1995 Justice as impartiality. Clarendon Press, Oxford, p 234–257.

Beauchamp TL, Childress JF 2001 Principles of biomedical ethics, 5th edn. Oxford University Press, New York.

Beauchamp TL, Walter L 1994 Contemporary issues in bioethics. Wadsworth, CA, Belmont.

Chambliss DF 1996 Beyond caring, hospitals, nurses, and the social organization of ethics. The University of Chicago Press, Chicago.

Davis AJ 1989 Clinical nurses' ethical decision making in situations of informed consent. Advances in Nursing Science 11(3):63–69.

Drought TS, Koenig BA 2002 'Choice' in end-of-life decision making: researching fact or fiction? The Gerontologist 42 (Special Issue III):114–128.

Engelhardt HT 1996 The foundations of bioethics, 2nd edn. Oxford University Press, New York.

Fan RP 1997 Three levels of problems in cross-cultural bioethics. In: Hoshino K (ed) Japanese and western bioethics: studies in moral diversity. Kluwer, Dordrecht, p 189–199.

Fowler MDM 1989 Ethical decision making in clinical practice. Nursing Clinics of North America 24(4):955–965.

Fromer MJ 1982 Solving ethical dilemmas in nursing practice. Topics in Clinical Nursing 4(1):15–21.

Holly C 1989 Critical care nurses' participation in ethical decision making. Journal of the New York State Nurses Association 20(4):9–12.

Hong Kong Hospital Authority Clinical Ethics Committee 2002 Hospital Authority guidelines on life-sustaining treatment in the terminally ill. Hospital Authority, Hong Kong.

Kohlberg L 1981 Essays on moral development. Vol 1: the philosophy of moral development. Harper & Row, San Francisco.

Kwong EWY, Pang MCS, Wong TKS et al 2005 Predicting pressure ulcer risk with the modified Braden, Braden and Norton scales in acute care hospitals in mainland China. Applied Nursing Research (in press).

Munhall P 1980 Moral reasoning levels of nursing students and faculty in a baccalaureate nursing program. Image 12(3):57–61.

Murphy C 1981 Moral reasoning in a selected group of nursing practitioners. In Ketefian S (ed) Perspectives on nursing leadership: issues and research. Teachers College Press, New York.

Pang MCS 2003 Nursing ethics in modern China: conflicting values and competing role requirements. Rodopi, New York.

Pang MCS, Chung PMB 2002 Nursing ethics in end-of-life care: the importance of respecting the patient's wish. Spirit 54:38–54 (in Chinese).

Pang MCS, Wong TKS 1998 Predicting pressure risk with the Norton, Braden, and Waterlow Scales in a Hong Kong rehabilitation hospital. Nursing Research 47:147–153.

Pang MCS, Sawada A, Konishi E et al 2003 A comparative study of Chinese, American and Japanese nurses' perception of ethical role responsibilities. Nursing Ethics 10:295–311.

Pang MCS, Chung PMB, Chung YMI et al 2004 The decision making of hand/tube feeding for patients with advanced dementia and its impact on their quality of life. Modern Nursing Education & Research 1(3):138–143 (in Chinese).

Pang MC, Volicer L, Leung WK 2005 An empirical analysis of making life-sustaining treatment decisions for patients with advanced dementia in the United States. Chinese Journal of Geriatrics 24(4):300–304 (in Chinese).

Parker RS 1990 Nurses' stories: the search for a relational ethic of care. Advances in Nursing Science 13(1):31–40.

Pence T 1987 Approaches to nursing ethics. Philosophy in Context 17:7–15.

Søderberg A, Norberg A 1993 Intensive care: situations of ethical difficulty. Journal of Advanced Nursing 18:2008–2014.

Swider SM, McElmurry BJ, Yarling RR 1985 Ethical decision making in a bureaucratic context by senior nursing students. Nursing Research 34(2):108–112.

Tao J, Lai PW (eds) 2002 Cross-cultural perspectives on the (im)possibility of global bioethics. Kluwer, Dordrecht.

Veatch RM 1998 Ethical consensus formation in clinical cases. In: ten Have HAMJ, Sass HM (eds) Consensus formation in healthcare ethics. Kluwer, Dordecht, p 17–34.

Viens D 1995 The moral reasoning of nurse practitioners. Journal of American Academy of Nurse Practitioners 7(6):277–285.

Yarling RR, McElmurry BJ 1986 The moral foundation of nursing. Advances in Nursing Science 8(2):63–73.

Further reading

Aroskar MA 1982 Are nurses' mind sets compatible with ethical practice? Topics in Clinical Nursing 4(1):22–32.

Fry ST, Killen AR, Robinson EM 1996 Care-based reasoning, caring, and the ethic of care: a need for clarity. Journal of Clinical Ethics 7(1):41–47.

Gilligan C 1982 In a different voice: psychological theory and women's development. Harvard University Press, Cambridge, MA.

Penticuff JH 1991 Conceptual issues in nursing ethics research. Journal of Medicine and Philosophy 16:235–258.

Chapter **9**

The application of principle-based ethics to nursing practice and management: implications for the education of nurses

Theresa Drought

Principle-based ethics is a powerful tool for examining ethically troubling situations. This chapter explores some cautions about the appropriate use of principle-based ethics, especially related to the preservation of the moral agency of the individual. I will explore the suitability of using this ethics theory when confronted with the phenomena of moral uncertainty, moral dilemma, and moral distress. The use of case studies for teaching principle-based ethics will be demonstrated with cases from clinical practice and nursing management.

INTRODUCTION

- What are the reasons for teaching ethics to nurses?
- What are the goals and purpose of the educational task?
- To what use will the knowledge be put?

Like physicians, nurses must:

> . . . *develop a clear understanding of the moral nature and requirements of the physician[nurse]–patient relationship including the importance of caring, presence, responsiveness and respect, the centrality of trust, confi-*

dentiality, non-judgemental regard, non-sexual regard, truth-telling, and informed consent. They also have to understand the moral importance of their relationships with peers and other professionals and how to reach agreement when they have different views. (Rhodes 2002 p 495)

The challenge in teaching ethics is to identify the means of inspiring in nurses these habits, traits, and attitudes. The goal is not to train nurses as philosophers but to instill in them the necessary skill, knowledge and – most importantly – habits of reflection and critical engagement with the intrinsically moral components of nursing practice (Stirrat 2003). The ethical focus for nurses is not just on problem solving; formulaic application of ethical theories will not provide ready-made answers for nurses. What the application of ethical theories can do is to reveal the complexities of the problem, which in turn will lead to better reasoned and more carefully considered choices of action. It is not necessary to find the one right action in a given situation, but to be able to identify the range of acceptable actions and to be able to articulate the reasoning behind any choice of action (Webb & Warwick 1999). Engaging practising nurses in this type of reflective practice will help to prepare them for the moral and emotional rigours of nursing's work.

In this chapter, I will explore how to apply ethical principles to particular situations. When carefully applied, principle-based ethics (PBE) can provide clarity about possible right actions. However, PBE should not be used to provide an algorithm for action. Instead, I will explore a method of analysis using PBE for cases in nursing care and management that will help nurses to appreciate and safely navigate through the complexities of the situation and identify the range of acceptable actions.

PRINCIPLE-BASED ETHICS FOR HEALTH CARE

Why is PBE a useful tool for developing the habits of moral reflection necessary for moral action in nursing practice and health care more generally? First, some sort of structure (method, language, concept) is useful when analysing complex situations. A means of organizing thinking and reasoning is helpful when confronted with complex and emotionally charged situations. Second, PBE is a familiar form of analysis. Individuals are often strongly motivated by certain principles to guide moral actions; we have all encountered PBE, perhaps unknowingly, in the common morality that we have learned since infancy. Familiar adages such as the golden rule ('do unto others as you would have them do unto you') are forms of principle-based ethics. Focusing on principles therefore reinforces and validates habits a nurse may already hold.

Tom Beauchamp and James Childress (1994) propose four principles to guide ethical deliberation in medicine and health care: autonomy, non-maleficence, beneficence and justice (see also Chapter 7). These principles are derived from 'the morality shared in common by the members of a society, that is, unphilosophical common sense and tradition' (Beauchamp & Childress 1994 p 100). The common morality comprises socially approved norms of conduct; acting in accordance with these principles will give rise to social approbation. Because of their basis in common sense, these principles tend to be very appealing to clinicians and of all bioethics theories, this theory has had the greatest influence and is most familiar to healthcare practitioners in the USA and further afield.

This notion of the common morality raises some immediate concerns, however. As Samantha Pang describes in Chapter 8, meanings and priority values may differ in different cultural contexts. Whereas the principle of autonomy holds great precedence within the USA's cultural context, ubuntu – the principle that the individual only exists within the context of the group; 'I am a person through persons' – makes autonomy something very different within the African context. There has been great debate about the universality of principle-based healthcare ethics and its appropriate application in cultural contexts outside of the Anglo-American context (Fagan 2004, Hayry 2003, Takala 2001). While the theory of PBE relies on the universality of the principles, the fact of universality has faced serious challenges. A discussion of these challenges and the concept of relativism more generally is beyond the scope of this chapter (see Macklin 1999, Wolfe 1996), but students should explore how they see the relevance of PBE within their own cultural context as well as how they understand the principles outlined here.

The principles of autonomy, beneficence, non-maleficence and justice are not the only principles an individual might apply, nor do these principles preclude the application or value of other rules that are widely considered to be beneficial in the healthcare setting. However, principles are considered to be prima facie obligations; they provide a moral basis for the duty to act regardless of any other concerns:

- To respect the integrity of the individual by allowing self-determination
- To try to provide benefit in the medical encounter
- To avoid doing harm
- To treat individuals in a fair and just manner

can all be traced to commonly accepted moral imperatives. These are the principles I will use here and apply in the healthcare setting. This is in contrast to rules – such as veracity, fidelity and confidentiality – that are strongly valued but do not carry the prima facie obligations of principles. Rules create an all-things-considered duty; they should be followed if the appropriate grounds supporting the action outweigh any that might count against it. Similarly, professional codes of ethics place obligations on nurses and create expectations and guidance for appropriate actions but do not create prima facie obligations comparable to those outlined in a principle-based theory of ethics. Principle-based ethics does not preclude the consideration of other values; it does, however, require that the consideration of principles be of primary concern.

Applying theory to practice

Exercise 1

Questions for discussion:

1. Are these four principles the most relevant for guiding nursing practice?
2. What other values do the students identify as operating within their practice settings?
3. Are there any other values that students would consider to impose prima facie duties?

SOME CAUTIONS WITH PRINCIPLE-BASED ETHICS

As this book demonstrates, there are many approaches to ethics and PBE is only one tool of many. Each approach carries its own benefits and limitations. One particular caution with PBE is the possibility for individuals to disengage from the action. Principle-based ethics seems to promise clarity, moral certainty and an elimination of ambiguity. If principles create a prima facie obligation then they must provide a clear explication of the right course of action. An uncritical application of PBE risks separating individuals from the action in important ways. Individuals are tempted to shift the focus of concern away from worrying about their own obligation to act correctly within a given situation, towards simply discerning what the principles demand of them. It protects an individual from the agony of uncertainty about what to do and replaces that concern with a seemingly intellectual exercise in discovering moral certainty. Is this moral certainty at the expense of moral agency? Larry Churchill describes PBE's appeal as part of the human need to think that we are good people who can know and do the right thing. He warns that 'Adopting these theories and their dogmas will keep us hovering above the action like a god, parsing principles with great agility but in a way that is irrelevant to ethics as lived experience' (1994 p 329). Although somewhat appealing, this position is very different from the experience of the individual in the midst of an ethically challenging situation and could limit what actions are considered to be available to the individual. Worse, it can give justification to actions that the individual would otherwise reject.

Principle-based ethics provides an easy label for a complex process of reasoning that is actually contextually based and value laden. Principle-based ethics is a tool for examining how to proceed in situations of profound human consequence; it is not a template for action. It is through human reasoning and deliberation that the individual discerns the right thing to do. Without this level of reflection, discretion (the application of carefully reasoned consideration) is unavailable to the individual (Toulmin 1981). Principle-based ethics provides a means of categorizing, analysing and understanding what is at stake; it does not eliminate the need for careful reasoning as to what the principles mean for action for particular individuals in particular situations. Principle-based ethics should never be utilized as a substitute for or to eliminate the use of discretion by a moral agent.

Applying theory to practice

The following are composite case studies drawn from a variety of clinical situations. For that reason, inferences or references to any actual patient or nurse should not be made.

Case 1

Joyce Anderson always said she wanted everything to be done to keep her alive. 'Being alive is always better than the alternative' she said. Her son and daughter took her at her word. Now she has developed advanced dementia from multiple strokes, she doesn't recognize her children, can't walk or speak, and resists hand feeding. She has considerable difficulty swallowing. She has pulled out several percutaneous gastric feeding tubes and considerable healing is required before another can be placed. She has a nasogastric feeding tube, which she pulls out several times a day, causing repetitive trauma to her nasal passages. Her family feels compelled to insist on continued tube feeding based on her previous statements. They insist that the nurses keep her hands firmly tied at all times, in spite of the patient's near constant crying and moaning when she is tied down. Sufficient chemical sedation to relieve the crying and pulling at tubes leaves her airway at risk. When she is not restrained she is less upset, however. It is not clear that tube feeding will prolong her life, given her other conditions, but it is clear that she is unable to take in sufficient calories under the current conditions. A long-term plan of care requiring constant physical restraints is the best chance of keeping a feeding tube intact, but she seems to be quite miserable when restrained. The nurses feel that tying her down in this way violates their obligation to treat her with respect and dignity and causes her undue suffering and distress.

Discussion

A simplistic application of PBE might be to determine whether tying Mrs Anderson down can be justified. Applying the four principles would look like this:

- Autonomy: Tying her down honours her statements made when competent. Although she now seems miserable when tied, she is no longer competent. Tying her can be justified based on her autonomous statements made when competent.
- Beneficence: Receiving artificial nutrition and hydration may be a benefit as she is not receiving sufficient calories now. Without tube feeding she will die in a relatively short period of time. From what we know of her values, she considers that being alive will always provide benefit. Receiving artificial nutrition can therefore be justified on this principle.
- Non-maleficence: Tying her down seems to cause her some harm, as evidenced by her crying and moaning; however it also avoids the harm she would certainly encounter if she was not artificially fed. The harm is not intended but is an unfortunate by-product of what is needed to benefit her. Tying her down can be justified on the basis of this principle.
- Justice: There are no prominent justice concerns in this case. It is possible that repeatedly replacing the nasogastric tube and attempting hand feeding takes a great deal of the nurses' time. Placing the patient

in firm restraints may free the nurses up to have more time to meet the needs of other patients. However, that consideration is not a compelling justification for the treatment of this patient.

This approach uses principles to justify a proposed action. It does not allow other actions to be considered. It privileges the woman's former expressions of desires over her current embodied experience. Nor do these justifications take into account the experience of the nurse who must take the woman's hands in her own, tie them to the chair, and listen to her crying and moaning for hours on end. The appeal to principles will not assuage the nurse's unease and sense of inhumanity – the experience of doing something wrong to another human being – and strips the nurse of a sense of moral agency. However, saying that the action is justified because an argument supporting it can be based on principles could be used to truncate the deliberative process and provide a false sense of comfort in an otherwise uncomfortable situation. The proper use of principles calls for a more complex and challenging reflection on the many moral concerns present in the situation.

NURSING AS A MORAL ENDEAVOUR

Nursing as a moral endeavour confronts nurses with challenges on many levels. As Steven Edwards points out in Chapter 7, many nurses are unaware of the moral dimensions of nursing practice. In addition, they may not have the words or familiarity to name what they are experiencing in moral terms. The moral concerns of nursing relate equally to what nursing does as to what nursing is (Taylor 1998). Nurses act for patients but they must also keep in mind the social and political place occupied by licensed nurses: why it is that nurses are authorized to act for patients and the ends to which that action is intended. This means that moral reflection is required for discerning what to do for others, as well as knowing how one is to be, what are proper motivations for action, and what are the consequences of the action for nurses and the profession, independent of patients (Donnelly 1994).

This focus on 'what nursing is' is especially important because without a clear articulation of the nurse as an individual with moral agency, with standing within the greater society as well as within the profession of nursing, the nurse risks instrumentality, becoming merely the means to another's ends (Liaschenko 1995). In most situations, the ends of the patient are equally the ends of the nurse. However, ethical reflection must take into account the complexity of the interests and concerns of the individuals involved in and affected by any action; this includes the nurse, the profession, future patients, and the greater society, as well as the individual patient.

The nurse acts for the patient by being an advocate for the patient. Principle-based ethics provides one support for the practice of nurse advocacy. One purpose of nursing is to protect patients from harm, to see that they are treated fairly, and to promote and protect their autonomy. The principle of autonomy privileges the patient's perspective of benefit and harm in most situations. However, the sole aim of nursing is not to advocate uncritically for whatever a patient may request. There must be some congruency between the aims of the patient and the aims of the nurse. Patients may not put unlimited demands on nurses or on the larger healthcare system. Similarly, the aims of the nurse should be properly aligned with the social position and professional role of the nurse.

Applying theory to practice

Case 1: Discussion

Return to Case 1 to re-examine it. Of concern in any analysis is how the moral agency of individuals involved in the situation is affected. In this case, if the nurse goes along with the proposed plan of treatment, she or he risks being used instrumentally to provide for the goals of the patient at the expense of the nurse's own sense of professional obligation and proper use of professional skills. Due consideration of the nurse's moral agency would seem to require a different course of action because the professional goals (to treat patients with dignity and respect) are at odds with the patient's personal goals (being kept alive in whatever state by whatever means necessary). This is not simply a case of competing interests since harm to the nurse's moral agency results. Principle-based ethics can allow exploration of the relevant moral concerns of various individuals involved in a given situation.

Examining the nurses' position in the light of principles might look like this:

- Autonomy: Autonomy is based on the concept of respect for persons. Although Mrs Anderson's previous wishes would seem to support tying her down, respect for her current position requires the nurses to consider also her current actions and concerns. Although she does not have the capacity to make her own decisions, she is telling the nurses something by her repeated removal of tubes and fights against hand feeding. Being tied down seems to cause her a great deal of distress that she does not experience when untied. It is impossible to say that these actions constitute an informed refusal; however, they should cause the nurses to ask if ignoring them constitutes disrespect of her person.
- Beneficence: The tube feedings are meant to benefit Mrs Anderson; however, research calls into question whether tube feeding in her situation actually prolongs life. For the nurses, the actions they must undertake to provide artificial fluid and hydration for her seem to cause harm and disrespect, rather than provide benefit. It is hard to defend a practice that appears so hurtful on the grounds that it is perhaps beneficial.
- Non-maleficence: These nurses are discomfited by their commitment not to do harm and the harm they perceive to be doing in their treatment of Mrs Anderson. Given the questionable benefit she will receive from the treatment, that harm becomes difficult to defend. Other means to maintain her well-being and preserve her dignity that are not so harmful for her should be explored.

● Justice: There is another type of harm to be considered that has ramifications for justice: that is the harm that results when healthcare providers become inured to the suffering of their patients. Justice requires that we treat similar patients similarly; by ignoring Mrs Anderson's cries and moans with the justification that it is what she wanted and it is good for her, nurses may ignore the distress of other patients and employ similarly dismissive justifications.

USING PRINCIPLES TO ADDRESS THE MORAL ASPECTS OF NURSING

Andrew Jameton (1984, 1993) and others have described the phenomena of moral uncertainty, moral dilemma and moral distress in nursing practice. These classifications can be a useful means of discriminating between the types of moral quandaries and discomforts that nurses may confront. Moral uncertainty describes the situation where nurses feel that there are moral issues involved and probably feel some level of discomfort but do not really know or understand the source of the discomfort or what action, if any, is called for. Moral dilemma describes the situation in which nurses are confronted with the need to choose between two equally undesirable courses of action. Moral distress arises when nurses have made a judgement about the right course of action but are unable to act on that judgement. The distress may arise either because nurses do not choose to act on the judgement or because nurses are constrained from acting by external forces. Another source of moral dis-ease has recently been described, that of moral residue. This is perhaps the most insidious and damaging form of moral distress. George Webster and Françoise Baylis define moral residue as 'that which each of us carries with us from those times in our lives when in the face of moral distress we have seriously compromised ourselves or allowed ourselves to be compromised' (2000 p 218). The effects of moral residue can be devastating over the course of a nurse's career.

In moral uncertainty, nurses are morally troubled but do not have a clear notion of the issues at stake. In a situation of moral uncertainty, nurses can choose among several preliminary courses of action: First, what nurses may need to do is simply engage in some moral reflection. While this seems an easy answer, the demands placed on nurses in the clinical setting do not make the time or space for reflection readily available. It is important that nurses are encouraged – during training, early in their career, as well as when they have become proficient in practice – to value and take the time, on a routine basis, to consider the moral aspects of their practice. Second, nurses may explore the situation with colleagues to discern the issues and options available in a troubling situation. Inculcating the value of habitual moral reflection and exploration will prepare nurses for managing situations of moral uncertainty and moral dilemma as well as helping them to avoid situations of moral distress and moral residue. Principle-based ethics can be useful in helping nurses to move past an emotional response towards identifying and naming the concerns that have been raised by the situation. Identifying the role of the four principles in the situation may provide clarity for nurses and relieve the uncertainty.

Moral dilemmas can occur in at least two forms: in the first, there is some evidence to indicate that one action is morally right while at the same time there is some evidence to indicate that the action is morally wrong, but the evidence on both sides is inconclusive. In the second case, individuals believe that they are morally required to take one course of action and at the same time are morally required to take another course of action incompatible or at odds with the first. Case 1 is an example of the former type of dilemma. In situations of moral dilemma, it is important to remember that reasonable people can come to different conclusions about the right course of action. PBE provides a shared language for individuals to explore their justifications and rationale. A formal exploration using PBE may allow individuals to see more clearly what is at stake and to decide what might be a more preferable action.

Moral distress results when nurses have made a judgement about a right action but either do not follow through on that action or are constrained from acting on it. Moral distress can have very real and detrimental effects on individual nurses and on the profession as a whole. It leads to feelings of powerlessness, helplessness, and apathy. Moral distress has been positively linked to cases of burnout and is frequently cited as a reason for leaving the profession (Joint Commission on Accreditation of Healthcare Organizations 2002; Sumner & Townsend-Rocchiccioli 2003). Many situations encountered by nurses have the potential of inducing moral distress in nurses. However, it is important to examine the issue of agency and how nurses are or are not culpable or blameworthy in the situation:

- In what instances do nurses have a choice in the matter?
- In what instances are the circumstances beyond the nurses' control?
- Do nurses have a realistic opportunity to refuse to participate in the concerning situation?

This type of examination can allow nurses to recognize opportunities for moral action and choice and discern them from those in which the nurses' agency is limited. Principle-based ethics is useful in framing that examination and providing a reference for the source of the nurses' distress. The issue of limited agency of nurses has been widely discussed in response to Rod Yarling and Beverly McElmurry's seminal work (1986). However, the fact of agency and culpability does not preclude nurses from feeling bad about the results of or participation in a given situation. The ability to articulate such culpability may help nurses to manage moral distress better and minimize the effects of moral residue.

Applying theory to practice

Exercise 2

1. Engage students in identifying situations of moral concern from their clinical experience. Categorize the situations as ones of moral uncertainty, moral dilemma or moral distress.
2. Using PBE, explore the issues involved in each case.
3. Explore the range of approaches available to nurses in addressing each type of situation.

TECHNIQUES FOR TEACHING PRINCIPLE-BASED ETHICS

It is widely agreed that the case-based approach for teaching ethics is most effective (Clark 2002, Macklin 1993, Malek et al 2000; see also Chambers 2000 for a discussion of the problematic notion of case representation). Cases engage learners in a way that abstract concepts alone cannot, by allowing immediate application to clinically relevant situations. The goal in using cases is twofold: to allow learners to experience the reasoning process; to simulate the real world settings the students are likely to encounter. Students should not be encouraged to find the one right answer but to engage in a cogently argued and full discussion of the possibilities and then to reach a defensible decision for action.

Using a grid to organize analysis with PBE can be useful, as shown below. Looking at the principles from the perspective of the various stakeholders can help to develop a fuller analysis. An important component of the analysis is to be sure to identify what concerns might be left out or misrepresented by using PBE alone.

Stakeholder	Autonomy	Beneficence	Non-maleficence	Justice	Other concerns

After analysis, a range of acceptable options that meet the requirements of the principles should be identified. A decision for action and justification for that action can then be articulated.

PRINCIPLE-BASED ETHICS IN CLINICAL PRACTICE

In clinical settings there is often a tendency to think that ethics concerns only the decisions made by or about patients. However, the framing of the issue of ethical concern will determine what is seen as relevant in the situation as well as who is seen as having moral standing. Using PBE to examine the situation from the perspective of multiple stakeholders can help to avoid biases in the analysis. The ethics of clinical practice must serve all involved in the clinical setting: patients, families, healthcare providers and healthcare systems. All are rightful participants in ethically troubling clinical situations. Ethics is a means of determining right action that can be accepted by diverse groups.

Applying theory to practice

Case 2

Steven was born by caesarean section at 36 weeks' gestation with severe intrauterine growth retardation. He weighed 1750 g at birth. He was vigorous at first, but at 2½ weeks he began to have difficulty with feeding and temperature regulation. Testing revealed a rare combined metabolic defect. An ultrasound of his head revealed massive hydrocephalus that was confirmed by CT exam. There was no evidence of ventricular obstruction or increased intracranial pressure, but positive evidence of profound cerebral atrophy was found. While it is difficult to assess the prognosis for this type of injury in an infant, the physicians felt that this level of cerebral atrophy would be commensurate with at least moderate if not severe cognitive disability, including the possibility of blindness, deafness, cerebral palsy, epilepsy, poor motor control and poor potential for speech development. Additionally, control of the metabolic condition would be challenged by any infectious process or increased physiological stress creating the possibility of further neurological damage. Long-term effects of the treatment (strictly limiting his diet to a specially prepared formula) are essentially unknown because his metabolic condition is exceedingly rare but the physicians felt he could survive a few years at best with considerable disability and suffering. Steven's parents are very concerned for the welfare of their son and for their family. They are concerned that the considerable demands of Steven's care may interfere with meeting the needs of their 3½-year-old daughter. However, their primary concern is that Steven does not suffer needlessly. After discussion of his treatment and prognosis, the mother and father are faced with an ethical dilemma: Continuing the special feeding will continue Steven's life for an unknown but short period of time (months to a few years) with considerable disability and suffering; stopping the special feedings will mean his metabolic condition will lead to his death in a period of weeks to months.

Stakeholder	Autonomy	Beneficence	Non-maleficence	Justice	Other concerns
Steven	An infant is not capable of formulating any autonomous interests of his own. This principle will not have a prominent role in this case. The infant's interests can only be considered in light of benefit and burden.	Life is generally a benefit; it is not known if Steven can appreciate life in any way, which does not mean it is not a benefit. Special feedings could keep him alive, but risk increased suffering by prolonging the dying process.	Special feedings will prevent further neurological damage but will not undo what has already occurred. They will not prevent further deterioration from other insults. Feeding him regular food will accelerate his neurological decline, but his dying will not be prolonged.	The special feedings are quite expensive and not readily available in the community. It may be appropriate to consider whether significant resources should be expended on a child who will experience considerable disability and a protracted dying process.	The child's prognosis is that he will die with or without the special feedings. It is unclear if the child will experience suffering given the degree of neurological damage.

Continued

Stakeholder	Autonomy	Beneficence	Non–maleficence	Justice	Other concerns
Parents	Although the parents will make decisions for Steven, they do not act autonomously; they act in his best interests.	As above. The parents are concerned about what constitutes the benefit; is it to prolong his life, probably in an institutional setting, or is it to accept his death and take him home for the short remainder of his life?	As above. Parents also want to avoid harm to the family. Steven's care demands have the potential to destabilize the family structure or to limit the ability of the older sibling to get the attention she may need.	How does one balance the needs of the family against the needs of the infant?	Since this is a true dilemma, there is no good outcome possible for this child; considering the child within the family may be especially appropriate.
Healthcare team	As above.	As above. Personal values of staff may make the determination of benefit clearer to some.	Staff may feel complicit in the child's death and decline by knowingly giving regular feedings that cause further neurological deterioration.	Staff may be especially concerned about the resource issues.	Staff values may affect their attitude about what constitutes benefit and harm.

This type of analysis does not give an easy answer and space precludes a more in-depth discussion. However, setting the issues out in a grid that lets nurses examine the special concerns of different stakeholders allows access to the ethically relevant issues. Options for action can then be developed that take the ethical issues into account. No easy answer emerges in a case like this; however, the process requires a conscious justification of the action chosen.

ORGANIZATIONAL ETHICS – THE NURSE IN MANAGEMENT

As traditionally utilized in the USA, PBE has been almost exclusively applied to patient care situations involving one-on-one relationships between the provider and the patient. Hospital ethics committees, physicians and nurses may be well versed in the principles discussed here, but there is often a disturbing disconnection between the expectations placed on clinician behaviour and the behaviours exhibited by the institutions within which they work. Stanley Reiser (1994) points out the difficulty this creates when institutions stress the ethical principles clinicians are to adhere to while creating an organizational climate within which justice, autonomy and basic respect for persons is missing. Nurses cannot effectively support the principle of autonomy for patients if the healthcare providers are treated in a tyrannical way. Staff cannot create a culture of beneficence for patients if staffing patterns, human resource issues and general management is one that is completely unconcerned about the employees or is systematically unjust.

Business ethics is a necessary component of running any healthcare organization and is not the topic of this chapter. While efficiency, cost-effectiveness and productivity are necessary principles of business, they are not sufficient in the healthcare setting. There must be some coherence between the long-standing and traditional principles guiding patient care and professional practice and the ethical environment established within the healthcare setting (Spencer et al 2000).

Applying theory to practice	*Exercise 3*

The managers of each department are told they need to cut their budget by 5% in the coming year. Use PBE to analyse the moral implications for the various parties who might be affected. Based on your analysis identify some basic guidelines managers could use in identifying an ethical means of cutting the budget.

Discussion — Analyse possible concerns using PBE.

Stakeholder	Autonomy	Beneficence	Non-maleficence	Justice	Other concerns
Future patients	Any decision should serve to protect individual integrity and promote patient autonomy. Patient choice and input on their care should be preserved.	The primary purpose of any nursing unit is to provide benefit to patients through nursing care. Any budget cuts should preserve that function.	Any budgetary decision should anticipate possible harms and minimize any real harms patients might experience.	Cuts should be made as fairly as possible; no patient group should be singled out to bear the burden of the cuts without reasonable justification.	Creativity should be utilized to cut costs without adversely affecting patients.
Nursing staff	Nurses share the same concerns as above. Any budgetary measure should not impinge on the nurses' autonomous practice.	Nurses should feel comfortable that they will be able to continue to benefit their patients.	Nurses should not be required to act in ways contrary to the interests of their patients.	Same concerns as for patients. Reasoning for budgetary decisions should be made explicit to all. Individual nurses should not be held accountable for practice changes required by management decisions.	Nurses are accountable for their practice but do not control the resources needed for that practice. They lack auton-omy in many ways; sensitivity to the concerns of nurses can create an environ-ment more conducive to the ethical provision of health care.

Continued

Stakeholder	Autonomy	Beneficence	Non-maleficence	Justice	Other concerns
Institutional administration	As above.	Financial solvency is a necessity if the institution is to be able to provide any benefit. Good stewardship is a means of providing benefit.	Harming patients is bad for business. Good stewardship requires managing resources well and preserving the ability to provide patient care.	Same as above. Justice in the larger business practices and within the institutions is also of concern.	Institutions are accountable for good business ethics; concerns for healthcare ethics may be in conflict with other business concerns.

Using PBE, managers could develop certain guidelines for any budgetary proposal. The following is an example:

1. Patient involvement in their care should be protected.
2. The provision of beneficial care and the ability of nurses to provide that care should be preserved.
3. Possible harms resulting from any budgetary cuts should be identified and minimized.
4. Reasoning behind any budget change and measures taken should be made explicit to all affected parties.
5. No group should unfairly bear the burden of any budget change.
6. Staff should have input into any decision. Staff support will be an imperative.

While these may seem simplistic, they could be utilized by managers to evaluate the acceptability of any proposal and identify ethically defensible measures to be taken. They create a useful template against which to measure any budgetary decision.

CONCLUSION

Principle-based ethics is a familiar and accessible means of examining ethically troubling clinical situations. In spite of this, there are many challenges to its appropriate use:

- Principles are defined as prima facie obligations. However, this can present challenges within differing cultural contexts.
- Care should be taken when using PBE to see that concerns about what nurses ought to do are not considered at the expense of concerns about how nurses are to be.
- Principle-based ethics can present the temptation to look for justification of an action rather than a robust analysis of what might be the range of ethically appropriate actions.
- Principles of autonomy, beneficence, non-maleficence and justice can be applied to actions affecting groups and organizations as well as decisions about one's own actions.
- Principle-based ethics should never be used to supplant or minimize the moral agency and discretion of individuals.

The purpose of teaching ethics in nursing is threefold: (1) to develop habits of moral reflection; (2) to encourage creative and responsible problem-solving; and (3) to allow nurses to engage with their fellow human beings in a caring and thoughtful manner when approaching issues of profound human consequence. Principle-based ethics is a powerful tool in that endeavour. However, it should never be taught as if it is the only tool. It is merely one of many ways to promote the type of dialogue and reflection required for us to live in human fellowship together.

References

Beauchamp TL Childress JF 1994 Principles of biomedical ethics. Oxford University Press, New York.

Chambers T 2000 Why ethicists should stop writing cases. Journal of Clinical Ethics 11(3):206–212.

Churchill LR 1994 Rejecting principlism, affirming principles. In: Dubose ER, Hamel RP, O'Connell LJ (eds) A matter of principles: ferment in US bioethics. Trinity, Valley Forge, PA.

Clark PG 2002 Values and voices in teaching gerontology and geriatrics: case studies as stories. Gerontologist 42:297–303.

Donnelly WJ 1994 From principles to principals: the new direction in medical ethics. Theoretical Medicine 15:141–148.

Fagan A 2004 Challenging the bioethical application of the autonomy principle within multicultural societies. Journal of Applied Philosophy 21(1):15–31.

Hayry M 2003 European values in bioethics: why, what and how to be used? Theoretical Medicine and Bioethics 24:199–214.

Jameton A 1984 Nursing practice: the ethical issues. Prentice-Hall, Englewood Cliffs, NJ.

Jameton A 1993 Dilemmas of moral distress: moral responsibility and nursing practice. AWHONN's Clinical Issues 4:542–551.

Joint Commission on Accreditation of Healthcare Organizations 2002 Health care at the crossroads: strategies for addressing the evolving nursing crisis. Joint Commission on Accreditation of Healthcare Organizations, Oakbrook Terrace, IL.

Liaschenko J 1995 Ethics in the work of acting for patients. Advances in Nursing Science 18(2):1–12.

Macklin R 1993 Teaching bioethics to future health professionals: a case-based clinical model. Bioethics 7: 200–206.

Macklin R 1999 Against relativism. Oxford University Press, New York.

Malek JI, Geller G, Sugarman J 2000 Talking about cases in bioethics: the effect of an intensive course on health care professionals. Journal of Medical Ethics 26:131–136.

Reiser SJ 1994 The ethical life of health care organizations. Hastings Center Report 24:28–35.

Rhodes R 2002 Two concepts of medical ethics and their implications for medical ethics education. Journal of Medicine and Philosophy 27:495–510.

Spencer EM, Mills AE, Rorty MV, Werhane PH 2000 Organization ethics in health care. Oxford University Press, New York.

Stirrat GM 2003 Education in ethics. Clinical Perinatology 30(1):1–15.

Sumner J, Townsend-Rocchiccioli J 2003 Why are nurses leaving nursing? Nursing Administration Quarterly 27:164–171.

Takala T 2001 What is wrong with global bioethics? On the limitations of the four principles approach. Cambridge Quarterly of Healthcare Ethics 10(1):72–77.

Taylor CR 1998 Reflections on nursing considered as moral practice. Kennedy Institute of Ethics Journal 8(1):71–82.

Toulmin S 1981 The tyranny of principles. Hastings Center Report 11:31–39.

Webb J, Warwick C 1999 Getting it right: the teaching of philosophical health care ethics. Nursing Ethics 6:150–156.

Webster GC, Baylis FE 2000 Moral residue. In: Rubin SB, Zoloth L (eds) Margin of error: the ethics of mistakes in the practice of medicine. University Publishing, Hagerstown, MD, p 217–230.

Wolfe SM (ed) 1996 Feminism and bioethics: beyond reproduction. Oxford University Press, New York.

Yarling RR, McElmurry BJ 1986 The moral foundation of nursing. Advances in Nursing Science 8:63–73.

Further reading

Beauchamp TL, Childress JF 2001 Principles of biomedical ethics. Oxford University Press, New York.

Childress JF 1982 Who should decide: paternalism in health care. Oxford University Press, New York.

Dubose ER, Hamel RP, O'Connell LJ (eds) 1994 A matter of principles: ferment in US bioethics. Trinity Press, Valley Forge, PA.

Fry S, Johnstone MJ 2002 Ethics in nursing practice: a guide to ethical decision making. Blackwell, Oxford.

Herrera CD 2000 Patient vignettes in bioethics literature. Journal of Clinical Ethics 11:213–218.

Lie RK, Schotsmans PT et al (eds) 2002 Healthy thoughts: European perspectives on health care ethics. Peeters, Leuven.

Redman BK, Fry ST 2000 Nurses' ethical conflicts: what is really known about them? Nursing Ethics 7:360–366.

Chapter 10

Virtue ethics

Louise de Raeve

Lord give me grace, on this and every day,
To do my work the best and simplest way;
And to remember that in all I do,
The very smallest task is seen by you.

Grant to me courage, Lord, when things go wrong,
To stop and think, and not rush blindly on.
And though the task I'm set, may not seem fair,
May I remember, that Thou too, art there.

Give me a humble heart, that I may know,
That things worth while, are not just things that show.
For though efficiency and skill mean much,
The greatest gift of all, is human touch . . .

(From *A Nurse's Prayer* by Alwyn M. Law)

INTRODUCTION

This prayer brings out the emphasis on motive, attitude and character on which the virtue perspective of ethics focuses. Rather than asking questions about what is the good or right thing to do, where one might then consider duties or rights or assess the consequences of action, virtue ethics turns to moral character and asks 'Who is the good man or woman?' This enquiry then deepens into consideration of those moral qualities (virtues) that might be required to justify such a description and an educative slant appears in the further question, 'can such qualities be inculcated or taught and if so, how?' The virtue perspective does not ignore questions of moral action (what should we do?) but its preference for the question 'How should we be?' deals with action via the moral exemplar of what the good man or woman would do. There is no particular reason why it has to have a religious underpinning, although Jesus Christ, the prophet Mohammed and Buddha would all be moral exemplars of the good man. However, what religion may provide is a culturally cohesive (because widely agreed) account of the good woman or man. In secular and multi-faith, multi-cultural societies, there may be less agreement. As will be seen later, this may pose a problem for the virtue ethicist.

HISTORY

Aristotle, the classical Greek philosopher, is the person first credited with developing a rounded account of the virtues to provide a unique moral perspective. To understand both its relevance and irrelevance to contemporary thought, it seems important to understand something of the social context with which Aristotle was familiar and which he addressed in his writing and teaching. By European standards, Athenian society was small and homogeneous. Its structure depended on slavery and this was something that Aristotle never questioned. His enquiry stems from a political concern about how the state can best educate and help its citizens to realize a good life: a project that sees ethics and politics as fundamentally the same and which necessitates some specification of what 'the good life' is (Field 1966 p 72). According to Aristotle, what all people seek, consciously or unconsciously, is *eudaimonia*, which can be translated as 'happiness' but is better understood as 'well-being' or 'flourishing'. His ethical perspective is therefore teleological, i.e. focused on ends, which in turn appears to emphasize a functionalist account of human nature (what produces this end?). This teleology gives the virtue perspective some superficial affinity with consequentialist (outcomes-based) moral theories such as utilitarianism, but the difference is also radical because there is no expectation that there should be any kind of quantitative calculation of benefits over harms and, once identified within a virtue framework, the virtues have intrinsic rather than instrumental value. In other words, from within the virtue perspective, there is not a simple, linear means–ends relationship of the virtues to overall human flourishing. To illustrate this in a nursing context, one might conclude that a kind attitude to patients is an important virtue for the nurse because it promotes both the flourishing of patients and also the professional satisfaction of the nurse. However, kindness is not merely valued for what it leads to, as it would be within a utilitarian conception of the virtues. It is of immediate, intrinsic value to nurse and patient at the moment of its expression. One might say that here the ends are contained within the means, which is a circular rather than a linear picture.

Returning to Aristotle, there is reason to think that it would not have been difficult in Athenian society to identify the 'good life' because of the homogeneity of that society. Assuming this to be so, the question then turns to what moral qualities of character would be most conducive to achieving this. What should the state educate or inculcate in its citizens? GC Field interprets Aristotle as follows:

> We can only, then, reach a good character at the end and as a result of a period of training of a certain length. And when we have attained good character, it means that we are of such a nature as to perform good acts spontaneously . . . At the beginning of our life's training we perform such acts under the direction of another, and from other motives than for their own sake, chiefly, no doubt, for the sake of rewards and the fear of punishment. And by doing them we become of such a character as to do them spontaneously. This is the work of education. But it is only possible because there is really there from the beginning some sort of underlying impulse towards the good, because in some sense we 'naturally' take pleasure in good acts (for that is almost the definition of good acts). (1966 p 80–81)

It should be apparent that this emphasis on spontaneity and on the love of the good captures our intuition that there is something morally preferable about the person who does a good deed in a good spirit, without pausing to reflect or calculate, rather than the person who merely acts out of a sense of duty. It might be claimed that a person who keeps a promise out of respect for the rule 'promises must not be broken', has a thinner grasp of morality than one who keeps a promise out of respect for and recognition of the value of promises in human life and specifically this promise in this particular life.

Field (1966) proceeds to consider Aristotle's idea of what exactly is the test of a 'good act' and this introduces the Aristotelian idea of the *mean*. This is an idea of moderation whereby 'good action is that which avoids the excess or the defect and strikes the mean between them' (Field 1966 p 81). An illustration of this would be anger, where in a particular situation it might be important to be able to be angry but at the same time not overly angry. One might speak of being 'appropriately angry'. This does not make 'anger' a virtue, but appropriate anger might be a necessary component of courage, which is a virtue.

We are not called good or bad, we are not praised or blamed, by reason of our emotions or capacities. It is rather what we choose to do with them that entitles us to be called virtuous or vicious. Virtuous choice is choice in accordance with a mean (MacIntyre 1967 p 65).

One can see how Aristotle would have had to insist on understanding particular issues in particular contexts in order to know if the mean had been achieved. As Alasdair MacIntyre (1967 p 66–67) states: '. . . knowledge of the mean cannot just be knowledge of a formula, it must be knowledge of how to apply the rules to choices'. Aristotle's ethics therefore opposes universal statements about what sort of actions are good or bad to do. From a more contemporary reading, one can see that it could claim to provide an alternative to the universal prescriptivism of duty-based ethics.

This idea of the mean seems more clearly applicable to some emotions rather than others. It is not controversial to talk of appropriate levels of anger but this idea is not so comprehensible when considering an emotion such as envy or love. MacIntyre (1967) criticizes this aspect of Aristotelian thought for being inadequately developed, and possibly, as a systematized account of the virtues, it is doomed to failure. Nevertheless, what it reveals is the relevance of the emotions to moral life. In this the virtue perspective, even in its classical form, is far removed from the heavy focus on rationality of Kantian ethics and Kantian suspicions of the emotions because they can lead us astray. What one sees in Aristotelian thought is an attempt to connect feeling and thinking through this notion of the *mean*. Whether it works or not as an idea, it invites development of understanding of the emotions, as being of intrinsic importance to any conception of morality.

THE CONTEMPORARY PICTURE

In Western moral philosophy there has been a recent renewal of interest in Aristotelian thought about ethics. This does not mean that in preceding centuries Aristotle had no influence. On the contrary, via St. Thomas Aquinas' (c. 1226–1274) interpretation, there has been a far-reaching influence on Roman Catholic theology. However, European accounts of the nature of morality have branched away from theological accounts and both the duty-based ethical explanation of Immanuel Kant (1724–1804) and the outcomes-based utilitarian ethics of John Stuart Mill (1806–1873) are determinedly secular in nature.

Several factors in contemporary life have led to some dissatisfaction with these two perspectives as constituting an adequate account of morality, in either isolation or combination. The growth in healthcare ethics may have contributed to this disillusionment, because it has compelled moral philosophers and healthcare practitioners to work closely together in the examination of moral dilemmas in specific contexts (Nussbaum 1992). This focus on particularity rather than generality has revealed the value but also the limitations of ethical explanations that aim to address general rather than particular states of affairs. For example, in his first maxim, Kant instructs us '. . . never to act otherwise than so *that I could also will that my maxim should become a universal law*' (original emphasis) (Field 1966 p 23). This means that if in any particular situation, I think it morally right to do *x*, I must agree that it would be morally right for everybody to do *x* when in the same or relevantly similar situation. With their exposure to the individuality of patients, nurses tend to be particularly aware that no moral situation is exactly the same as any other. There may be just as many morally relevant differences as similarities in specific situations, even in those that could be said to embrace the same overall theme, such as 'truth-telling' or 'consent'. This tends to expose the limitations of any general, formulaic response to the making of moral decisions.

Feminism has also played its part in producing women philosophers, such as Annette Baier (1993), who ask questions about how morality gets started developmentally, thereby bringing together an interest in philosophy and moral psychology. This has led to a new focus on the moral life in families and therefore in parent–child relationships. A hitherto much neglected area of philosophy has been the nature of the emotions. It would be a mistake to portray this as only the province of women philosophers or to suggest that all women philosophers are feminists, but it would appear that feminism helped to propel these developments forward. These new areas of inquiry have been grouped under various headings but they include: feminist ethics, caring ethics, relational ethics and virtue ethics.

More will be said about the first two of these in other chapters in this book. Relational ethics can be subsumed under caring ethics, although not all advocates of this position would necessarily agree with this. Vangie Bergum (1999) is someone who writes from this perspective. Virtue ethics, however, could be seen as capable of addressing these concerns. The Aristotelian position emphasizes the development of good moral character. It allows for the particularity of context, is non-formulaic in approach and has an interest in the contribution of the emotions to moral life. However, since there is a world of a difference between contemporary society and that of pre-Christian Athens, it is preferable to call contemporary virtue theorists neo-Aristotelians. They are using and adapting Aristotelian thought to current circumstances. Two such writers are Martha Nussbaum (1992, 1993) and Alasdair MacIntyre (1975, 1985), although they do not share the same stance.

MacIntyre (1975, 1985) is concerned that the virtue perspective depends on sufficient social agreement concerning who constitutes the good man or woman, or, in health care, the good doctor or nurse. He is pessimistic that in multi-cultural, morally plural societies, this agreement may not exist, thereby leaving no moral means for arbitrating between clashing perspectives. He is particularly concerned that in health care there may be such differences between patients' values and the health carers' values that it becomes impossible for a doctor or nurse to act virtuously, no matter how sincere the attempt. An illustration of this would be with a paternalistic approach. Here the health carers believe that they know what is good or best for patients and that this is fundamentally independent of any view the patients may have. In the past, patients may have matched this view, believing that professional health carers did indeed know best and decisions should be left to them. The system works only for as long as ideas of patient autonomy are not present. When they appear, the system can no longer operate, and patients and health carers have to connect differently. This may work to both parties' continuing and even increasing advantage. However, if the value of patient autonomy is pushed to its extreme, as a consumer view of health care would be inclined to do, this can undermine the value of professional judgement and the professional person's self-expectation by profoundly compromising the freedom to make such judgements. The 'good' from a consumer and professional perspective may ultimately be irreconcilable. If this is not acknowledged openly, it is likely that attempts at resolution will be based on the exploitation of power.

Nussbaum (1992) is much less pessimistic. She believes that while there may be differing and competing conceptions of the good life, the good man or woman, etc. there are 'thick' (richer) and 'thin' (poorer) versions of these. For example, a 'thin' account of courage might equate with fearlessness. A 'thicker' account might suggest that a courageous person is not so much the person who feels no fear but the person who can be brave in spite of fear. This is a different account from the 'thin' version but it is also a more complex and hence richer portrayal of courage.

Despite cultural variety, Nussbaum would maintain that there is an underpinning universality to understanding the good life, human flourishing (Aristotle's *eudaimonia*), etc. and this enables discrimination between competing accounts. She is, in this respect, a moral realist rather than a moral relativist, believing that morality is founded on something shared by all human beings. This gives a kind of objectivity to moral debate, even if this is not the scientific objectivity of facts that can be established by observation of the practical world. Nussbaum states:

> I believe . . . that an ethics of virtue, understood in the way the ancient Greeks understood it, will emphasize the importance of friendship, moral emotions, and precise attention to contextual particularity; but it will also lead to an intense concern with human universality, with normative principles of broad applicability, and with the material prerequisites of human flourishing. (Nussbaum 1992 p 9)

IS VIRTUE ETHICS A THEORY?

This is a very interesting question. Given the neo-Aristotelian focus on the importance of understanding particular contexts, there is a case for saying that the virtue perspective is deliberately anti-theoretical. Irrespective of what can be said generally about them, all particular situations are ultimately unique. However, if Nussbaum is right and it is possible to talk about universal conceptions of a flourishing life and of corresponding thick and thin descriptions of the virtues, the case for a theory looks promising. First, however, it is necessary to establish what one might expect of a moral theory.

As Hugh Upton (1993) states, one might expect that a moral theory should at least do two things. It needs to say something about 'which actions are right' and 'it should as far as possible explain, in the sense of helping to make intelligible, our evaluation of actions, telling us something of what gives actions moral worth and in what way they are made right or wrong' (Upton 1993 p 190). He points out that this does not mean that only actions are the focus. If this were so, the virtue perspective would be disqualified from being a theory from the outset. Any viable moral theory has to encompass action, but it can have additional concerns, character being of central interest for virtue theorists.

It is beyond the province of this chapter to consider whether there can be an overarching moral theory at all and whether any contender for this position succeeds. This is an exploration that Upton (1993) pursues. The more limited focus here is whether or not the virtue perspective can be considered to be a moral theory, i.e. one theory among other contenders.

Richard White (1991) divides the virtue perspective into two categories. The first makes the virtues derivative and thus provides a 'weak' account of them. They are conceived of as being those qualities of character that facilitate good action as identified by either the utilitarian calculation of outcomes or the deontological (duty-based) reference to moral law. The latter is seen as either God-given, for example the Ten Commandments, or as of prima facie truth, identifiable via a highly logical and secular form of thought (as it was for Kant). White (1991) remarks:

> In general, I think it would be true to say that many discussions of morality restrict the role of virtue to that of a mere means directed towards the end of fulfilling the law: courage is a virtue because it gives us the strength to fulfil difficult obligations, temperance is a virtue because our passion might otherwise make us forget our obligations, and so forth. (1991 p 220)

He goes on to add that in his view, this 'is an inadequate characterization of true virtue, since it transforms virtue into a mere technique that is not praiseworthy in itself, but only insofar as it helps us to perform our duties' (White 1991 p 220). In the utilitarian context, this would be to maximize the general welfare. It would also mean that the virtue perspective, as understood in this 'weak' sense, cannot be a moral theory in its own right because it is entirely dependent on these other theoretical perspectives.

White (1991) then proposes that there is also a 'strong' account of the virtues that places them at the centre of morality, making them by definition non-derivative. He is not suggesting that this makes the virtue perspective the only useful account of morality, thereby denying the importance of duties and consequences in moral thinking. Rather, he suggests that the virtues occupy the centre-stage of morality as they are of intrinsic value to us, thereby making them a 'basic category of morality' (White 1991 p 226).

This gives rise to the question of how we recognize the virtues and if and how we can discriminate between pseudo and authentic manifestations of them. White (1991) talks about 'moral beauty' and the example set by 'paradigm individuals'. He says:

> For it seems to me that what we most admire in a virtuous individual is not so much devotion to principle, but the perfection of a particular existence, and the cultivation of virtue in unique and unrepeatable ways. Such moral 'beauty' is most obviously manifest in the lives of such 'paradigm individuals' – to use Jaspers' term – as Christ, Buddha, Socrates, or Confucius. (White 1991 p 225, citing Jaspers 1962)

This leads White to conclude that the 'strong' version of the virtues is in fact a-theoretical. He states:

> *We cannot have a 'theory' of virtue because virtue is not something that could ever become a matter of routine. It cannot be prescribed, for the order 'Be virtuous!' is itself a ridiculous command. Any attempt to discover virtue by analysing the principles embodied in the lives of virtuous individuals will therefore diminish the value of the whole, since the virtuous life is unique and unrepeatable. Such a life must be understood as being like a work of art. It is grounded in a particular moral tradition, which it transcends at the same time by the sheer force of its moral necessity. The study of morality should thus address itself to the life histories of paradigm individuals. . . . (White 1991 p 229)*

From this position, White (1991 p 229–230) then promotes the importance of the parable (e.g. New Testament accounts of the teachings of Christ that use metaphors and stories rather than direct instruction) and also of 'literary and dramatic portrayals of virtue' as being the only ways in which virtue can be taught.

White's position has had some prominence in considering whether or not the virtue perspective in morality can be said to be a theory and his position commits the 'strong' virtue account to an a-theoretical stance, for conceptual reasons. It remains questionable, however, how best to describe the positions that Nussbaum and MacIntyre adopt. Would they, for instance, agree with White?

It would seem that they would not entirely agree. Nussbaum (1993 p 248) stresses the importance of an idea of moral progress that would lead to finding 'the correct fuller specification of a virtue', a process which, like Aristotle, she believes can be achieved by the careful examination of human problems, choices and rational debate. This does not sound like a completely a-theoretical position and indeed she later adopts a kind of 60:40 stance in favour of virtue theory by saying:

> *The Aristotelian virtues involve a delicate balancing between general rules and a keen awareness of particulars, in which process, as Aristotle stresses, the perception of the particular takes priority. It takes priority in the sense that a good rule is a good summary of wise particular choices, and not a court of last resort. (Nussbaum 1993 p 257)*

This position seems to imply that in as far as the virtue perspective requires consideration of general rules, it can be said to be theoretical. However, in as far as the uniqueness of particular situations always outweighs this, it remains fundamentally a-theoretical. This would mean that while one might be able to refer to a theoretical dimension of the virtues, it is incoherent to talk of a 'virtue theory', if by this is meant a systematic and complete account of the virtue perspective. From this point of view, no general statements can be made that would fully capture the meaning of good action.

MacIntyre (1975) notes that some virtues are prevalent at some periods of history and then decline: chastity and temperance would be illustrations; and some may occur in one culture and not another. Despite this, he maintains that there are some virtues he calls 'central invariant virtues' which would occur in all cultures. These are justice, courage and truthfulness. He accepts, however, that these will be interpreted differently in different cultures and does not believe that there would be enough consistency of interpretation to form a theory of morality. He is, therefore, extremely sceptical that there could be a comprehensive virtue theory.

WHO IS THE GOOD NURSE?

A response to this question is developed more fully in the two following chapters. It is, however, possible now to see the lines of enquiry that might contribute to an answer. We could for instance carefully examine the lives of paradigm individuals in nursing, with Florence Nightingale and Mary Seacole as two among many contenders. We could attempt to describe and analyse the key virtues in nursing, on the assumption that MacIntyre is right, that 'practices' such as nursing (see glossary for this meaning of 'practice') involve values and virtues that are unique to them. This might entail careful scrutiny of the work already done in medicine in this field by authors like Edmund Pellegrino (1995) and Edmund Pellegrino and David Thomasma (1993). Any such exploration would have to consider relevant similarities and differences between nursing and medicine and seek to capture these in the description of the virtues arrived at. Such work might need cross-cultural comparisons between nurses, in an attempt to see if richer or thicker understandings of the virtues in nursing could be arrived at and accepted via rational debate. Answers in the affirmative would confirm Nussbaum's (1993) position. Negative answers would support MacIntyre's (1975) pessimism.

The work that Madeleine Leininger (1991) and her colleagues have been doing is relevant to this. They have examined cross-cultural understandings of care and they believe that, despite divergence, it is possible to arrive at a universal understanding of the nature of care in nursing. A criticism of this view might level the accusation that the agreement discovered is in fact imposed by the more dominant group (the American vision) and that the cultural hegemony apparently 'discovered' is American imperialism in disguise. A more generous interpretation would link Leininger's work with Nussbaum's (1992, 1993) ideas, seeing the former as empirical endorsement of the latter.

It is not obvious that 'care' is in itself a virtue and, as we can do many bad things carefully, there is nothing about 'being careful' that implies moral worth or approbation. One needs to know the context to see what, if any, moral value should be ascribed. However, in health care, when we speak of 'care', we tend to take this as short hand for 'good care'. This therefore becomes an evaluative rather than simply descriptive concept and tends to imply an attitude of 'being caring', in addition to consideration of the actual care delivered. In itself, 'being caring' may be a rather 'catch all' concept, standing for a cluster of virtues yet to be specified.

These could include: honesty, kindness, patience and courage. It is debatable whether or not care is a virtue (see Allmark 1998). One view would be that it is not a virtue in itself but because of the moral context of health care, i.e. the commitment to the patients' good, 'good care' is inevitably linked with both technically competent care and those virtues of character that form a 'caring attitude'.

According to Pellegrino (1995), identifying such virtues in nursing would first require the establishment of a theory of nursing that specified the ends (*telos*) aimed for. In the case of all health care, this would be the good of the patient and would require attending to 'three phenomena of the healing relationship' which are 'the fact of illness, the act of profession, and the act of medicine (healing)' (Pellegrino 1995 p 267).

The fact of illness requires careful analysis of what it is to be a patient, including appreciation of the vulnerability and dependency of patients. Pellegrino (1995 p 267) sees the act of profession as being '. . . an act of implicit promise making that establishes a covenant of trust'. The act of healing has to focus on the particular patient, using all the skills and abilities at the nurse's disposal but directed at the *telos* of health care, which is 'the cultivation and restoration of health and the containment or cure of disease' (Pellegrino 1995 p 267). The virtues he singles out as being of particular relevance to health care are: fidelity to trust and promise, benevolence, effacement of self-interest, compassion and caring, intellectual honesty, justice and prudence (Pellegrino 1995 p 269–270). His starting point is medicine but his assumption seems to be that these virtues are relevant to all healthcare professionals.

It would seem likely that, to some extent at least, Pellegrino is right about this, but it is a position that might be better argued for than merely assumed. While there are obvious similarities of aim between nursing and medicine, there are many differences in the two practices. Generally, for instance, nurses have much more extended contact with patients than doctors and this can often be of a physical kind, such as washing and dressing patients. This may mean that what it is appropriate for doctors to do with patients is not the same for nurses, and vice versa. Such differences, however subtle, are likely to have an impact on moral ideas about what is a proper attitude to patients in specific contexts. A nurse might easily extend his or her role to encompass massage for a patient but a doctor doing so might infringe professional boundaries. While both professions can adhere to a virtue of benevolence, precisely how this is interpreted within different healthcare practices may be different.

WHICH VIRTUES ARE RELEVANT FOR NURSING?

This seems to be relatively unexplored territory. There is a lively 'concept clarification' movement among nurse researchers that seems to be driven by an attempt to try and standardize nursing language nationally and internationally. Such efforts may be useful for the more technical and scientific aspects of nursing, for example, the standardization of approaches to wound care. However, with regard to the more emotional and obviously moral aspects of practice, i.e. the relational dimension, such research may be worryingly reductive. A sociological approach to language analysis tends to be uncritically assumed in research of this kind.

It may be that no examination of conceptual meaning can occur without making some assumptions about the nature of language, but this sociological approach seems to assume that the most common way a concept is used is its core or central meaning, and that other meanings are therefore peripheral. Such a move tends to simplify conceptual complexity by diminishing the importance of peripheral meanings. John Paley (1996) has argued convincingly against this approach and this creates an argument for good philosophical analysis of the 'softer' (non-scientific) concepts in nursing that include 'the virtues'.

Some work of this kind exists and articles by Ruth Schröck: *A question of honesty in nursing practice* (1980) and *Conscience and courage – a critical examination of nursing conduct* (1990) are examples. Gerald Winslow (1984) took a historical position in his article *From loyalty to advocacy: a new metaphor for nursing*, which demonstrates the way in which the virtue of loyalty seems to have become less significant as the professional as well as the wider culture changed over time. Betty Winslow and Gerald Winslow (1991) have also written an interesting article on *Integrity and compromise in nursing ethics*. In addition, it is important to acknowledge the work of Sally Gadow (1980) on 'existential advocacy'. While she makes no direct reference to a virtue perspective, her writing on this subject reflects the central importance she gives to the development of a certain kind of attitude in nurses.

More recent contributions come from Peter Allmark (1998) in his analysis of whether or not caring can be said to be a virtue in nursing, my own analysis of trust and trustworthiness in nursing (de Raeve 2002), the relational ethics work of Vangie Bergum (1999) and the Aristotlelian–Thomistic (following Thomas Aquinas) realism of Beverley Whelton (2002). Much remains to be done. In the two chapters that follow, I will not presume that the virtue position is a theory. I will use other terms, such as 'position' or 'perspective' in an effort to keep this issue open.

CONCLUSION

This chapter has attempted to give an overview of the nature of the virtue position in ethics from the perspective of its historical development, commencing with classical Greek thought through to a contemporary Western view. The relevance of these ideas for health care and for nursing specifically have been described. It may not be possible to claim that the virtue perspective is a moral theory that could capture, in one explanatory system, the whole of morality and there are grounds for claiming that it cannot be a theory at all. Nevertheless, it may have an essential, non-derivative place in ethics. We value the virtues as being good in themselves and not merely because in any functional sense they bring about good states of affairs, which they may also do. The relationship between the virtues and the Aristotelian *telos* of *eudaimonia* need not be conceived of as a linear relationship from means to ends.

There are, however, strong criticisms against the virtue perspective. Some of these have been alluded to. For example, there may be a problem in deciding between competing illustrations of paradigm individuals and competing descriptions of the virtues, particularly in a multi-cultural society. I will consider these and other objections more fully in the next chapter.

References

Allmark P 1998 Is caring a virtue? Journal of Advanced Nursing 28:466–472.

Baier A 1993 What do women want in a moral theory? In: Larrabee M (ed) An ethic of care. Routledge, New York, p 19–32.

Bergum V 1999 Ethics as question. In: Kohn T, McKechnie R (eds) Extending the boundaries of care: medical ethics and caring practices. Berg, Oxford, p 167–180.

de Raeve L 2002 Trust and trustworthiness in nurse–patient relationships. Nursing Philosophy 3:152–162.

Field G 1966 Moral theory. Methuen, London.

Gadow S 1980 Existential advocacy: philosophical foundations of nursing. In: Spicker S, Gadow S (eds) Nursing images and ideals. Springer, New York, p 79–101.

Jaspers K 1962 Socrates, Buddha, Confucius, and Jesus (The great philosophers vol 1) (trans. Manheim). HBJ, San Diego. In: White R 1991 Historical perspectives on the morality of virtue. The Journal of Value Inquiry 25:217–231.

Leininger M (ed) 1991 Culture care diversity and universality: a theory of nursing. National League for Nursing Press, New York.

MacIntyre A 1967 A short history of ethics. Routledge and Kegan Paul, London.

MacIntyre A 1975 How virtues become vices: values, medicine and social context. In: Engelhardt HHT, Spicker S (eds) Evaluation and exploration in the biomedical sciences. D Reidel, Dordrecht-Holland, p 97–111.

MacIntyre A 1985 After virtue. Duckworth, London.

Nussbaum M 1992 Virtue revived. Times Literary Supplement July 3:9–11.

Nussbaum M 1993 Non-relative virtues: an Aristotelian approach. In: Nussbaum M, Sen A (eds) The quality of life. Clarendon Press, Oxford, p 242–269.

Paley J 1996 How not to clarify concepts in nursing. Journal of Advanced Nursing 24:572–578.

Pellegrino E 1995 Toward a virtue-based normative ethics for the health professions. Kennedy Institute of Ethics Journal 5:253–277.

Pellegrino E, Thomasma D 1993 The virtues in medical practice. Oxford University Press, New York.

Schröck R 1980 A question of honesty in nursing practice. Journal of Advanced Nursing 5:135–148.

Schröck R 1990 Conscience and courage – a critical examination of professional conduct. Nurse Education Today 10:3–9.

Upton H 1993 On applying moral theories. Journal of Applied Philosophy 10:189–199.

Whelton B 2002 Human nature as a source of practical truth: Aristotelian–Thomistic realism and the practical science of nursing. Nursing Philosophy 3:35–46.

White R 1991 Historical perspectives on the morality of virtue. The Journal of Value Inquiry 25:217–231.

Winslow G 1984 From loyalty to advocacy: a new metaphor for nursing. The Hastings Center Report June:32–40.

Winslow B, Winslow G 1991 Integrity and compromise in nursing ethics. The Journal of Medicine and Philosophy 16:307–323.

Chapter 11

A critique of virtue ethics

Louise de Raeve

A scenario

John had been in hospital with diarrhoea for days. He was very emaciated and his bowel was in poor shape. The surgeon told John that he was going to have to do an operation and explained the operation briefly. The anaesthetist was going to come in later with the junior doctor, to get consent. When the junior registrar [a qualified, middle-ranking, specialist doctor] came in, it was someone who John did not know very well and John said that he was not going to have the operation. The doctor said 'You have to have this operation or you will die.' John replied 'I'd rather die.'

It was some time later when I was helping him to the toilet for the twentieth time that day I was able to ask him some questions about what he understood by the operation. It was quite clear that he was horrified by anything to do with faeces. He had just about managed to control the nightmare of having nurses wash and wipe him during the episode of this illness but the thought of his wife and family having to see anything so disgusting was more than he could bear and he felt he would rather die.

He went on about giving up football. When we were alone in the room I asked him if he had thought about what sex would be like after the operation. He did not speak at first then started to pour out a stream of expletives about how it would feel trying to make love when he stank, and had a bag of faeces dangling from his stomach. No-one had discussed it with him and, through the stoma nurse, I got another man who had a stoma to come and talk to him. Someone else could have raised it with him but with me, a married woman of his age, I suspect he felt safe to test my reaction and make the opening, which I took. He consented to go to theatre that evening.

The above scenario was taken from *The value of nursing* (Royal College of Nursing 1992 p 24). It can be interpreted in at least two different ways. These will be described in turn and distinguished as 'account 1' and 'account 2'.

Account 1   The patient, John, refuses the operation. This was an autonomous decision; there is no suggestion of incompetence. The nurse, who has a different set of values, thinks that the patient should have the operation and sets about making him change his mind which, by subtle pressure she succeeds in doing. John's subsequent change of heart has been forced upon him. Such nursing manifestly lacks professional integrity because the power of the nurse's position is exploited to manipulate the patient into conforming to the nurse's vision of what should happen to him.

Account 2   A nurse responds sensitively to John's predicament. She does not take what he says at face value but, by her interest, presence and sensitive questioning, she engages with the emotional dimensions of the patient's situation. This enables him to be less fearful, to distinguish more accurately between his imagined fate and his likely fate and he subsequently changes his mind, deciding to have the surgery.

Readers might like to consider with which account they would align themselves and why. Those whose intuitions support account 1 are going to conclude that John's nurse is far from being a virtuous nurse and, if one uses Alasdair MacIntyre's (1975) illustration from social work and accepts his formulation, she is positively corrupt. MacIntyre says:

> *Sometimes, for example, social workers are taught to become 'friends' with their clients in order to gain their confidence so as to manipulate them more effectively. Now it is of the essence of friendship as a virtue that one cannot become a friend from such a motive and with such an intention. What the social worker is being taught is to do and to speak as a friend would do and speak, but in such a way that what is produced is a counterfeit version and not authentic friendship. It is because the social worker's version is a counterfeit of the virtue and one calculated to deceive the innocent that it is a vice and not merely a neutral quality.* (MacIntyre 1975 p 106)

In complete contrast to the above, those who support account 2 might agree that while there is no such person as a perfect nurse, John's nurse is as near perfect in her nursing as one could hope for. Here is the virtuous nurse at work, demonstrating the complexity of nursing in its requirement to combine practical and emotional care (Nichols 1993). John responds by changing his mind and consenting to have the surgery, thereby endorsing the authenticity and utility of this nurse's engagement with him.

It would appear that while there is enough common ground between those who support account 1 and those who support account 2 for each camp to see that there is a genuine moral disagreement between them, there is little ground for optimism that this could easily be settled one way or the other. If one appeals to ideas of the paradigm individual, then two different paradigms as to who is the virtuous nurse seem to be implicit in the dilemma. Those adhering to account 1 would seem to have in mind a nurse who puts patient rights and autonomy, conceived of as a right, at the front of the care agenda. Such a nurse would be wary of influencing patients in any way. Those supporting account 2 might see less certainty. From their point of view, autonomy is understood less as a right and more as a process that is dependent on relationships and inter-subjectivity: a position Sally Gadow (1980) has argued for. Robert Louden (1993) states: 'We ought, of course, to do what the virtuous person would do, but it is not always easy to fathom what the hypothetical moral exemplar would do were he in our shoes . . .' (Louden 1993 p 195).

It might be crucial to know what John felt about his nurse's response both before and after his surgery, but even this could be interpreted differently by the two positions. Positive appreciation of the nurse's intervention could be interpreted by account 1, as further evidence of the extent to which the nurse had successfully duped John into believing that what she thought was good for him, really was good. From the position of account 2, positive appreciation would be read as a warm endorsement of the moral worth of the nurse's engagement with her patient.

CAN VIRTUE THEORY HELP TO RESOLVE THIS DILEMMA?

If the virtue approach was a theory, one might hope for a theoretical resolution of the above dilemma, leading to a practical resolution. However, a case has been made in the previous chapter for saying that the virtue perspective offers a crucial and perhaps central understanding of moral life, but it falls short of providing a theory of morality. This is because it avoids the general and thus theoretical, in favour of a focus on particular and unique individuals existing at distinct times in discrete contexts. However, if one accepts the a-theoretical position, it is hard to see how the virtue perspective has much to offer in trying to resolve any moral dilemma. A theory can be relied on to contain some prescriptive statements about what morality requires, such as 'do that which maximizes happiness/welfare' in the case of utilitarianism. By contrast, an a-theoretical position looks as if it will be speechless. Nevertheless, having something useful to say about a dilemma does not have to equate with providing a blueprint for its resolution. These issues will be developed further in the sections that follow.

MACINTYRE'S POSITION

It would appear that the dilemma posed by accounts 1 and 2 resonates with illustrations given by MacIntyre (1975 p 98–99) and that his conclusion might be similarly valid. He states:

Given each set of premises, it is rational to move to each conclusion, but there is no argument available, no criterion available, no rational procedure to decide between rival and incompatible conclusions.

We appear therefore to have to make a non-rational choice between alternative positions, so far as our own moral judgments upon each issue are concerned, and to have to resort to non-rational persuasion if we are to affect the choices made by others. (MacIntyre 1975 p 99)

MacIntyre's position is based on a conception of the virtues that is linked to the Aristotelian idea of a *telos* (see Glossary, p. 362). This is a widely, if not universally held understanding of a person's true end and of what constitutes 'an essential human nature' (MacIntyre 1975 p 100). The virtues contribute towards this end but not necessarily in a means-to-ends, linear fashion. They can have intrinsic value, such as the virtues of kindness or compassion might be said to possess. MacIntyre argues that there are cultural-specific virtues that are 'those qualities which have been considered virtues in some times and places and not in others', for example, 'thrift, humility, charity, authenticity and friendship' (MacIntyre 1975 p 104). He also argues that there are 'central invariant virtues' such as justice, courage and truthfulness (honesty), which must have a place in all societies and cultures. They are necessary features of any society. In other words, without them there would be no society. He accepts, however, that there will be cultural variation in how these invariant virtues are interpreted and encoded and acknowledges that this will mean that:

. . . the central invariant virtues are never by themselves adequate to constitute a morality. To constitute a morality adequate to guide a human life we need a scheme of the virtues which depends in part on further beliefs, beliefs about the true nature of man and his true end. But about these matters cultures have of course varied and disagreed. (MacIntyre 1975 p 104)

MacIntyre suggests that, within medicine, virtues are 'not to be derived in any simple way from the invariant human virtues' but rather they emerge from special beliefs about the value of preserving human life, 'about the special character of the physician–patient relationship and about professional autonomy' (MacIntyre 1975 p 105). He proceeds to outline three social presuppositions that had underpinned the traditional medical virtues (1975 p 108):

1. The supreme value placed on human life and the preservation of it.
2. The existence of a shared morality between doctor and patient that was endorsed by the wider society and made it safe for each party to assume that their attitudes towards life and death would be roughly similar. This meant that in trusting the physician, the patient did not feel he or she was relinquishing moral autonomy.
3. '. . . The activities of the physician or surgeon took place within a given social order, but were not themselves able to shape or be responsible for shaping that order' (MacIntyre 1975 p 108).

It is MacIntyre's view that social change has meant that none of these presuppositions still pertains and that this places physicians, and by extension nurses, in a 'tragic dilemma'. The dilemma is a result of our social change in the direction of 'secular, liberal pluralism which leaves us resourceless in the face of moral problems' (MacIntyre 1975 p 109). He claims that this results from a change in medicine's presuppositions, thereby rendering vicious what was once virtuous, and problematic what was once unproblematic (see the quotation on p 110 for an illustration of how a virtue can become a vice).

For MacIntyre the virtue perspective cannot provide a meta-account of morality to enable a rational resolution of the moral conflict delineated by accounts 1 and 2. What it can do is provide a detailed explanation of why this is not possible. Such an explanation should help us to endure the pessimism of this situation and not opt for superficial and inherently bogus 'solutions' to this and other dilemmas. This is an inherently 'relativist' (see Glossary) as opposed to a 'realist' (see Glossary) conclusion. In other words, we are faced with having to agree to differ or, alternatively, to using non-moral powers of force and persuasion in areas of severe moral conflict. The hope might have been to resolve moral disputes by appealing to shared moral truths (which some would consider to be facts) and rationality. For realists, these truths are believed to be common to all moral positions, no matter how conflicted.

NUSSBAUM'S POSITION

Martha Nussbaum is less pessimistic than MacIntyre. If one imagines moral realism and moral relativism being at opposite ends of a continuum, her position would be weighted more towards moral realism than his more relativist conclusion. How might she understand the conflict between account 1 and account 2? Referring to Aristotle, Nussbaum (1993) states:

> For it is obvious that he was not only the defender of an ethical theory based on the virtues, but also the defender of a single objective account of the human good, or human flourishing. This account is supposed to be objective in the sense that it is justifiable by reference to reasons that do not derive merely from local traditions and practices, but rather from features of humanness that lie beneath all local traditions and are there to be seen whether or not they are in fact recognised in local traditions. And one of Aristotle's most obvious concerns was the criticism of existing moral traditions, in his own city and in others, as unjust or repressive, or in other ways incompatible with human flourishing. (Nussbaum 1993 p 243)

This interpretation of Aristotle promises the possibility of a resolution of the conflict expressed by accounts 1 and 2. It invites one to look deeply at what might be meant by human flourishing in John's position, then at what virtues might be expected of a nurse to promote this, and at what might be said to be 'thinner' or 'thicker' descriptions of these (see Glossary). It is accepted that there may be competing 'thin' descriptions of the virtues required but the belief is that, via moral endeavour, a 'thick' description can be arrived at. This view contains a belief in ethical progress, envisaged as an ongoing quest. Nussbaum states:

> When we understand more precisely what problems human beings encounter in their lives with one another, what circumstances they face in which choice of some sort is required, we will have a way of assessing competing responses to those problems, and we will begin to understand what it might be to act well in the face of them. (Nussbaum 1993 p 248)

In examining account 1 and account 2, it is possible to see that in spite of their differences, they share considerable common ground. This is not surprising since they both arise within a western tradition of nursing. Account 1 has, however, a more libertarian flavour than account 2. What adherents of either account are likely to endorse is the idea that patient consent should be voluntary, i.e. uncoerced, and informed. They are also likely to agree that achieving this state of affairs in a hospital context is difficult. John is physically very ill and probably very exhausted. He is not in the best shape for making a decision about anything, let alone something as momentous as the surgery he is offered. He is dependent on care. Those looking after him are well and in positions of power over John in the hospital context. This raises questions about how voluntary John's consent or dissent can be in such circumstances. It also raises questions about how to help him with this decision, on the assumption that adherents to either account 1 or account 2 would agree that making a decision to have major surgery is not like choosing which cereal packet one prefers in a supermarket. If one accepts this, then saying to John: 'Here are the facts, the choice is yours' could be to abandon him, as Gadow (1980) has argued. On the other hand, engaging with him raises questions about how to do this in a way that will support his autonomy and will not subtly coerce him. This seems to be the nub of the disagreement between account 1 and account 2, the former seeing coercion where the latter does not.

At this point, a suggestion could be made to see which position the majority of nurses supported. This indeed would give normative weight to one position over the other, but such a stance would merely feed those who criticize virtue ethics as being traditionalist and inherently conservative: a point that Nussbaum (1992) levels against MacIntyre's position. There is also nothing more moral about a position the majority support as opposed to a position the minority support, simply because one wins on a calculation of numbers. Moral argument is needed to demonstrate the superiority of one account over the other, or to present a third account that might be a synthesis of the best in account 1 and account 2. However, in so far as account 1 presents a challenge to account 2 (the latter seeming to square roughly with the nurse's own evaluation of what she did), it could be argued that the onus is on account 1 to provide evidence for interpreting the situation in this way. What can count as moral evidence is not up to individuals to decide privately; it is a public matter and in any such discussions the rule of contradiction must also apply. Together, these would provide further common ground between account 1 and account 2. Both positions, for example, would accept that the nurse cannot be both coercive and not coercive in the same expression at the same time, and both positions would rule as irrelevant to this particular context as described, John's religious faith or the lack of it (although this could be highly relevant in some other contexts).

One sees that the virtuous nurse is asked to care for the patient physically and emotionally in such a way that where there is any doubt about what to do, the nurse errs on the side of life. The nurse must also strive to preserve the patient's dignity and compassionately seek to enable the patient to arrive at determining his or her own good, rather than imposing the nurse's view of this. In the scenario described, it would seem that the nurse felt that John's initial rejection of surgery was not a truly autonomous decision, in the sense that it seemed hasty and made without sufficient time for thought. On the other hand, it is also likely that the nurse did think that John should have the operation, so she cannot be said to be a neutral player in the story. Being a person who professes (professional) something tends to rule out neutrality. Did the nurse coerce John or sensitively allow him to explore what was at stake for him, so that he could make a decision that was not primarily a reaction to fear?

If one had before one all the arguments supporting both accounts, and one also knew about John's own views on the matter, it may be that a clear case would emerge for preferring one account over the other on moral grounds. However, provided no contradiction is involved, not everyone would be logically obliged to see it this way. Interpretations of events are not themselves factual truths, although they may be more or less accurate, more or less illuminating, and more or less helpful, according to the task in hand.

For Nussbaum, even if one accepts that to have a view at all is to interpret and that in morality therefore, there is no such thing as ethical truth independent of some interpretation or other, this does not mean that judgements cannot be made about different interpretations. She says:

> Certain ways in which people see the world can still be criticised exactly as Aristotle criticised them: as stupid, pernicious, and false. The standards used in such criticisms must come from inside human life. (Frequently they will come from the society in question itself, from its own rationalist and critical traditions.) And the inquirer must attempt, prior to criticism, to develop an inclusive understanding of the conceptual scheme being criticised, seeing what motivates each of its parts and how they hang together.
> (Nussbaum 1993 p 260–261)

Interpretations may be reliant on facts that can be shown to be false, thereby weakening or even falsifying the interpretation. For example, those who wanted to justify slavery could not continue to support this with an appeal to the inferiority of intelligence of black Africans, once this was shown to be a false claim. Similarly, it might be difficult for British people to sustain their cultural habit of smacking children (justified as a corrective that does no harm) if this can be shown adversely to affect children psychologically. In a Moslem culture it may be awkward to vindicate female circumcision, if this can be shown to cause physio-logical and emotional damage to women, since the Qur'an has no instruction to torture or damage women.

In the scenario described at the beginning of this chapter, it would be a fact in the case if John were to state that he did or did not feel coerced by the nurse and similarly, it would be a fact for the nurse to state whether or not, on reflection, she felt she had been coercive. It would be odd if these facts made no difference in evaluating the respective truth of account 1 and account 2. However, because of the way in which facts themselves are subject to evaluation, it is still possible for the same fact (e.g. John says he does not feel he was coerced) to be read differently. Some might believe him and take what he says to be true, others might think that John believes this and that is certainly a fact, but that neverthe-less he is deceived about himself. He is unconscious of the possibility that he has been coerced (using perhaps the analogy of how subliminal adver-tising works). However, there would come a point where to keep doubt-ing John's and his nurse's claim that the interaction between them had nothing to do with coercion, would become increasingly untenable in the face of their intersubjective agreement, without other supporting evi-dence. It might not be illogical to keep sustaining such a view, but it would be likely to appear obdurate and finally pointless.

One could also argue that there is something very healthy, albeit diffi-cult, about account 1 and account 2 adherents having to have a dialogue with each other. The critique supplied by account 1 of account 2 has to be taken seriously and in so doing it provokes deeper reflection. It is also possible that those initially endorsing account 2 come to see that the sit-uation is not quite so simple and that it is very difficult for nurses, no matter how hard they try, not to have some coercive impact on patients. This is because of the difference in power relations between nurse and patient and because, not surprisingly, nurses tend to believe in the value of what medicine offers. Nurses, however, may feel that in being con-scious of the impact of this, they are in a position to ameliorate its effect on patients and can genuinely work towards helping patients to discover what it is *they* want to do. In adopting this view, John's nurse would have conceded some ground to account 1, thereby modifying her original position (account 2).

From the above, one can see that while moral debate can sometimes reach an impasse and adherents to different views just have to agree to differ, the struggle to justify one's own view and to listen to different views with respect may be painfully enriching. It can lead to changes of position, the abandonment of positions, and sometimes a commonsense agreement as to the most probable interpretation to take, or the one that seems most generous or most hopeful, as perhaps in deciding to give people the benefit of the doubt, etc. This is a kind of moral pragmatism that provides sufficient moral certainty to permit action, without fixing the debate in terms of discovery of truth. In so far as this is a familiar sit-uation in health care, with irresolvable dilemmas being the exception rather than the norm, it may be the case that MacIntyre's pessimism needs to give ground to the more optimistic position expressed by

Nussbaum. Nussbaum's belief in a grounding of the virtues in what it is to be human is perhaps intuitively a better fit.

SUMMARY OF THE ARGUMENT

So far, I have been concerned with an exploration of whether or not the virtues can be said to offer an interesting and helpful way of understanding and resolving differences of view about the best course of action in health care. No claim is made that the virtue perspective is the only useful way of looking at such issues, but the question is, is this helpful and illuminating in a different and complementary way to other moral perspectives? The general case for this was presented in the previous chapter, but in this chapter, I have narrowed the focus to consider a particular healthcare scenario involving disagreement. In considering this case, it has been possible to describe and evaluate some of the criticisms used against the virtue position. These are:

1. That the idea of appealing to a paradigm individual is not very helpful because there is a question of who to appeal to, particularly where there may be different paradigms implicit in a conflict.
2. Some ways of thinking about the virtue perspective, particularly those articulated by MacIntyre (1975), invoke pessimism because of the relative nature of the virtues, conceived of as grounded in specific cultures. There may be universal virtues (such as justice, courage and truthfulness) but these too have different 'shades' of meaning in different cultures and any such commonality as exists would not be enough to ground any universal system of morality. In multi-cultural contexts, we are likely to find ourselves increasingly unable to resolve moral disagreements.
3. Locating the meaning of the virtues in cultures and 'practices' (see Glossary) can lead to a criticism that the virtue perspective is inherently conservative and traditionalist. This is a criticism that Nussbaum (1992) levels against MacIntyre, although he anticipates this objection and responds to it (MacIntyre 1984).
4. Nussbaum's (1992, 1993) version of virtue theory (and for her it is more a theory than not) relies on the Aristotelian idea of a *telos* for its sense. Nussbaum believes that the virtues can ultimately be grounded in universal understandings about humanity. This provides a theoretical underpinning for the intuition that both within and between cultures it is possible to arrive at a degree of shared understanding about 'thinner' or 'thicker' accounts of the virtues and about better or worse ways of seeing the world and understanding human beings within that world. This view is only as solid as its underpinning belief and is vulnerable to the counter assertion that there simply is no such universal *telos*.

Account 1 and account 2 can both be said to provide competing ideas of how the good nurse should respect patient autonomy. Could one of these accounts be considered 'thicker' than the other, or might a third account that combined the insights of both be preferable? What is clear is that the virtue perspective provides no 'off the peg' solution to this. Any ensuing moral agreement would be earned via painful moral debate of those involved. That a 'thicker' or 'richer' understanding could be arrived at and recognized as such by all involved would be evidence in support of Nussbaum's ideas. How far this could be said to operate between diverse cultures might be open to question. Some ideas do not translate between cultures. For example, I recently heard a European person remark that polygamy is 'having a bit on the side', but this is not the view of people living within a polygamous culture. It is a view of polygamy from the perspective of a monogamous culture; a view that seems to contain both censure and envy.

OTHER CRITICISMS OF VIRTUE THEORY AND THE VIRTUE PERSPECTIVE

In addition to the above criticisms of the virtue perspective, there are two others expressed by Louden (1993):

LOUDEN'S FIRST OBJECTION

Louden points out that because of its emphasis on moral agency rather than action, virtue theorists 'de-emphasize discrete acts in favour of long term, characteristic patterns of behaviour' (Louden 1993 p 194). He states:

> It has often been said that for virtue ethics the central question is not 'What ought I to do?' but rather 'What sort of person ought I to be?'. . . However, people have always expected ethical theory to tell them something about what they ought to do, and it seems to me that virtue ethics is structurally unable to say much of anything about this issue.

(Louden 1993 p 194)

He goes on:

> Virtue theory is not a problem oriented or quandary approach to ethics: it speaks of rules and principles of action only in a derivative manner. And its derivative oughts are frequently too vague and unhelpful for persons who have not yet acquired the requisite moral insight and sensitivity.

(Louden 1993 p 195)

This view has obvious implications for teaching nursing ethics since it suggests that the approach is not useful for the novice who has yet to develop the necessary insight. I will say more about this in the next chapter. Here, it is sufficient to point out that this conclusion is likely to be at odds with those virtue theorists such as MacIntyre (1975, 1984) and Nussbaum (1992, 1993) who, while not rejecting the value of other moral perspectives, give primacy of place to the virtues. In the previous chapter, GC Field (1966) was quoted as referring to how we 'naturally take pleasure in good acts' and how essential this is to learning morality, since rewards and punishments alone would never enable a person to grasp morality fully. Louden may be right that developmentally this affection for or 'love of the good' as Iris Murdoch (1985) would have called it, may take time to acquire, but nevertheless, it could be said to have an irreducible primacy of place in morality. Without it we may not recognize that we are in a moral situation. This capacity may also be something that cannot be adequately described within either a Kantian or utilitarian view of morality because for all their differences, they are both highly rational constructions of morality. The virtue perspective allows for the idea that reason has to work on something prior to itself. This could be called a receptivity, a sensitivity or an insight. The virtue perspective insists that this capacity is not simply a useful addition to moral thought but an intrinsic component of it.

LOUDEN'S SECOND OBJECTION

Louden (1993) proceeds with his critique. He suggests that there is a problem for virtue theorists in that '. . . we do not seem to be able to know with any degree of certainty who really is virtuous and who vicious' (Louden 1993 p 198). He explains that normally we try to infer character from observing behaviour, but that since virtue theorists are committed to the view that '. . . the moral value of Being is not reducible to or dependent on Doing', then '. . . the measure of an agent's character is not exhausted by or even dependent on the values of the actions which he may perform' (Louden 1993 p 198). Louden then creates a distinction between what he calls 'actional' virtues, which clearly relate to action and 'spiritual' virtues (such as self-respect and integrity) that '. . . do have a significant impact on what we do, but whose moral value is not wholly derivable from the actions to which they may give rise' (Louden 1993 p 198). He then wonders how we can recognize and evaluate these inner qualities if we cannot rely on external evidence. He is sceptical that we can and cites both Kant and Aquinas in support:

> . . . the real morality of actions, their merit or guilt, even that of our own conduct . . . remains entirely hidden from us. (Kant, cited by Louden 1993 p 199)

And:

> Man is not competent to judge of interior movements that are hidden, but only of exterior acts which are observable; and yet for the perfection of virtue it is necessary for man to conduct himself rightly in both kinds of acts. (Aquinas, cited by Louden 1993 p 199)

Contemporary understanding of the role of the unconscious in mental life would endorse this difficulty of reliably evaluating inner qualities and motives. John's nurse, for example, might simply be deceived about her moral motivation. She believes herself to be acting in John's best interests but perhaps she is really acting out of self-interest?

Louden (1993) concludes that as we cannot clearly differentiate the virtuous from the vicious, advocating an ethics of virtue lacks applicability. He concedes, however, that for Aristotle existing in a relatively small and homogeneous society, the story may well have been different. Must we share Louden's pessimism?

Louden is certainly right to draw attention to the difficulty of claiming to know another's state of mind and of claims to know one's own mind. The problem is that we are only too aware of how, on both accounts, we can discover that we were mistaken. Introspection is not a public procedure with agreed methods of verification, in contrast to the way uncertainty is dealt with in science, history or mathematics. Knowledge of other minds is inferred from speech, behaviour and the patterns that are established through knowing someone over time. In other words, there is evidence, but not of a systematic and easily traceable kind. There is therefore always the possibility that people who are thought to be virtuous, and even stand as paradigm examples, turn out not to be so in all aspects of their lives. Worse, we could be completely duped with a virtuous façade hiding something vicious, but the fact that this could be demonstrated, even posthumously, surely allows for some confidence in our capacity to distinguish virtues from vices. It could be argued that getting it wrong sometimes hinges on confidence in getting it right much of the time.

Louden's distinction between the 'actional' virtues and the 'spiritual' begins with him pointing out that there is no necessary connection for the virtue theorist between being a good woman or man and doing good deeds. This must be correct, for a kind person does not have to be kind on every occasion where kindness is possible, to be judged kind. However, it would be odd for a person judged to be kind never to manifest actions of kindness. Louden seems to assume that where there is no necessary or logical relationship between the ascription of a virtue and corresponding action, the link between the virtues and action must be a contingent or accidental one. Western philosophy drives this conclusion by the dichotomy it establishes between necessary and contingent relationships (see Glossary). A necessary relationship always operates; for example, the relationship between oxygen and water is a necessary connection (H_2O) because one can never have water without oxygen.

A contingent relationship sometimes operates and sometimes does not and even if the connection has always been observed, it is possible to imagine it not happening one day. The link between cooking food and eating must be a contingent one because cooked food is not always eaten (it may be thrown away, used merely for demonstration purposes or offered to deities). Nevertheless, it would seem to be part of the meaning of cooking food that ordinarily this is for someone to eat. This connection would appear to be more than a mere accident. Similarly, one might conclude that the relationship between the virtues and corresponding action is not strong enough to be described as a necessary connection but again the connection seems deeper than mere accidental association would allow for.

To state this and to accept the argument that there is not a necessary connection between them, one has to postulate a category in between 'necessary' and 'contingent'. This category has been called an 'intimate' or non-contingent connection. It indicates a stronger relationship than one of mere contingency, without the commitment to the logic of a necessary connection. If one accepts this (and this is open to philosophical debate) it can allow for quite a robust relationship between the virtues and corresponding action. This could weaken Louden's critique. Even the position of what he calls 'spiritual' virtues could be said to have an intimate connection to behaviour, once one has elaborated what must count for someone to be ascribed 'dignity' or 'self-respect'.

CONCLUSION

In this chapter I have presented several arguments criticising virtue ethics either as a theory or as a position. There are other criticisms and readers may be interested in a book such as that edited by Joram Graf Haber (1993). It contains abbreviated articles both for and against virtue ethics. In the analysis I have attempted both to describe the critique as clearly as possible and then to evaluate it, or at least indicate how it could be evaluated. Readers must obviously come to their own conclusion. It may be that neither MacIntyre's pessimism nor Nussbaum's optimism are very satisfactory in isolation from each other. MacIntyre seems to rule out creative moral debate between cultures, leading to increased understanding and fruitful moral change within a culture. Intuitively this seems mistaken. However, it may be the case that because we are culturally embedded creatures with no 'God's eye' view of other cultures, any such change is lived rather than being describable or prescribable in a theory or formula. For this reason, Nussbaum's idea of a universal theory of the virtues where there could be thick and thin descriptions of them agreed across cultures is not very promising. The problem is that the ascriptions of 'thick' and 'thin' pertain to a culture. Without having God's eye, how could this be evaluated neutrally between cultures? It would seem to presuppose some universal criteria of assessment. These conclusions re-enforce the view that ultimately virtue ethics is not a theory but an a-theoretical position. This would not, however, rule out the existence of theories of the virtues within specific cultures, where meaning can be given to the ascriptions 'thick' and 'thin'. This looked promising in the discussion about John's nurse. Such a conclusion would support those who argue that virtue ethics is inherently conservative because it tends to be locked in a particular cultural tradition.

The first objection raised by Louden – that the virtue perspective is not an approach that is helpful to novices because they may lack the required moral insight and sensitivity – could be correct. If he is right, this would mean that the virtue perspective is inadequate as the sole account of morality. It would not however, diminish the force of the virtue perspective as providing a useful and even unique commentary on the nature of morality. What might ensue is some careful thought about what moral education would require from a virtue perspective and I will develop this in the next chapter.

Louden's second objection is that, within the virtue tradition, it is impossible to distinguish virtues from vices with any degree of conviction.

This can be argued against by the introduction of a third category other than 'necessary' and 'contingent'. This is the category of an 'intimate' connection. The refutation of Louden's position is only as good as the strength of this argument.

References

Field GC 1966 Moral theory. Methuen, London.

Gadow S 1980 Existential advocacy: philosophical foundation of nursing. In: Spicker S, Gadow S (eds) Nursing images and ideals. Springer, New York, p 79–101.

Haber JG (ed) 1993 Doing and being: selected readings in moral philosophy. Macmillan, New York.

Louden R 1993 On some views of virtue ethics. In: Haber JG (ed) Doing and being: selected readings in moral philosophy. Macmillan, New York, p 191–204.

MacIntyre A 1975 How virtues become vices: values, medicine and social context. In: Engelhardt HT, Spicker SF (eds) Evaluation and exploration in the biomedical sciences. D Reidel, Dordrecht, p 97–111.

MacIntyre A 1984 After virtue: study in moral theory, 2nd edn. Duckworth, London.

Murdoch I 1985 The sovereignty of good. Ark Paperbacks, London.

Nichols KA 1993 Psychological care in physical illness, 2nd edn. Chapman and Hall, London.

Nussbaum M 1992 Virtue revived. Times Literary Supplement 3 July:9–11.

Nussbaum M 1993 Non-relative virtues: an Aristotelian approach. In: Nussbaum M, Sen A (eds) The quality of life. Clarendon Press, Oxford, p 242–276.

Royal College of Nursing (RCN) 1992 The value of nursing. RCN, London.

Chapter **12**

Teaching virtue ethics

Louise de Raeve

A nurse who subsequently became a psychotherapist writes:

> I stood at the end of the bed of someone with tubes coming out of every orifice. He was gripping so tightly to the bedframe that his knuckles were white. I felt giddy and faint. In my imagination the man was being tortured, a thought so terrible I could not even voice it to my friend, who was asking sensible questions about the temperature chart. Later as I sat recovering in the cool corridor, I felt foolish . . . (Anna Dartington 1994 p 103, writing of her first visit to a surgical ward as a student nurse)

> . . . They talked, not surprisingly, about the number of deaths on the ward, the liver transplant patients whom they lost after days or weeks of painstaking intensive care, the distress of the relatives, their own exhaustion. The most difficult thing to talk about was the resentment and even hatred they sometimes felt towards the patients who seemed to thwart their every effort and care. These were the alcohol- and drug-dependent patients who returned again and again to be repaired, with the single intention, or so it seemed to these nurses, to continue to connive at their own death. (Dartington 1994 p 106–107)

INTRODUCTION

Nursing is a stressful occupation. The rewards may be many and gratifying, as in the complete recovery of a sick child surrounded by a grateful family, but equally, as these quotations reveal, nursing exposes its practitioners to a gamut of emotions including shock, horror, resentment and sometimes hatred. The emotional reality of this world of the nurse can be grasped or ignored in the teaching of ethics, but to ignore it may result in a practitioner with a good intellectual grasp of the subject being unable to let this understanding really influence their practice. This may then intensify feelings of guilt and increase what has been termed 'moral distress' (Jameton 1984). As Gavin Fairbairn and Donna Mead (1990) put it:

> . . . we have begun to think in terms of moral grief when we meet and work with those whose lives bear the marks of moral dilemmas. (Fairbairn & Mead 1990 p 22)

They add:

> When nurses experience moral dilemmas they lose the self that they thought of as caring, the self who does the right thing for patients, the self who will not do wrong to others, their whole self. They lose their integrity. (Fairbairn & Mead 1990 p 23)

They continue:

> We guess that many nurses never reach the final stage of the grieving process – acceptance. It is our contention that nurses need to be helped to achieve acceptance. (Fairbairn & Mead 1990 p 23)

Thus one sees that the approach adopted to teach ethics must be itself both a moral and philosophical matter.

For the virtue ethicist, the focus will be on how to teach or inculcate the virtues required of a good nurse. This presumes that we know and agree on what those virtues are and can give 'thick' as opposed to 'thin' accounts of them (see Glossary, p 362). In fact, as pointed out in the previous chapter, this work, while more advanced in medicine, has barely begun in nursing. This chapter, however, will proceed on the assumption that while there may be plenty of room for disagreement about who is a virtuous nurse and what virtues such a person must demonstrate and in what way, it is much easier to agree on who is a failing nurse or a person found wanting in important respects. This allows for a starting point, and what follows in this chapter will focus more on the structure or process of teaching virtue ethics than on the content. This is because if one is to be consistent within the virtue theory approach, the educator will inevitably be looked to as a moral exemplar, with respective failings and strengths noted. Virtuous behaviour and sensitivity cannot be learned by didactic methods: a point that will be elaborated in the rest of this chapter. If they can be taught at all, it will be through student-focused and participative forms of experiential learning. The injunction 'Be quiet!' is clear enough, but the instruction 'Be kind!' has no such clarity. One must first understand the complexity of being kind and unkind in different contexts and then grasp what is salient about the specific context referred to, to have any idea of what 'being kind' might mean in that context. Different interpretations may lead to disagreement with others.

CAN GOODNESS BE TAUGHT?

On the assumption that we can specify to some extent what this goodness is, this question remains an extremely challenging one. If answered in the negative there would be no teaching of the virtues, although it might still be worth teaching moral principles and duties and operating sanctions of reward and punishment to try to compel compliance. However, as was pointed out in Chapter 10, an understanding of morality based on obedience and compliance alone could be said to be so lacking that it does not count as a proper grasp of morality at all.

If the question is answered in the affirmative, it seems in danger of being a highly omnipotent claim and if it were true, one assumes that the government would have purchased the expertise long ago to reduce the prison population and to treat people with a psychopathic personality.

Another answer to the question seems to be the position of 'cautious affirmative' that most people adopt on this matter. This view holds that it is possible to improve or enhance someone's natural affinity towards goodness. Is there such an affinity? According to GC Field (1966), and quoted in the first chapter on the virtues (Chapter 10), an Aristotelian conception of moral education is based on the idea that '. . . there is really there from the beginning some sort of underlying impulse towards the good, because in some sense we "naturally" take pleasure in good acts (for that is almost the definition of good acts)' (Field 1966 p 80–81).

This is a belief, but moral psychology may be able to provide some evidence for or against it. Accepting this belief would still raise the question of whether or not this 'impulse towards the good' is innate, and even if it is, whether or not certain unfavourable life experiences can deaden it forever. Christian theology's insistence on the possibility of redemption for all would be one answer. What is likely, however, is that although moral psychology could be used to provide evidence to support or contradict various positions concerning how best to teach morality, as a form of human inquiry, it too will be underpinned by general moral beliefs about human beings and their relationship to good and evil.

HOW MIGHT GOODNESS BE TAUGHT?

In the preceding two chapters different ideas have arisen about this question. Richard Louden (1993) was quoted in the critique chapter (Chapter 11) as saying that because 'virtue theory is not a problem oriented or quandary approach . . . its derivative oughts are frequently too vague and unhelpful for persons who have not yet acquired the requisite moral insight and sensitivity' (Louden 1993 p 195). The implications for nursing would seem to be that student nurses are too much moral novices in the context of nursing to be expected to use independent judgement and initially need to be guided by clear rules and principles of conduct. This idea reflects a parental model of moral education and would also accord with Patricia Benner's (1984) ideas of the level of functioning of novice practitioners. This view is a potential problem for the virtue theorist, if it is maintained that the virtues are the only coherent perspective that explains morality. It is unproblematic for a view that accords equal or even key importance to the virtues, while allowing for the relevance of other moral perspectives.

Teachers of moral theory who endorse a virtue perspective have often argued that while knowledge of moral principles, duties and rules may be imperative, no rule or principle in and of itself can dictate when it is supposed to be applied or what weighting to give to each if several are relevant. For these tasks, both an appreciation of the uniqueness of the context and a grasp of its general features (if any) are required. The capacities that help to ensure this are moral sensitivity and acuity of moral vision. This argument supports the claim made by Richard White (1991) in Chapter 10 that the virtues are a 'basic category of morality' and that they have an irreducible primacy of place. In the context of moral sensitivity and acuity of perception, one might be referring to the virtue of compassion, among others.

MORAL SENSITIVITY AND ACUITY OF MORAL PERCEPTION

Lawrence Blum (1991) gives the following illustration:

> John and Joan are sitting riding on a subway train. There are no empty seats and some people are standing; yet the subway car is not packed so tightly as to be uncomfortable for everyone. One of the passengers is a woman in her thirties holding two relatively full shopping bags. John is not particularly paying attention to the woman but he is cognizant of her. Joan, by contrast, is distinctly aware that the woman is uncomfortable. Thus different aspects of the situation are 'salient' for John and Joan. That is, what is fully and explicitly present to John's consciousness about the woman is that she is standing holding some bags; but what is in that sense salient for Joan is the woman's discomfort. That an aspect of a situation is not salient for an agent does not mean she is entirely unaware of it. She could be aware of it in a less than fully explicit way. (Blum 1991 p 702)

He goes on to say:

> In this situation, the difference between what is salient for John and Joan is of moral significance. Joan saliently perceives . . . the woman's good (i.e. her comfort) as at stake in a way that John does not. Joan perceives a morally relevant value at stake, while John does not. (Blum 1991 p 703)

Blum observes that it is perfectly possible to imagine Joan pointing out to John the woman's discomfort or simply asking if he shares her perception, for John to come to see what Joan sees. However, in so far as this initial 'not seeing' may be a characteristic of John and repeated on many occasions, it is possible to describe this as a 'defect of character'; 'He misses something of the moral reality confronting him' (Blum 1991 p 704).

Extrapolating simplistically from this example to the world of nursing, it is possible to say that we want more Joan-types than John-types, since we need nurses who are quickly sensitive to the moral reality (which will include much suffering) of patients. This is an issue for recruitment but in so far as this chapter is about education, how might we teach John-types to have a greater moral sensitivity and how might we help Joan-types preserve theirs? The two illustrations given at the beginning of this chapter are instructive. In the first illustration one could say that there is nothing lacking in this student's sensitivity to the patient's predicament. What she needs is help to bear it so that she can think about it to inform her care, rather than be overwhelmed. In relation to the liver unit example, one might say that here perhaps Joan-type nurses have reverted to John-type behaviour because the strength of their feelings is interfering with their capacity to perceive the full complexity of the moral reality surrounding them. This could include coming to understand that many of these patients are both physically and mentally ill or disturbed. In their addictive behaviours of alcohol abuse, etc. may lie histories of great emotional deprivation, combined with an implicit if not explicit ambivalence towards respecting and preserving their own lives. Intense self-hatred may be part of their inner worlds, thereby providing a context in which body repair might be viewed with considerable ambivalence.

The nurses in the account are in touch with feelings of hatred. Perhaps this emanates from the frustration of the nurses' own need to be useful and helpful, combined with the nurses becoming unconscious recipients of the patients' unconscious hatred of those who try to help them. This is a complicated idea and for those who might like to read further, suggested texts are Keith Nichols (1993), Isabel Menzies Lyth (1988) and Anton Obholzer & Vega Zagier Roberts (1994).

ENHANCING MORAL SENSITIVITY AND ACUITY OF MORAL PERCEPTION IN NURSES

This section begins with a disclaimer! There is a proverb in English that you can take a horse to water but you cannot make it drink. To turn again to the example of John and Joan, John might be perennially unable to see what Joan sees, unless she is there to point it out to him and, even then, there may be some 'John's' in the world who cannot really see it when shown. These would represent two differing types of moral blindness. It is possible that both might be open to change through some form of psychological therapy but they are likely to be very resistant to ordinary educative processes. It seems important therefore not to assume too much about how effective any of the following strategies are likely to be. Proceeding cautiously, what might such strategies involve?

LEARNING BY EXAMPLE

The word 'strategies' is to some extent ill-suited for the task. This is because what follows is less about techniques in education and more about a way of thinking and being in education. If I think back to my own entry into nursing, I recall the senior staff nurse on my first ward. She was competent and capable, able to contain rather than spread anxiety in difficult situations and treated staff and patients alike in a kindly, humorous way. She clearly loved her job and was good at it. Students assigned to her tutelage considered themselves lucky. We instinctively knew her worth and tried to learn from her, not just by absorbing her instructions, but by trying to model ourselves on her. Such modelling can be simply at the level of copying, but to be of much use in the future, it has to be internalized and become part of oneself. This process requires unconscious positive identification and this cannot happen if there is not a genuine relationship of mutual respect between the persons concerned.

The two previous chapters refer to paradigm examples. Here, there may be no grounds for viewing an ordinarily excellent nurse as a paradigm example. However, following and identifying with people who set an example simply through being good and kind in what they do is an important way of learning what it is to be a virtuous nurse. Unfortunately, however, one might have to reckon with the possibility that if my staff nurse had been brusque and unkind, some students might have internalized this as the model of nursing and come to behave similarly. There is a great degree of moral responsibility therefore for those who manage and teach in what Paul Halmos (1969) has called the 'human service professions', to 'practise what they preach'. Otherwise there is a danger that the implicit rather than the explicit model of nursing on offer will be the one internalized by novices.

STUDYING THE HUMANITIES

A relatively recent development in the UK (which follows a longer history in the US) is the introduction of the humanities into medical and nursing curricula. The aim is to use the humanities' potential to have a humanizing effect on students, but what the rationale and the limitations of this idea might be require further elucidation. Beginning with the limitations first, Robin Downie (2001) writes:

> . . . enthusiasts for the medical humanities often say that the aim is to produce doctors who are more compassionate or who have empathy. But it is not clear that such aims can be achieved through the study of the humanities and certainly they cannot be evaluated. To be versed in the humanities is not the same as being humane, a point often illustrated by referring to Nazi officers.
>
> (Downie 2001 p 205)

He continues:

> I shall therefore suggest more concrete and realistic aims which those in the humanities might be in a position to help students and doctors achieve. In general terms, the hope would be to introduce students and doctors to a range of concepts and methods, other than narrowly scientific ones, which can assist with the understanding of human beings and their interactions and with doctor–patient communication.
>
> (Downie 2001 p 205)

Downie makes it clear that he is using this term 'humanities' inter-changeably with the 'arts' and that he has in mind such subjects as: 'archaeology, drama, the fine arts, history, languages, literature, medical history, music, philosophy, theology and so on' (Downie 2001 p 204). Downie then proceeds to specify in what ways studying the medical humanities may be helpful and he lists among these the development of moral sensitivity. He states:

> The teaching of medical ethics has tended to fall into the hands of philosophers. But philosophers are interested in general principles and theories which have limited appeal to medical students because of their abstract nature. On the other hand, literature or film can make a much more powerful impact on moral awareness because of its immediacy. Like medicine itself literature deals with the detail of cases. Indeed, there is a danger that philosophy actually blunts moral awareness because students become caught up with terms such as 'deontology' or 'patient autonomy' or with the technicalities of moral argument which blind them to the reality of the situations they will be dealing with.

> (Downie 2001 p 207)

This resonates with the point made in Chapter 10 that if the virtue per-spective is tied to an idea of reverence for and development of capacities to see the 'irreducibly particular' aspect of situations, people and things, it resists generality by definition and must in this respect be a-theoretical, as White (1991) suggested. Ann Gallagher develops some of these points in Chapter 20.

THINKING BEFORE ACTING: ENHANCING REFLECTION THROUGH CLINICAL SUPERVISION

Developing one's moral sensitivity is likely to be something of a dou-ble-edged sword, particularly in the world of suffering patients and inadequately resourced healthcare services. Students sometimes com-plain that increasing moral awareness does not make their lives easier and, from this perspective, moral blindness or insensitivity could seem quite an attractive state if the alternative is to feel overwhelmed by human pain. However, in the human services professions one could argue that this state of mind in the provider is potentially damaging and even dangerous to the recipient. John-types may do well working in a laboratory or as sales personnel but they are not an asset in areas of health care where contact with patients is required. Their failure to see much of what is going on around them means that they have very limited reasons for action when compared with Joan-types. Concerning the subway illustration described earlier, Blum comments:

> John's perception provides him with no reason to offer to help the woman. Whereas, in involving the woman's good, Joan's perception of the situation already provides her with a reason for action not based in her self-interest or projects. (Blum 1991 p 703)

Nothing requires that Joan must act. She might be carrying too many heavy bags of her own to help, but she has at least to think and justify to herself one course of action or inaction as opposed to another.

In Dartington's (1994) description of her reactions as a new student, one sees that the capacity to think and act meaningfully has been temporarily lost because the emotional impact of what was seen and imagined overwhelmed her. Without some way of being helped to bear and think about such an experience, there is a risk that such a nurse may lose her sensitivity and become more John-like as time goes on. What might enhance the capacity to think and act thoughtfully (rather than impulsively) in a way that preserves rather than blunts moral sensitivity? It must be something that allows for a connection to be made between thoughts and feelings. One, and only one, way of trying to do this is by instituting clinical supervision.

Clinical supervision in nursing has been much misunderstood and the term itself invites suspicion by the word 'clinical', which might suggest something cold, rational and technical and by the idea of 'supervision', which can invite notions of criticism, judgement, and a management-led, fault-finding enterprise. If it is not carefully established, it could amount to any or all of these things, but for those who believe in its utility, it has a very different purpose.

Supervision is a working alliance between a supervisor and a worker or workers in which the worker can reflect on [him- or] herself in her working situation by giving an account of his or her work and receiving feedback and where appropriate guidance and appraisal. The object of this alliance is to maximize the competence of the worker in providing a helping service. (Proctor 1988, cited by Joyce Scaife 2001 p 2)

A definition with a slightly different emphasis follows:

> *Clinical supervision is a regular, protected time for facilitated, in-depth reflection on clinical practice. It aims to enable the supervisee to achieve, sustain and creatively develop a high quality of practice through means of focused support and development.* (Bond & Holland 1998, cited by Rolfe et al 2001 p 79)

These are two of many definitions of clinical supervision, none of which seems universally satisfactory although all capture important aspects of supervision. What is important is that the 'feedback' is not delivered in an instructive and didactic mode, as if the supervisor had all the answers. Rather, when the supervisee and supervisor jointly search for deeper meaning and fuller understanding, then the supervisee's difficulties and successes can be mutually explored in his or her work. This process can be conducted one-to-one or in small groups. For it to work, it requires the protected and regular allocation of time and place and the committed attendance of supervisor and supervisee(s). A climate of trust has to be created and this cannot happen without confidentiality and, when absolute confidentiality cannot be promised, joint acceptance of when and why this is the case. How successful the enterprise is at discovering deeper meaning and fuller understanding will depend on the ability of the supervisor, the willingness of the supervisee to risk disclosure, and the nature of support for the process that the employing institution of either party is willing to offer (unless it is a completely private contract).

Just as there are many definitions of supervision, there are also many ways of structuring it and thinking about the process and content. This is influenced by the differing affinities of supervisors to different psychological theories explaining human emotion and human interaction. The resulting proliferation of models and frameworks seems reminiscent of the early days of nursing theory. One needs to search for what is most useful to one's purpose and not be overwhelmed. Francesca Inskipp and Brigid Proctor (1993, 1995) developed the Supervision Alliance Model that identifies three responsibilities for the supervisor and the supervisee. These are:

- Formative (the tasks of learning and facilitating learning)
- Normative (the tasks of monitoring, and self-monitoring, standards and ethics)
- Restorative (the tasks of refreshment)

Beginning with the last, the *restorative* responsibility is an attempt to offer nurses a place where distress, emotional exhaustion, fury, etc. can be listened to, accepted and understood before reflection on how these feelings might be managed in a way that enhances, rather than impedes the care of patients. Although the immediate focus is the welfare of the nurse, the ultimate justification for such attention is that it will benefit patients. This link seems as impossible to prove as the link between enhanced moral sensitivity and increased compassion in care that Downie referred to in the section on the humanities. Research has demonstrated that clinical supervision can be said to benefit nurses (Berggren & Severinsson 2000, Bowles & Young 1999), although this view is not without its critics (Yegdich 1998). Efforts have also been made to find a connection between clinical supervision for staff and improved patient care, for example Kristiina Hyrkäs and Marita Paunonen-Ilmonen (2001). Such research demonstrates positive trends but, so far, falls short of being conclusive. In spite of this there are experiential and theoretical grounds for believing that patient care must benefit from nurses receiving good clinical supervision. This point will be developed in the remainder of this chapter.

The *normative* dimension of supervision makes it perfectly plain that there is an important aspect of supervision in nursing that has to be concerned with limits, standards, rules, laws and principles. The codes of conduct reflect moral and legal values and principles of the cultures in which they have been developed. Not everything a nurse does is acceptable, no matter how well intentioned, and it is not unknown for some nurses to be deliberately cruel. This can be explored in supervision but not ultimately condoned or colluded with.

It is in the *formative* dimension, however, or perhaps more correctly, the *formative* in conjunction with the *restorative*, that one can most fully appreciate the connection between supervision and the virtues. The context of Dartington's (1994) description of the nurses on the liver unit, quoted at the beginning of this chapter, needs elucidation. These nurses were offered a chance to sit in a group and talk with a trainee psychotherapist functioning as the supervisor. Only five out of a possible 12 nurses elected to attend but for those who did: 'Acknowledging and understanding their hatred of their patients for (as it seemed to them) refusing to get better could help them not to retaliate by ignoring the patients' distress' (Dartington 1994 p 107).

Julia Fabricius (1991) gives an account of a small group of six student nurses that she facilitated. It met regularly, for an hour at a time. The aim was to offer these students a supportive and emotionally containing structure, by providing a space and place for them to talk about their experience of their work in a free, non-prescriptive and unstructured way. It is a model of clinical supervision in progress, although Fabricius does not use this description herself. This is a section from the account she provides. It may be helpful to know that these students were people in their late teens.

> *. . . Without more ado, Bridget said that yesterday they had had three deaths. One of the deaths, of a patient called Edith, was expected, she thought . . . One patient, Mrs. Brown, Bridget went on, was very ill but was not expected to die. Bridget had come on duty and seen the curtains round Edith and thought she had probably died, but then she was told that Mrs Brown had died at 6 that morning. The staff-nurse, Susan, was terribly upset because the doctor had blamed her for bad care. Then the third patient, a lady who was unconscious after a stroke, died. It was Bridget herself who suddenly saw she was not breathing, and she felt terribly guilty that the patient had died alone like that, and no-one had even noticed at first. Bridget helped to lay this patient out, her first time. She really wished she had not – it was awful putting the sheet over her face and moving her onto the trolley like a lump of meat. The curtains were pulled round all the beds while each of the bodies was removed. And no-one told the other patients what was happening – although they must have known. For the rest of the morning, Bridget said, she neglected her other patients and she felt particularly bad about one who needed 2-hourly toileting. She was too occupied with trying to keep a brave face.*

> *After almost no pause, Christine said: 'We had three deaths running too.' At this point I felt 'Oh, no, not another three.' There seemed to be more than enough distress already for 1 group in 1 hour and I felt that more would be really intolerable. Also I noted that Christine had said this in a slightly throw-away manner, as if to say, 'Three deaths are nothing – one can cope with these things.' So I commented that maybe they were all trying to keep a brave face here, and that it must feel like the only possible course in order not to be overwhelmed. This led to some discussion about Bridget's experience, how one might manage things better with the other patients, and so on . . .*

> *In the discussion that centred on Bridget's experience, I was strongly aware of my memory of Bridget having told the group previously of her*

father's death from a heart attack about a year before, although no-one mentioned this. I commented that people must be remembering her telling us about this and wondering what to say. Fiona, who was always quiet, took this up, saying how awkward one felt not knowing whether to mention such things; and Bridget told us that it had made her think about her father and she had telephoned her mother to find out if he had been wrapped up like that. Her mother had said not. We were able to relate their difficulty in mentioning Bridget's father to the difficulty of talking to the other patients about the patients who had died, and to see how for Bridget it was actually a relief that it was mentioned . . . (Fabricius 1991 p 103–104)

This passage can be interpreted in different ways. It may, however, be useful to state that the underlying theoretical position of the facilitator is a psychodynamic one. This means that the focus is on the emotions with the aim of trying to make explicit some of the semi-conscious or unconscious aspects of what is being discussed in the group. It is not group therapy; the focus is on the work, but some unconscious dynamics may be interpreted by the facilitator, if judged relevant to the group's purpose. In this account the facilitator makes use of the feelings engendered in her and reflects these back to the group for consideration. The skill lies in being able to do this in a way that facilitates thought rather than defensive retreat. Only those participating in the experience could ultimately say whether or not they found it helpful. However, one can see that what was hitherto enacted (neglecting other patients) or reflected on in isolation (the link between dead patients and a dead father) has now been given words and is being mentally digested through a shared experience. This offers containment as an alternative to enactment. One can also see how the formative function (better responses to the needs of the other patients) of supervision does not emerge as a prescription but as a consequence of the prior acknowledgement of distress. It could therefore be said that the formative function is dependent on sufficient restorative work having preceded it. This provides one illustration and explanation of the point made at the beginning of this chapter, that teaching the virtues cannot be done meaningfully in a didactic way. It also links directly with the quotations by Fairbairn and Mead (1990) about the necessity for helping nurses to grieve.

CONCLUSION

In this chapter I proposed that maintaining and enhancing moral sensitivity and acuity of moral perception are key aims in teaching the virtues. I suggested that three different approaches may facilitate this development. These are:

- Learning by example, a perspective that has links with the idea of apprenticeship
- Studying the humanities
- Enhancing reflection via clinical supervision

There is no suggestion that any of these approaches should be mutually exclusive and indeed it is likely that a combination of all of them might be expected to yield the best outcome. This is speculative and research might be helpful to see whether there is any justification for confidence in this claim. Research is unlikely to be conclusive in this field but it might indicate trends. However, it would have to presume operational agreement on the meaning of concepts such as 'moral sensitivity' and 'acuity of moral perception'. These are moral concepts whose meaning is as open to debate as any other concept in our moral language. Fixing the meaning may both facilitate research but also bias the result: an interesting problem where research concerns values rather than facts.

References

Benner P 1984 From novice to expert: excellence and power in clinical nursing practice. Addison-Wesley, Menlo Park, CA.

Berggren I, Severinsson E 2000 The influence of clinical supervision on nurses' moral decision making. Nursing Ethics 7:124–133.

Blum L 1991 Moral perception and particularity. Ethics 101 (July):701–725.

Bowles N, Young C 1999 An evaluative study of clinical supervision based on Proctor's three function interactive model. Journal of Advanced Nursing 30:958–964.

Dartington A 1994 Where angels fear to tread. In: Obholzer A, Roberts VZ (eds) The unconscious at work. Routledge, London, p 101–109.

Downie R 2001 Medical humanities: means, ends, and evaluation. In: Evans M, Finlay I (eds) Medical humanities. BMJ Books, London, p 204–216.

Fabricius J 1991 Running on the spot or can nursing really change? Psychoanalytic Psychotherapy 5(2):97–108.

Fairbairn GC Mead D 1990 Ethics and the loss of innocence. Paediatric Nursing 2(5):22–23.

Field GC 1966 Moral theory. Methuen, London.

Halmos P 1969 The problem of sincerity in the personal service professions. In: Freeman H (ed) Progress in mental health: proceedings of the seventh international congress on mental health. JA Churchill, London, p 309–317.

Hyrkäs K, Paunonen-Ilmonen M 2001 The effects of clinical supervision on the quality of care:

examining the results of team supervision. Journal of Advanced Nursing 33:492–502.

Inskipp F, Proctor B 1993 The art, craft and tasks of counselling supervision. Part 1, making the most of supervision. Cascade Publications, Twickenham, UK.

Inskipp F, Proctor B 1995 The art, craft and tasks of counselling supervision. Part 2, becoming a supervisor. Cascade Publications, Twickenham, UK.

Jameton A 1984 Nursing practice; the ethical issues. Prentice-Hall, Englewood Cliffs, NJ.

Louden R 1993 On some vices of virtue ethics. In: Haber J (ed) Doing and being: selected readings in moral philosophy. Macmillan, New York.

Menzies Lyth I 1988 Containing anxiety in institutions: selected essays, volume 1. Free Association Books, London, p 43–114.

Nichols K 1993 Psychological care in physical illness, 2nd edn. Chapman and Hall, London.

Obholzer A, Roberts VZ (eds) 1994 The unconscious at work. Routledge, London.

Rolfe G, Freshwater D, Jasper M 2001 Critical reflection for nursing and the helping professions: a user's guide. Palgrave, Basingstoke, UK.

Scaife J 2001 Supervision in the mental health professions: a practitioner's guide. Brunner-Routledge, Hove, UK.

White R 1991 Historical perspectives on the morality of virtue. The Journal of Value Inquiry 25:217–231.

Yegdich T 1998 How not to do clinical supervision in nursing. Journal of Advanced Nursing 28:193–202.

Chapter **13**

The care perspective in healthcare ethics

Chris Gastmans

INTRODUCTION

Care ethics evolved out of the Kohlberg–Gilligan debate on moral psychology and from the work done by social scientists such as Joan Tronto in the USA and Selma Sevenhuijsen in the Netherlands (Gilligan 1982, Sevenhuijsen 1998, Tronto 1993). For philosophical–ethical research regarding care and its application in health care, the works of Warren Reich and Margaret Little in the USA, Stan van Hooft in Australia, Henk Manschot, Marian Verkerk and Guy Widdershoven in the Netherlands, are seminal (Little 1998, Manschot & Verkerk 1994, Reich 1995, van Hooft 1995, Verkerk 2001, Widdershoven 2000). The care perspective in health care has until now been primarily applied within nursing (Gastmans et al 1998, van Hooft 1999; see also Chapter 15), in the care of elderly people (Widdershoven 1999), mental health (Verkerk 1999), in prenatal diagnosis and abortion (Gatens-Robinson 1992, Loots 2002) and in the care of persons with disabilities (Lindemann 2003, Parks 2003).

Care ethics is criticized in the literature as hopelessly vague and ambiguous (see Chapter 14). There is confusion about what care is and what contributions a care ethics has to make to the field of moral theory in general and healthcare ethics in particular. Therefore I shall begin by analysing the concept of care. Next, the contribution of the care approach to the process of ethical decision making in health care will be illustrated by analysing a case study. Finally, some guidance for further developing the care approach in healthcare ethics will be formulated.

CARE AS HUMAN PRACTICE

One of the main criticisms of the care approach is that the meaning of care has not been made clear (see Chapter 14). Before coming to a more precise conceptualization of care, therefore, I start this part of the chapter with an exploration of some characteristics of the phenomenon of care, considered as a human practice.

DIMENSIONS OF CARE

According to Tronto (1993), the concept of care can be described as a fundamental way of life that expresses itself in specific actions and attitudes that focus on maintaining, continuing and repairing our world, so that we can live in it as well as possible. That world includes our bodies, our selves and our environment (fellow human beings, animals, nature, etc.), which we try to interweave in a life-sustaining web. Tronto only speaks about care when there is talk of a motivation to care and when it is accompanied by an activity. The presence of this latter is especially important. Most authors who developed a conception of care before Tronto defined care mainly as an emotional state of mind that was necessary in order to care (Noddings 1984). The conception of care as an emotion rightly gets the reproach of being too utopian. It is not possible for nurses to develop personal relationships with all patients, for any number of reasons. Tronto points out that placing the accent on emotion also brings with it the fact that care is easily privatized and sensibilized, something she wants to avoid.

Care is a complex concept; therefore many care ethicists formulate the characteristics of care that describe the phenomenon of care, rather than give one central definition of care. Tronto (1993) distinguishes four dimensions of care:

The first is 'caring about': worrying about someone or something, being troubled, paying attention to. Concern about the state in which a fellow human being finds himself or herself is the point of departure of care. The corresponding ethical attitude is 'attentiveness'. Attentive nurses take up a receptive position with respect to the patient; they are challenged to step out of their own personal reference system in order to take up that of the patient, so that they can better understand the patient's real-life situation (Gastmans et al 1998). Without an attitude of attentiveness the request for care is not noticed.

The second dimension of care is 'taking care of': looking after, providing care. This may not mean actually carrying out any tasks of caring. One only takes responsibility for improving the condition of the other person. 'Responsibility' is thus the corresponding ethical attitude.

The third dimension of care concerns the actual 'caregiving'. This dimension of care requires the necessary 'competence'. Attentiveness to the needs of another and taking responsibility for those needs, but not succeeding in an effective and adequate way to meet those needs, means that the goal of care has not been reached.

Finally, there is the dimension of 'care receiving'. The focus here is on the person receiving care and not on that of the caregiver. Good care demands feedback and the verification that the caring needs are actually being met. So that care can be received, the receiver has to show an attitude of 'responsiveness' towards the caregiver. Simply saying 'thank you' could express this attitude of responsiveness. It also suggests the need to keep a balance between the needs of the caregiver and that of the care receiver.

These four dimensions indicate that good care demands more than just good intention; good care should be understood as the practice of combining activities, attitudes and knowledge of the situation.

CARE AS RECIPROCAL PRACTICE

The practice of caring always takes place within the framework of a relationship where the caregiver and the care receiver are reciprocally involved. One can only begin to speak about care when the caregiver as well as the care receiver give care together. Even when the person receiving care cannot verbally or consciously express a request for care, his or her presence alone is the motivation for a human being to care for this person in need. If the person receiving care is conscious, then the process of care can only be considered as 'completed' if the care offered is affirmed (Noddings 1984). The fundamental reciprocity of a relationship of care can be found in the dynamic interaction of giving and receiving care (Widdershoven 2000).

Because care is also fundamentally about an attitude of involvement, reciprocity consists of verifying that the care given meets the needs of the care receiver. This means that care receivers have to be taken seriously as human beings in the specific life situation in which they find themselves, and of their experience of that situation. The characteristic of reciprocity also protects care from being used for paternalistic and narcissistic ends when caregivers abuse their power.

The characteristics of relatedness and reciprocity should be understood against the background of a broader societal context. Not only are caring practices positively appreciated because they are worthwhile for caregivers and care receivers alike, they also gain meaning from their embeddedness in societal practices as a whole. The healthcare system is a good example of such a social practice because it represents a joint effort aimed at the realization of the collective goal of health care for all. The caregivers do not just begin a relationship with the care receivers and vice versa, but also begin relationships within an institutional and societal context by forming teams of caregivers, relatives of patients, healthcare institutions and healthcare systems. In such institutional and societal frameworks, certain visions exist of what care is and what care should be, such as equal access to health care for all. Such visions contribute to determining how care is given.

ACTIVITIES AND ATTITUDES

The four dimensions of care according to Tronto illustrate most convincingly that empirical acts of care, as well as caring attitudes, form part of the integral practice of care. Attentiveness, responsibility, competence, and responsiveness are the essential attitudes that those involved in the process of care must acquire if care is to be optimal. Caring attitudes should be cultivated in people because they need to discern how to care (Carse 1991) as well as be attentive to what happens around them. Care-givers need to detect situations where the 'life-sustaining web' is weak. Thus a caring person clears the way to be 'touched by' and subsequently to be 'concerned' by the situation of anyone in need of care.

Attitudes also have an expressive function in that the quality of ethical actions does not only depend on the content of such actions, but also on the manner in which the actions are carried out (Carse 1991). An example is a nurse who helps an older person with hygiene care. The nurse does not only have to carry out the technical activities of such care correctly. He or she has to approach the older person in a respectful manner. A caring person should be able to listen, ask questions, have a conversation, pay attention to the other person's well-being, as well as be attentive and responsive. These are the qualities that make a human being a caring person.

CARE AS A VIRTUE

The general description of the phenomenon of care as a human practice brings me to a more precise conceptualization of care as a virtue. Characterizing care as a virtue allows me to distinguish care from other psychological phenomena, such as emotions, from which it has not always been well differentiated. For this analysis, I rely mainly on the work of Stan van Hooft (1995, 1999) and Laurence Blum (1980, 1994).

COGNITIVE, AFFECTIVE AND MOTIVATIONAL COMPONENTS OF CARE

In analysing care more closely, I will distinguish a cognitive, an affective, and a motivational component (Gastmans et al 1998, van Hooft 1995, 1999). When a caring person is directly involved in the well-being of another individual, care has a cognitive dimension. A truly caring attitude will not tolerate indifference and ignorance. Someone who has inadequate medical or nursing knowledge or is not competent to translate this knowledge into practice is not a caring nurse. A caring nurse collects as much data as possible about the situation of the patient and about the means that can eventually contribute to the improvement of the patient's situation.

Having knowledge of the situation of the person in need of help is an important condition but is not enough to qualify someone as a caring person. Caring behaviour is not the result of a purely rational wish for another person's good (Blum 1994). As well as gathering and making available any relevant information, the caring nurse needs to be emotionally touched by what happens to the patient, in both a positive and a negative sense.

The caring nurse can empathize with situations of pain and suffering. Yet this empathy always stands in relationship to any professional behaviour.

Care involves motivation: wanting to help the other person. The caring nurse must be motivated to respond to the appeal of the patient. Care stimulates these perceptions, leading to a judgement about what should be done, and then motivating the nurse to act accordingly. The desire for the good of the other is common to all care. This desire prompts beneficent actions when the nurse is in a position to engage in it (Blum 1980).

On the basis of these cognitive, affective and motivational components of care, van Hooft (1999) suggests therefore that care can be understood as a virtue. When care is understood as a virtue, it encompasses all the aspects of human behaviour, such as knowledge, emotions, motivations, and the ethical thinking that go along with it. In this way, caring is seen as an overarching quality that gives action its moral character (van Hooft 1999). Precisely this integration of reason, emotion, and motivation in care as a virtue is an important argument against ethicists like Helga Kuhse (1997; see Chapter 14), who see care mainly as an emotional state of mind that is a necessary but not sufficient component for care-givers in order to act morally and make moral judgements. van Hooft writes:

> *Caring does not consist in emotion alone and so to act on emotion alone is not to act in a caring manner. One acts from the virtue of caring when all the features mark one's action as I have elaborated, including that of judgement and understanding. It is a mistake to think of caring just as an emotion and then to suppose that the feeling of that emotion justifies any action that that emotion motivates.* (1999 p 199)

THE DISTINCTION BETWEEN CARE AS A VIRTUE AND EMOTIONAL INVOLVEMENT

So far, I have described the positive way in which care as a virtue consists of a cognitive, an affective and a motivational dimension. It is also important to state clearly that care as a virtue is not subject to the vagaries of other psychological phenomena from which it has not always been well differentiated (Gastmans et al 1998). In the first instance, care as a virtue should be distinguished from transitory emotions, personal feelings or moods. As part of a happy, joyful, and exuberant mood, I may be feeling very expansive and generous and may therefore be more inclined than I would normally be, for instance to give money to people in need around me. Such a mood may well pass, causing my generous feelings to disappear (Blum 1980). The virtue of care that motivates us to caring behaviour cannot be fleeting, nor linked to the passing moment. On the contrary, virtues must be lasting. It is important to warn against the danger of an emotivist concept of care that would reduce caring involvement to some form of sentimentality. The bearer of the virtue of care is primarily concerned with the factual and existential condition of a real individual and is motivated to do something about it (Blum 1980).

Second, the virtue of care should be distinguished from positive, personal feelings that one might have towards someone else. The bearers of the virtue of care and the bearers of positive personal feelings have in common that they are oriented to promote the well-being of others. They differ from each other, however, in the strength and lasting character of the desire to promote this well-being of the other. My positive feelings towards a good friend can be considered as an altruistic emotion. It is not certain that this emotion is based on a strong desire for acts of care that take time, trouble, and effort, and will mean inconvenience and perhaps sacrifice on my part. The motivational strength to continue a benevolent engagement is much stronger in someone who possesses the caring virtue than in a person who simply maintains an emotional link with someone based on positive experiences (Blum 1980). Thus, for example, nurses whose activities are inspired by the virtue of care are prepared to make great efforts to improve as much as possible the living conditions of a patient. In this example, caring is an important motivational factor for nurses, and they will actively try to exhibit this in their practice.

Virtues such as care are further distinguished from personal feelings as having different origins. Nurses find motivation for their caring behaviour by being involved in the well-being of patients. The positive feelings that people experience towards others originate, by contrast, in their involvement in various personal features of the person whom they experience as pleasant, enjoying their sense of humour, vitality or integrity. For these reasons, it is indeed possible that one could feel affection for another person without being prepared to act altruistically for that person's benefit (Blum 1980).

It is also quite possible to be engaged in caring behaviour for someone or a group of people without feeling seriously emotionally attracted to certain personal features of that group of people or without maintaining a close personal relationship with any one person or persons. What motivates nurses to caring behaviour is not the fact that they feel attracted to certain personal features of a patient, but rather the material and existential condition in which patients finds themselves. Being emotionally attracted to personal features of the person cannot be considered as the principal condition of caring behaviour (Blum 1980). Examples of this are the many altruistic engagements that are undertaken for the benefit of minority groups, such as immigrants, refugees, people from developing countries, people with AIDS or who are mentally ill. Caring behaviour towards the members of these groups does not necessarily originate in personal affection of the caregiver for personal features of the care receiver. Being emotionally attracted to personal features of others cannot be ruled out in advance either. Caring behaviour is not mainly concerned with personal affective attraction to people, enjoying their presence, being drawn to them, and so forth. Much more important is that caring behaviour is motivated by the actual situation in which the other finds himself or herself, or in his or her well-being.

THE PROCESS OF ETHICAL DECISION-MAKING

So far, I have tried to present a clear conceptualization of care. However, care ethics should not be reduced to a theoretical discussion about its main concepts. On the contrary, a characteristic of the care approach in healthcare ethics is its orientation to clinical practice. The main focus is the ethical aspects of the actual situation, paying attention to all relevant clinical factors involved, such as the patients' expectations, pains, fears, etc., as well as the professional and personal experiences of the caregivers. Clinical decisions, especially those at the end of life, could not be considered as decisions that are purely based on clinical facts, but they need a normative–ethical interpretation. Questions of dignity and meaningfulness transcend the clinical–technical discourse and require an ethical judgement in which all parties can enter into dialogue. An ethical interpretation of a clinical reality uses specific methods, concepts, and a series of arguments. In this part of the chapter I want to explore the care approach as a specific perspective from which ethical problems are detected, interpreted and solved. I will illustrate the care perspective based on the process of ethical decision-making as it relates to artificial feeding and hydration of an elderly patient.

The case of Denise	Denise was 85 years old and had for the past 7 years been a resident in a nursing home. The management considered that the primary goal of their nutritional policy was to delay artificial feeding and hydration as long as possible, and if possible, to avoid it altogether. Denise was recently transferred to a general hospital for hip surgery. Before the operation could take place, Denise suffered a cerebrovascular accident (CVA) that left her hemiplegic, aphasic and with an impaired swallowing reflex. She was transferred to the hospital's care of the elderly department where she remained a patient. The hospital had no ethical policy relating to medical decisions at the end of life. Without much consultation, artificial feeding and hydration by nasal drip was immediately started. It soon became obvious that the drip was making Denise uncomfortable; she had pulled it out three times. The nurses had ascertained that Denise experienced increasing periods of confusion. She could not speak but the nurses had managed to let her indicate yes or no by using simple gestures. Denise's only close relatives were two nieces and a nephew. The family confided in the team of caregivers that, just before her admission to hospital, Denise told them that she would rather be dead than completely dependent on the care of others. The family informed the team of caregivers in writing, after Denise had pulled out the drip for the third time, that it was their unanimous wish to withdraw tube feeding. Nurse A believed that granting the family's wish was an attack on her professional and moral identity. She deemed it possible that the family's decision stemmed from interested motives; their aunt was very affluent. The social worker, who had spoken several times with the family, could not quite exclude conflict of interests.

Denise's nephew told nurse A about his discontent with the so-called 'unanimous wish of the family'. In his opinion, his aunt's life was still valuable.

Denise's attending physician was more inclined to follow the family's wish. She thought that nurse A exaggerated the discomfort caused by the withdrawal of artificial feeding and hydration. The doctor also stated that this possible discomfort had to be weighed against the discomfort of continuing tube feeding. The attending physician was irritated by the conviction with which nurse A stated her opinion. She made it perfectly clear that in the end it is the doctor who decides.

It was therefore agreed that Denise should be asked if she wished tube feeding to be continued. Denise indicated by sign language to the attending physician and nurse A that she wished tube feeding to continue. The family was informed of Denise's wish. They refused to accept the fact that the hospital had not taken their wishes into account. They threatened to move their aunt from the hospital to the nursing home, where tube feeding would not be administered. They also demanded that this conversation with Denise should be repeated in their presence. Taking into account the recently expressed wish by Denise and the possible fatal consequences of not providing nutrition, the attending physician decided to resume artificial feeding and hydration until Denise had unequivocally expressed her wish in the presence of her family.

Some days later, Denise's cognitive abilities had seriously deteriorated. When her relatives and family doctor were present, she was asked if she wished to be artificially fed and hydrated, Denise reacted with a violent crying fit and restless plucking at the nasal drip. It was not clear to the caregivers whether they had to interpret this behaviour as a purely impulsive reaction or as a clear refusal. Consequently, all those involved reaffirmed their previous opinion. Nurse A was still of the opinion that administering nourishment was a moral duty. The attending physician asked herself whether continuing artificial feeding and hydration should not be considered futile treatment. The family demanded the immediate cessation of the artificial feeding and hydration and a transfer to the nursing home.

THE RELATIONAL EMBEDDEDNESS OF ETHICAL PROBLEMS

According to the care approach, ethical problems relate to the tensions between the responsibilities of people who live and work in a network of relationships. In the case of Denise, this relationship web consists in the first place of Denise herself, her two nieces and nephew, the attending physician, the nursing team, the directors of the hospital and the nursing home. The search for what is best for Denise is not solely focused on Denise's wishes as an isolated individual. To do justice to the relational identity of Denise, it is important to listen to the stories told by Denise, her family, her physician, her nurse and the institutional policy formulators because they outline the narrative context in which Denise's care has to take shape. Because of the very difficult decision that had to be taken, the relational network had been put under severe pressure. To reduce the pressure, a solution had to be found that satisfied all parties. The fact that all concerned could claim certain rights was not a deciding factor. Attention should not be paid to Denise's claim alone, or the possible claim of her family, or her caregivers, or indeed the balance between all these claims, but to the relational bond. The relationships that all the parties have with one another have a strong influence on the opinions expressed in this case. The care approach therefore demands great skill from all those involved in ethical decision making when interpreting the viewpoints that manifest as stories: healthcare ethics reveals itself as a form of narrative and interpretative ethics.

CLINICAL–ETHICAL DECISION MAKING AS AN INTERPRETIVE PROCESS

The care approach gives much attention to interpreting the different viewpoints of all those involved with the ethical problem. These viewpoints are never completely clear to the people concerned, especially when they are confronted with a life-threatening situation. Even those who voice certain opinions are never totally aware of all the contents or consequences of their opinion. Denise's wishes therefore cannot be considered as a given, with the contents easily deducible from the case study. Neither is it clear to those involved what must be done for Denise throughout the consecutive stages of her care. What Denise would have wanted under the specific circumstances needs to be construed based on what we know of her life, previous pronouncements and actual reactions to concrete proposals. This information reaches us indirectly and through the mediation of the third parties who knew Denise more or less well. From conflicting stories communicated by them and from background information provided by a social worker, it becomes clear that this information is not impartial. On the contrary, the disagreement of Denise's nephew illustrates that the concrete relational bonds that the family members have with their aunt influence all viewpoints. There is no direct access to Denise's wishes.

What does apply are the wishes and viewpoints expressed by those concerned with her care. These cannot be considered as a given, but they need to be gradually construed and then interpreted. The wishes of nurse A are an example. What does she really want? On what information is her opinion based? Does she want to continue the tube feeding at all cost or does she not want to let Denise down? I assume that she wanted the latter because of her strong commitment to Denise. However, one could also imagine her radically changing her opinion if she was to receive and be receptive to recent clinical findings on the therapeutic value of artificially feeding and hydrating terminally ill patients (Finucane et al 1999, Gillick 2000). These studies show that, under similar circumstances, artificial feeding and hydration cause more harm than good to the patient and that other forms of palliative care more accurately show a caring attitude to the patient. Taking into account the possibility of incomplete and/or incorrect information on the part of nurse A, I assume that the nurse's wishes are dynamic and thus continually explored. It is only through the process of joint exploration that the wishes of nurse A gradually become clear. The position of nurse A makes very clear that caring nurses need to express the right emotions and attitudes and also need the right knowledge and empirical evidence in order to translate their caring attitude into a caring activity. It is therefore a pity that the attending physician did not take time to have a conversation with nurse A during which she could have clarified the recent clinical findings on artificial feeding and hydration of which she was presumably aware. The physician avoided such a conversation by stating that 'in the end it is a doctor who decides whether or not artificial feeding and hydration will cease'. By using an argument of power, the ethical question of what is in Denise's best interest slips into the background in favour of the pseudo-ethical question of who has the right to decide. The goal of the process of interpretation, which is to clarify ethical viewpoints, is abruptly broken off and replaced by an external item about decision-making authority.

THE INSTITUTIONAL DIMENSION OF CARE

Care ethics is mainly seen as an ethics of individual relationships between family members, neighbours, colleagues, friends, etc. (Jecker & Reich 1995). A careful reading of Denise's case makes it clear that the doctor–patient relationship cannot be seen as an isolated form of interaction. On the contrary, it is situated in the wider care process, which is enacted in the work of a team of caregivers who are also part of a health-care institution. The institutional context of the nursing home and the hospital where Denise resides is partially outlined in the existence of concrete opinions and policies on care or lack of it. Denise's case is to a large extent marked by the tension between the existence of a carefully thought out policy on nutritional care at the nursing home on the one hand, and the lack of such a policy at the hospital on the other hand.

A good observer of the clinical–ethical dialogue will quickly note that the process and outcome of ethical reflection is influenced not only by these institutional factors, but also by external factors such as the position of power between doctors and nurses, the working relationship within the team and in the hospital, etc. This means that the position caregivers have in an institution is crucially important for the way in which they deal with ethical problems and participate (or not) in ethical consultations. In the case here presented, one can suspect that in view of the physician's irritation with nurse A, she will only moderately appreciate the assertive attitude of nurses in the ethical debate. Is the attending physician convinced by the contribution supplied by an interdisciplinary ethical dialogue in the search for what is humanly possible for Denise? This difficult ethical dialogue between all those concerned with the case illustrates how ethical problems are predominantly anchored in institutional and professional dimensions. Ethical problems in health care occur in an atmosphere of powerlesness, efficiency and cost-effectiveness, pressure at work, (in)competence, scarcity of human and financial resources, etc. This atmosphere determines what ethical problems are expressed and how they are dealt with. As a consequence, a care approach to healthcare ethics should not be reduced to a one-to-one ethics, but has to incorporate the broader institutional and societal context where healthcare practices are located.

POSSIBILITIES FOR FUTURE DEVELOPMENT

In this final part I shall investigate three possible directions that I consider to be of great importance for the future development of care ethics. These possibilities could also be considered as my partial answers to some major misunderstandings that lie behind the criticisms of care ethics.

A VIRTUE APPROACH TO CARE

The critics of an ethics of care (Kuhse 1997; and see Chapter 14) argue that care alone is an inadequate basis on which to make ethical decisions. Despite the fact that these ethicists admit that care is necessary for caregivers to remain sensitive to the moral characteristics of the clinical situation, they say that this is not enough to secure a moral activity. They argue for objective and principle-based ethical thinking that can ensure that people behave correctly and that they are able to justify such behaviour in terms of a public ethical discourse. A care-based ethical perspective, according to them, would not be able to meet these demands: care is a stage wherein one is sensitive to the needs of the patient, but ethical behaviour flows out of ethical reasoning. Against such a viewpoint, I argue, together with van Hooft (1999) that care as a virtue encompasses all aspects of moral behaviour, that is, the emotions, motivations, knowledge and ethical reasoning itself.

Care as a virtue means that emotion and reason are intrinsically linked. Thus, care no longer needs an external practical reason to justify moral behaviour. In this sense, Kuhse fails to see that ethical deliberation can be present in care, and care as virtue also implies a basis of knowledge out of which moral behaviour can occur. She argues that 'ethical behaviour' means that one behaves in agreement with universal principles. Against this I argue that only morally justifiable actions arise out of actions that flow from the virtue of care. After all, the virtue of care is an ethical orientation of the individual. This orientation encompasses the motivations and emotions as well as rationality, which is to say that it is an aspect of the internal life of an individual that is expressed in his or her behaviour. The virtue of care encompasses for example the nurse who is concerned about doing the right thing, with the right degree of sensitivity, with the right knowledge and skills, at the right time. The caring behaviour of this nurse does not need an external rationality to give it an ethical qualification.

FROM THEORY TO PERSPECTIVE

Does the conceptualization of care as a form of virtue bring with it a need to see a care ethics as virtue ethics? If yes, why do we then still speak about a care ethics and not just about a virtue ethics (Veatch 1998)? These questions are linked to the great confusion that exists about care ethics and about what exactly care ethics adds to the field of moral theory (Verkerk 2001). The conceptualization of care as a virtue does not necessarily lead to envisioning care ethics as virtue ethics. I claim that a care ethic stands on its own, as Marian Verkerk (2001) and Margaret Little (1998) have argued, as a 'moral perspective or orientation' from which ethical theorizing can take place. This will mean that care ethics is more a stance from which we can theorize ethically rather than a full-blown ethical theory in itself. An orientation can always be described in terms of emphasis on concern and discernment habits and tendencies of interpretation and selectivity of skills. Concern and discernment relate to worrying more, e.g. about the dangers of 'abandoning' a patient rather than the dangers of interfering too much. The habits of interpretation related to the tendency, say, to read 'the' moral question presented by a situation in terms of responsibilities rather than rights. Selectivity of skills relates to having developed the capacity to attune to difference and particularity rather than an ease of abstraction (Little 1998). Most of these characteristics of acting, taking responsibility and of the particularity of the care perspective are illustrated in the case study of Denise. In short, care ethics as a perspective makes it possible for care to be conceptualized as a particular moral virtue, without claiming that it has to be interpreted as a moral theory with prior claims so that we can compare and assess it easily.

CARE ETHICS AND HEALTH CARE

From the beginning, when a care ethics was being written about, a certain affinity existed between it and with nursing ethics. The field of nursing care was found to be well qualified to illustrate the worth of the care ethic. More than the life-and-death decision making that gets so much attention in medical ethics, nurses focus their attention on the entire caring process that people undergo. Nurses are in close interaction with all involved, not just the physicians, but also other nurses and family members, and they continually have to make small and large decisions to maintain the character of dignity of the patient in every situation in which they find themselves. A care ethics with the emphasis on 'responsibility for', 'connectedness to', 'involvement with' and 'communication', seems very suitable to interpret ethical problems in nursing practice, and to provide solutions.

This bond between care ethics and nursing ethics cannot just reduce care ethics to nursing ethics. Based on the analysis of the case of Denise, it would be hard to argue that only nurses have to be careful, open and attentive. More and more authors emphasize a re-evaluation of care, not only in the field of nursing but also in medical practice (Binstock & Cluff 2001). A relationship of care and trust is essentially what the patient–physician relationship consists of. The work *Extending the boundaries of care: medical ethics and caring practices* (Kohn & McKechnie 1999) is an example of this. The book puts emphasis on examples of how the care perspective can function in medical practice. The elements of contextual and narrative appreciation, communication, dialogue, and involvement are all considered as elements of moral deliberation. These elements also have a central role in the analysis of the case of Denise, which cannot be characterized as a nursing ethics case. Although it is certainly true that nursing ethics does make use of insights from care ethics, it is clear that the care perspective cannot be reserved for the nursing care sector alone (Verkerk 2001).

CONCLUSION

In this chapter I have tried to illustrate the contribution of the care perspective to healthcare ethics. Most of the confusion that has plagued discussions of the care framework in ethical theory is due to the fact that it has not always been well differentiated from other phenomena. Therefore, I started with an analysis of the concept of care. However, much work still has to be done on a fundamental level in order to develop a sound theoretical basis for care ethics. In that sense, further analysis of the concept of care as a moral virtue is needed. A clear examination of care ethics as an ethical perspective that is differentiated from other ethical theories and not exclusively oriented towards nursing care, should also be further encouraged.

References

Blum L 1980 Friendship, altruism and morality. Routledge & Kegan Paul, London.

Blum L 1994 Moral perception and particularity. Cambridge University Press, Cambridge.

Carse E 1991 The 'voice of care': implications for bioethical education. Journal of Medicine and Philosophy 16(1):5–28.

Cluff LE, Binstock RH (eds) 2001 The lost art of caring: a challenge to health professionals, families, communities, and society. The Johns Hopkins University Press, Baltimore.

Finucane T, Christmas C, Travis K 1999 Tube feeding in patients with advanced dementia. Journal of the American Medical Association 282:1365–1370.

Gastmans C, Dierckx de Casterlé B, Schotsmans P 1998 Nursing considered as moral practice: a philosophical–ethical interpretation of nursing. The Kennedy Institute of Ethics Journal 8:43–69.

Gatens-Robinson E (1992) A defence of women's choice: abortion and the ethics of care. Southern Journal of Philosophy 30(3):39–66.

Gillick M 2000 Rethinking the role of tube feeding in patients with advanced dementia. New England Journal of Medicine 342:206–210.

Gilligan C 1982 In a different voice: psychological theory and women's development. Harvard University Press, Cambridge, MA.

Jecker N, Reich W 1995 Contemporary ethics of care. In: Reich W (ed) Encyclopedia of bioethics. Simon & Schuster/MacMillan, New York, p 336–344.

Kohn T, McKechnie R (eds) 1999 Extending the boundaries of care: medical ethics and caring practices. Berg, Oxford/New York.

Kuhse H 1997 Caring: nurses, women and ethics. Blackwell, Oxford.

Lindemann K 2003 The ethics of receiving. Theoretical Medicine 24:501–509.

Little M 1998 Care: from theory to orientation and back. Journal of Medicine and Philosophy 23:190–209.

Loots C 2002 Expecting a child with a disability: clinical ethical reflections on prenatal diagnosis and selective abortion. In: Gastmans C (ed) Between technology and humanity: the impact of technology on health care ethics. Leuven University Press, Leuven, p 81–94.

Manschot H, Verkerk M (eds) 1994 Ethiek van de zorg: een discussie (Care ethics: a discussion). Boom, Amsterdam.

Noddings N 1984 Caring: a feminine approach to ethics and moral education. University of California Press, Berkeley.

Parks J 2003 Envisioning a kinder, gentler world: on recognition and remuneration of care workers. Theoretical Medicine 24:489–499.

Reich W 1995 Care. In: Reich W (ed) Encyclopedia of bioethics. Simon & Schuster/MacMillan, New York, p 319–344.

Sevenhuijsen S 1998 Citizenship and the ethics of care: feminist considerations on justice, morality and politics. Routledge, London.

Tronto J 1993 Moral boundaries: a political argument for an ethic of care. Routledge, New York.

van Hooft S 1995 Caring: an essay in the philosophy of ethics. University Press of Colorado, Denver.

van Hooft S 1999 Acting from the virtue of caring in nursing. Nursing Ethics 6:192–193.

Veatch R 1998 The place of care in ethical theory. Journal of Medicine and Philosophy 23:210–224.

Verkerk M 1999 A care perspective on coercion and autonomy. Bioethics 13:358–369.

Verkerk M 2001 The care perspective and autonomy. Medicine, Healthcare and Philosophy 4:289–294.

Widdershoven G 1999 Care, cure and interpersonal understanding. Journal of Advanced Nursing 29:1163–1169.

Widdershoven G 2000 Ethiek in de kliniek: hedendaagse benaderingen in de gezondheidsethiek (Ethics in the clinic: current approaches in healthcare ethics). Boom, Amsterdam.

Further reading

Cates DF, Lauritzen P 2001 Medicine and the ethics of care. Georgetown University Press, Washington DC.

Gastmans C 2002 Tube feeding and assisted oral feeding in demented patients with eating difficulties: a clinical ethical approach. In: Gastmans C (ed) Between technology and humanity: the impact of technology on health care ethics. Leuven University Press, Leuven, p 197–216.

Gilligan C 1982 In a different voice: psychological theory and women's development. Harvard University Press, Cambridge, MA.

Kuhse H 1997 Caring: nurses, women and ethics. Blackwell, Oxford.

Tronto J 1993 Moral boundaries: a political argument for an ethic of care. Routledge, New York.

van Hooft S 2004 Life, death, and subjectivity: moral sources in bioethics. Editions Rodopi, Amsterdam & New York.

Chapter 14

Past caring.
The limitations of one-to-one ethics

John Paley

INTRODUCTION

Perhaps the most difficult problem associated with offering a critique of the 'ethics of caring' is that it is extremely difficult to say what the 'ethics of caring' is. Much of the nursing literature is vague on this point, and many authors prefer to celebrate caring rather than interrogate it. There is much talk about caring being a moral ideal (Watson 1985), a virtue (Fry 1989), a moral imperative (Morse et al 1990), an ethical ideal (Warelow 1996) and so on. However, none of this is particularly illuminating, and it leaves all the significant questions unanswered. For example, is caring just one 'ethical ideal' among others? On the face of it, there are plenty of other moral values relevant to nursing, including some that are rarely mentioned in discussions of ethics. It would be morally wrong, I assume, to give treatment that empirical evidence had shown to be harmful, or to infringe deliberately against hygiene protocols. Yet the nursing literature is silent about the 'ethics of evidence'; and I have never come across any reference to 'transpersonal hygiene moments'. Quite how these various 'moral imperatives' are supposed to balance out, and whether caring is supposed to be the overriding value in cases of conflict, remains deeply unclear.

However, our assessment of the 'ethics of caring' will depend on what claim is being made. If the idea is that caring (whatever account we give of it) should be the dominant value, the one that takes precedence over all the other 'moral imperatives' in nursing, then that is a bold and interesting suggestion. It is also implausible and urgently in need of arguments to support it. If, however, the idea is that caring is just one of several 'virtues', none of which has pride of place, then that is a far more credible proposal. However, it is also much less interesting, to the point that it is difficult to see what all the fuss is about. This ambiguity is going to bedevil any attempt to make sense of 'caring ethics', and make a final evaluation very difficult.

Nevertheless, I shall mount an attack on 'the ethics of caring' despite this handicap. In the next section, I will set the scene for a discussion of normative ethics by examining a second ambiguity. I will then present a strong version of the 'caring thesis' – that is, the 'ethics of attachment'. This version is distinctive and enterprising but, I think, mistaken. The next step, therefore, will be to formulate a weaker and more plausible version, the 'ethics of the one-to-one', although I will subsequently argue that even this weaker version is inadequate. I turn next to meta-ethics, and examine the ontological and empirical reasons for thinking that an ethics of caring is viable. The literature regularly appeals to Martin Heidegger's ontology and to Carol Gilligan's 'different voice' in support of the 'caring' ideal, so I will consider these two sources in particular. Finally, I will ask whether there is any prospect of deriving 'caring' from either an ethics of principle or utilitarianism. I suggest that there is . . . but only at a price. The price is: reason rules.

THE MEANINGS OF 'CARE'

It is commonly suggested that the nursing literature recognizes two senses of the verb 'to care', one of which refers to providing a service, the second of which refers to an 'attitude of mind'. For example, Helga Kuhse has noted that nurses distinguish between 'looking after or providing for the needs of the other' and 'an emotional response – concern for the other, emphasis on relationship' (Kuhse 1997 p 146–147). The terminology varies. Some writers talk about the 'instrumental' and 'expressive' senses of 'care' (Lea et al 1998); others distinguish between a 'behavioural concept' and an 'emotional concept' of caring (van Hooft 2003). Anne Griffin separates an 'activities aspect' from the 'attitudes and feelings underlying them' (Griffin 1983). Margaret Dunlop describes the second sense – she claims it involves a form of love – as 'emergent', because there is 'little evidence that "caring" in the sense that it is now being used is a longstanding meaning of the word' (Dunlop 1994 p 28).

The 'ethics of caring', if there is one, is clearly predicated on this second 'attitude of mind', 'emotional', 'expressive', 'emergent' sense. However, there is a problem, and it must be unravelled before we can proceed. The second meaning is a mess. It runs together three different ideas and renders the 'ethics of caring' multiply ambiguous. We have already had one ambiguity, and this is another. Fortunately, to unpick the semantics is a relatively straightforward task.

Consider some of the attributes associated with the second meaning: relationship, openness, concern for the other, attachment, attentiveness, empathy, compassion, worry, listening, being careful and attentive to details, affection (Swanson 1999). This list includes three distinct clusters centred on (1) 'concern', (2) 'attentiveness', and (3) 'attachment. Allocating each term to its respective cluster, we find: (1) concern, worry, compassion, empathy; (2) openness, being careful, attentiveness, listening; (3) attachment, relationship, affection, fondness.

Prima facie, there are three senses here, not just one. There is a *motivational* sense, a *cognitive* sense and an *affective* sense, each of which is independent of the others. For example, it is quite possible to be motivated by a concern for other people's misfortunes, to be (in that sense) a 'caring person', without feeling any obligation to listen to them. This situation is unfortunately common. Equally, it is entirely possible to be attentive and careful in one's dealings with someone and still not have a relationship with the person concerned. This is, or should be, routine. So, referring back to the nursing literature, we can discriminate between, first, the fact that some people are bothered by the sufferings of others and want to do something about it (what Oppenheimer 2003 calls 'mattering'); second, 'a willingness to give the lucid attention required to appropriately fill the needs of others' (Manning 1992 p 61); and, third, a relationship between nurse and patient, which might be anything from 'moderated love' (Campbell 1984) to a deep, intimate encounter (Mayeroff 1971).

Putting these three senses together and calling them the 'expressive' sense, confuses the issue. For one thing, it prevents us recognizing that some of the questions posed about 'caring' do not have a single answer. For example: 'Can nurses be caring in fleeting encounters with patients?' It depends on which sense of 'caring' is intended. The answer seems to be: 'yes' in the motivational and cognitive senses, 'no' in the affective sense (how can one have a relationship when the encounter is fleeting?). A more significant question is: which of the three senses is implicated in the idea of an 'ethics of caring'? If the motivational or cognitive sense is intended, the 'ethics of caring' seems unobjectionable but unexciting, and it cannot be regarded as unique to nursing, because many health professionals are motivated by sympathetic concern and it would be difficult to argue that only nurses are careful and attentive. So it is the affective sense that is the most interesting, because it would presumably imply that it is a good thing for nurses to form personal relationships with their patients. This is an extremely strong claim and, if it could be justified, would certainly be unique to nursing. The 'ethics of attachment' is therefore the subject of the next section.

THE STRONG VERSION: CARING AS ATTACHMENT

In Dunlop's (1994) view the 'emergent' sense of caring 'seems to involve a form of love' (p 28), and several variations on this theme can be found in the nursing literature. There is a spectrum of positions. Some writers express a certain caution: 'it might not be too far-fetched to identify a dominant emotion in caring as a kind of love' (Griffin 1983 p 294). Other writers are more confident: 'Caring is loving' (Jacono 1993). As if to emphasize the implications of this, Olivia Bevis adopts Rollo May's definition of 'caring' as 'a relationship of dedication, taking the ultimate terms, to suffer for the other' (Bevis 1981 p 50). Then we find a metaphysical edge starting to creep in, with claims that caring is a 'form of loving oblative or other directed love, where co-presence in human encounter is a mystery rather than a problem to be solved' (Ray 1981 p 32). Jean Watson goes even further: 'In a transpersonal caring relationship, a spiritual union occurs between the two persons where both are capable of transcending self, time, space and the life history of each other' (Watson 1988 p 66). Here, I will keep to the moderate end of the spectrum: if the tentative position cannot stand up, the more colourful metaphysical versions will topple over as well.

I do not really need to criticize the 'ethics of caring' at length, because the job has already been done very well by several authors (Allmark 1995, Mackintosh 2000, Stockdale & Warelow 2000, van Hooft 1987, Warelow 1996). Three writers, in particular, have said everything that needs to be said on the matter (Curzer 1993, Kuhse 1997, Koehn 1998).

CARING AS UTOPIAN

It is unreasonable to expect nurses to develop a personal relationship with every patient, or even to experience affection towards every patient. 'We do not feel this attachment to others just because they are people' (Curzer 1993 p 57); and exhorting nurses to strive for such unattainable goals is 'setting the ideal of caring in nursing too high' (Kuhse 1997 p 149). Any serious attempt to invest this kind of emotion, indiscriminately, is likely to result in an acute sense of failure, compounded by emotional exhaustion (Maslach 1982).

CARING AS UNJUST

It is not possible to love every patient to the same degree. 'A caring worker cannot be in love with all his clients' (Downie & Telfer 1980 p 91). Inevitably, then, caring-as-attachment implies favouritism, and might open the door to 'unsavoury practices such as racism, sexism and ageism' (Curzer 1993 p 58). Moreover, attachment is a deeply unfair basis for nursing on purely practical grounds because the emotional energy invested in one patient will mean that much less is available for others. Consequently, patients will not have equal access to the nurse's attention.

CARING AND ACTING

As Howard Curzer points out, 'caring makes some desirable actions more difficult' (1993 p 56), and he cites causing pain as a result of treatment, and communicating bad news, as examples. Moreover, the 'ethics of attachment' can provide no guidance in particular cases, especially when competing principles are at stake. If a 43-year-old woman, paralysed for a year and kept alive by a ventilator, wishes to be allowed to die, what is the most 'caring' response? Healthcare staff told a High Court hearing in London that 'The patient is just asking us to kill her and that is something we would not wish to do' (Hall 2002). The presiding judge ruled that the patient's request be complied with.

CARING AS A VICE

The 'virtue' of caring can slide into one of several vices. 'In general, caring for a person seems to make paternalism easier and more frequent' (Curzer 1993 p 57). There is also a 'narcissistic component' in caring, which diverts attention away from patients and descends into a celebration of the nurse's own qualities as a 'caring' person. This is, in turn, associated with the 'caregiver's temptation to infantilize another person so that she can experience the joy of nurturing' (Koehn 1998 p 42).

SELF-SCEPTICISM

The slide into vice is not inevitable, but the 'ethic of attachment' provides no self-analytical check on the possibilities of projection, narcissism, voyeurism and other dubious motives. 'What all these vices have in common is the unconscious wish to exercise power over others ... to inflate one's self-esteem' (Paley 2002a p 31). So 'the ethic should have some feature or factor capable of engendering self-suspicion in the caregiver regarding his or her own motives' (Koehn 1998 pp 40–41). Unfortunately, it doesn't.

THE POLITICS OF CARING

The ethics of attachment risks reinforcing a narrow 'female virtue' stereotype, remaining largely silent about the subordination of women's interests (Grimshaw 1986, Hoagland 1991), and breathing 'new life into traditional ... perceptions of the limited role women and nurses can and should play in social life' (Kuhse 1997 p 164). Caring, in this sense, will inevitably tend to an acceptance of burdens and a reluctance to alienate: 'In these terms caring begins to smack strongly of self-sacrifice or perhaps even self-established exploitation' (Bowden 1997 p 124).

PATIENT ATTITUDES

The evidence suggests that patients do not seek the kind of relationship that this version of the 'ethics of caring' recommends. Almost all the empirical studies that try to assess patient priorities find that they place a 'trusting relationship' near the bottom of the list (Kyle 1995, Swanson 1999). For most patients, having friendly and helpful nurses is enough. Nurses who insist on 'caring as attachment' are, to this extent, ignoring the patients' wishes.

CHARACTERISTICS OF A WEAKER VERSION

On all these grounds, the strong form of the 'ethics of caring' looks implausible, even if it is regarded as just one 'virtue' among others, and absurd if it is taken to be nursing's dominant 'moral imperative'. However, it might be possible to formulate a weaker version, one that does not insist on a personal relationship (or even a spiritual union) between nurse and patient. I do not know what, specifically, this weak version of 'caring ethics' would actually recommend, or what its status would be, compared to other 'ethical ideals' invoked in the nursing literature. However, I can suggest characteristics it might have, derived from various sources in the literature, and evaluate those as a series of parameters governing nursing ethics. In this section, therefore, I will identify six such 'parameters', and then argue, in the next section, that they form an inadequate basis for ethics in any healthcare discipline.

AGENT-CENTRED

The 'ethics of caring' will be agent-centred (O'Neill 1996). This means that the focus of moral thought is the person acting, rather than the action itself or the consequences flowing from it. As in all forms of virtue ethics, the emphasis is on the qualities of the agent, not on the principles of action or the desirable nature of the outcome. So the characteristics of the 'caring nurse' will be regarded as more central than what the 'caring nurse' does, or what he or she is likely to bring about.

ONE-TO-ONE

Discussions of 'caring' usually refer to the relationship between nurse and patient. Caring is an 'ethical relationship', progressively in danger of being replaced by 'scientific technologies designed to meet the needs of populations rather than individuals' (Peacock & Nolan 2000 p 1066). Almost by definition, then, the 'ethics of caring' will concern itself with the association between one individual and another, and with what the nurse, in particular, brings to that association. I shall therefore say, in logical terms, that 'caring' is a one–one relation, and that the 'caring ethic' is itself an ethics of the one-to-one.

EMOTION

Even if we resist the notion of an ethics of attachment, because it is too extreme, the 'ethics of caring' still represents a commitment to emotion, as opposed to reason. What is ethically significant about the 'caring' agent is what he or she feels, not the logical rigour of his or her thought processes. 'Caring is an emotional response', according to Dyson (1997); and most care ethicists go further, expressing an outright distrust of reason. Patricia Benner, who stresses the key role of emotions, and the fact that 'embodied humans inhabit worlds imbued with meaning sensed and felt' (Benner 2000 p 10), is an obvious case in point.

DIFFERENCE

Most writers on 'caring' place great emphasis on the individual, on the unique and on what is context-related. 'Moral judgment is more contextual, more immersed in the details of relationships and narratives' (Benhabib 1986), so the 'care ethicist takes seriously the idea of individualism' (Koehn 1998 p 22). Each person, each situation, is unique. Rather than generalizing over types of circumstance, an ethics of the one-to-one will assign primary significance to the particularities and nuances of every encounter and require 'a responsiveness to a person that values their uniqueness and individuality' (Dyson 1997 p 197).

PARTICULARISM

An 'ethics of caring' will reject the idea of acting by reference to general principles, and will therefore be particularist (O'Neill 1996) in outlook. 'We do not say with any conviction that a person cares if that person acts routinely according to some fixed rule' (Noddings 1984 p 13). Caring deals with the concrete and the particular, in a way that transcends rigid imperatives. It appeals 'to the particular sensibilities, attachments or judgements of individuals in particular situations' (O'Neill 1996 p 13).

UNMEASURABILITY

It is sometimes said that 'caring' cannot be tested or measured (for example, Dunlop 1994, McCance et al 2001, Peacock & Nolan 2000). However, it is rather difficult to find any argument in support of this position. It seems to be assumed that 'caring' will resist measurement and quantification. For the 'ethics of caring', this implies that all claims about moral decisions will be essentially incontestable. Whatever understandings (of the patient) the nurse cites in support of his or her judgement, whatever personal qualities (in the nurse) are alleged to embody 'caring' values, they will have to be taken on trust. This is, perhaps, an ethics of the spiritual, the ineffable, the intangible.

WHY THE WEAKER VERSION IS INADEQUATE

The image that emerges from this characterization of the weaker version has a certain coherence, even though it is impossible to say what, in practice, the 'ethics of caring' is likely to recommend. Indeed, this is the point, since *particularism* implies that no general prescriptions are available, and that the only way to give this ethics expression is to tell stories of caring moments and relationships. The image is clearly one of a nurse with a specific sensibility, who encounters patients in their uniqueness, in ways that cannot be subject to principles or measurements. No wonder caring is said to be 'elusive' (Lea & Watson 1996, Morse et al 1990) or 'nebulous' (Greenhalgh et al 1998, McCance et al 1997). It seems almost wilfully slippery. That, arguably, is one objection to it. However, I shall suggest that it is inadequate for other reasons as well.

AGENT-CENTRED

Any ethical theory is obliged to give some account of the moral virtues. However, this obligation does not imply that ethical concern should focus primarily, or even exclusively, on character and sensibilities. Virtues can only be 'individuated by reference to characteristic, intelligible patterns of action' (O'Neill 1996 p 73). We describe people as 'caring' presumably because their *actions* are caring. Equally, we would be unimpressed by someone claiming to have a sympathetic nature if his or her actions were routinely unsympathetic. 'Caring' as a virtue is only interesting to the extent that the 'caring person' *acts* in particular ways. Unfortunately, as long as attention remains focused on the qualities of the nurse, we are not likely to discover what these ways are, except in the vaguest terms. Worse, there is a risk that an interest in the virtues of the nurse will become obsessive (Paley 2004b), and that what the patient actually wants will be ignored.

ONE-TO-ONE

The assumption that ethics involves a one-to-one relationship between individuals excludes an enormous range of moral considerations. What becomes of questions about our obligations to groups, and the responsibility to ensure that our treatment of different individuals is equitable? In nursing, these questions are no less significant than in any other sphere. Public health nursing, for example, is concerned with populations, epidemiology, health promotion, community development and so on. In that context, an ethics of the one-to-one looks threadbare. More generally, equal access to healthcare services is currently a priority in the UK (Appleby et al 2003) and other European countries (Mossialos & Thomson 2003). A 'one-to-one ethics' has little to offer to this kind of debate. Using the vocabulary of logical relations, the ethics of health care will involve not a one–one relation, but a one–many relation; and frequently, in multi-professional contexts, it will involve a many–many relation. We have to look beyond 'caring' for an ethics that meets this description.

EMOTION

An ethic of emotion provides no independent check on the experiences of the agent concerned. There is no space in this ethics for a distinction between 'how it seems' and 'how it is'. This is not to imply that feelings are irrelevant to the moral enterprise. However, to act on the basis of emotions and nothing else, makes it impossible to distinguish between 'finer feelings' and those of another kind. It is reason's job to vet emotion and intuition, to 'check that they are not simply camouflage for whim, folklore, fad or fancy', or 'any other form of parochialism, chauvinism or preconception' (Paley 2002b p 140–141). We are all vulnerable to pervasive illusions about ourselves and others (Wilson 2002), and an unrestrained ethic of emotion does nothing to correct them. This is why, in health care, there is so much emphasis on empirical evidence as the foundation of decision making. Evidence is, precisely, a way of ensuring that 'moral' and 'personal' knowing (Fawcett et al 2001) do not get out of hand.

DIFFERENCE

In privileging difference, the 'ethics of caring' overlooks the moral implications of the fact that, in certain important respects, people are the same. This is the Kantian approach, in which every person is a rational being, with equal worth and equal rights. A 'universalist' ethics is based on a 'commitment to the equal treatment of persons' (Holmes 1989 p 244). The essential point is that, when it comes to fairness, the idiosyncratic differences – the things that make people unique – are irrelevant (Mulhall & Swift 1996). It is this insight that, in the context of health care, grounds the idea of equal access, self-determination, patient rights and so on. Curiously, however, some writers try to have it both ways. For example, Sara Fry emphasizes the particularity of relationships but then incorporates 'a Kantian form of respect for persons' into her theory of 'caring' (Fry 1991 p 169). The resulting hybrid is then passed off as 'caring'. This manoeuvre illustrates a frustrating aspect of the nursing literature, as authors commonly describe as 'caring' anything they find attractive. This is another reason why the concept is supposedly 'elusive', and why it is impossible to say exactly what the 'caring ethics' is. It is infinitely elastic – partly because it is used to label whatever each author happens to approve of.

PARTICULARISM

Writers who embrace particularism seem to believe that the only alternative is action governed by rigid rules (for example, Peacock & Nolan 2000). Arguably, however, they confuse 'principles of universal form' with 'principles recommending uniformity'. This is a mistake. A principle such as 'Each should be taxed in proportion to ability to pay' is universal in scope but its implementation clearly depends on the individual case (O'Neill 1996 p 75). In private life, there is probably no reason why a particularist ethic should not prevail – if it can avoid principles, which is doubtful. In the professions, however, and particularly in health care, there is a strong case for transparency and the accountability that goes with it. A principle can be stated, appraised, evaluated. It is open to inspection, discussion and challenge. The 'ethics of caring', however, is a kind of private language. It resists examination by any authority other than the person who adopts it, and for this reason is unsuited to professional people employed in public-service organizations.

UNMEASURABILITY

This is the condition that renders any attempt to challenge the 'ethics of caring' impossible. Infinitely elastic, lacking in transparency, governed by nothing but sensibility, it is, finally, not subject to any empirical test other than 'relational narratives' (Gadow 1995). With a more accountable system of ethics, we can enquire whether, for example, utilitarian acts bring about an increase in happiness or whether principle-based acts increase equitability. The 'caring ethic' refuses this option; and it is ironic that some writers insist on the unmeasurability of caring while others complain about its 'invisibility. In any case, a mathematics of caring is quite feasible. Anyone who thinks it cannot be done is probably unfamiliar with non-linear mathematical modelling techniques. If marriage can be quantified (Gottman et al 2002), so can the 'caring relationship'. Creating mathematical models of caring would be the most effective way of putting an 'ethics of caring' to the test (Paley 2004a).

In summary, even the weak version of 'caring ethics' is inadequate. It might perhaps be acceptable in private life but it cannot serve as a public-service ethic because it ignores huge tracts of moral territory. These tracts represent the terrain in which liberal values, originating in the Enlightenment, took root (Holmes 1989). These are the values that deal in rights, transparency, equity, justice, fairness and the ordering of a society in which individual claims compete. So the 'ethics of caring' is another anti-liberal train of thought, translated to a healthcare context. At best, it needs to be propped up by liberal principles; at worst, it is an irrelevance in a world that has not yet managed to ensure (as routine) equal access to health care, respect for patient's wishes, patient rights, informed consent, patient involvement in decision making, privacy, confidentiality, evidence-based treatment and a raft of other basic rights and equities.

THE META-ETHICS OF CARING: HEIDEGGER

I come now to the various attempts to ground an 'ethics of caring' in ontology and anthropology. This might seem unnecessary, given that even the weak version of caring-as-a-normative-ethic is inadequate. However, if there is a persuasive meta-ethical reason for supposing that *some* version of the 'ethics of caring' can be sustained, that would motivate an attempt to find it. For reasons of space, I will review only two of the several possible meta-ethical arguments. In this section, I will consider appeals to Martin Heidegger's ontology (Heidegger 1962); in the next, I will turn to Carol Gilligan's findings on gender differences in moral reasoning (Gilligan 1982).

Heidegger's work is notoriously difficult, but I will try to avoid technicalities in this discussion (Paley 2000). The basic idea is surprisingly uncomplicated. It is this: The most essential fact about human beings is that things matter to them. I propose not to worry about exactly what 'essential' means in this context, nor how we determine what is essential and what is not, nor why Heidegger thinks this statement is true. I shall just take it that, according to Heidegger, the most fundamental characteristic of human beings is that they *care* about things; and I will assume, for the sake of argument, that this claim is accurate.

The key word presents itself immediately: care (in German, *Sorge*). However, we must avoid leaping to conclusions. The essential fact to which Heidegger is directing our attention is that people are never indifferent to what is around them. They have priorities, preferences and desires. They have projects, and make plans. However, these priorities, plans and projects vary considerably from person to person. We all care about different things. Each of us has a different permutation of things-that-matter. Some people care about making money, others care about the environment; Hitler cared about *Lebensraum* (Allmark 1995, Dunlop 1994).

Sorge is clearly not the kind of caring nurses have in mind (however we interpret that). Nurse-caring is just one of the innumerable forms that *Sorge* can take. Heidegger's view is that we all, necessarily, have *Sorge* for something; that is what being human means. However, he is not interested (in his book *Being and time*) in any particular manifestation of it. Any attempt to derive nurse-caring from *Sorge* is therefore doomed to failure.

Nor does it help that *Sorge* has two aspects, *Besorgen* ('concern') and *Fürsorge* ('solicitude'). The first applies, broadly, to things; the second applies, equally broadly, to people. However, *Fürsorge* is morally neutral. People matter to us in a way that things, in general, do not; but this 'people-mattering' includes an enormous range of attitudes and emotions, many of which have nothing to do with nurse-caring. We care about people (in the *Fürsorge* sense) when we envy them, resent them, manipulate them or compete with them. Equally, we care (*Fürsorge*) about people when we love them, look after them and try to help them. You cannot care, in this sense, about inanimate objects. You cannot, for example, envy a hammer, or fall in love with a doorknob. The conclusion is much the same. The kind of caring that interests nurses is just one manifestation of *Fürsorge*. One, that is to say, among countless others.

It is impossible to derive an 'ethics of nurse-caring' – or an ethics of any kind – from *Being and time*, a conclusion confirmed by Heidegger himself. In asking whether ontological thinking has any ethical implications, he observes: 'The answer is that such thinking is neither theoretical nor practical . . . Such thinking has no result. It has no effect' (Heidegger 1993 p 259). The position could hardly be stated more clearly.

This has not prevented many nurse writers appealing to Heidegger in support of the 'ethics of caring'. A recent example: 'caring is a collection of human activities that assists others (Heidegger 1962/1997)' (Kapborg & Bertero 2003 p 184). This sort of appeal is common practice, although it is perhaps more usual to *imply* that Heidegger's 'care' is the same as nurse-caring. One article, for example, in the middle of a discussion of 'caring in nursing', notes that 'Heidegger views caring as a motivating force' (Cheung 1998 p 226). There are many similar instances in the nursing literature (Bevis 1981, Bishop & Scudder 1990, Leininger & Watson 1990, Roach 1984).

In any case, Heidegger is an odd choice as a patron saint of 'caring'. He was a member of the German Nazi Party for elevan years, aspired to become the philosopher of Nazism, and his political record at the

University of Freiburg (1933–1934) is appalling (Farias 1989, Fritsche 1999, Philipse 1998). One can abstain on the question of whether Heidegger's Nazism renders the phenomenology of *Being and time* suspect, but still think that his unofficial appointment as a moral authority on *caring* is an aberration.

THE META-ETHICS OF CARING: GILLIGAN

The appeal to Heidegger as a meta-ethical source for the 'ethics of caring', although somewhat vague, is understandable in the following terms. Heidegger claims that *Sorge* (including *Fürsorge*) is the core of what it is to be human. If that is correct, and assuming that *Fürsorge* has an ethical resonance (which I have argued it does not), it is tempting to suppose that an 'ethics of caring' is more fundamental than any alternative conception. This is a strange idea, because it would make an ethics out of something that we cannot help doing anyway. If caring really is the 'human mode of being' (Roach 1984), there cannot be much sense in recommending that people *should* care, because (on this view) they already do. It is like proposing an ethics of breathing, and recommending that people ought to breathe.

The appeal to gender (Gilligan 1982) does not have the same implications. Gilligan claims that women (or some women) have a different ethical 'voice'. Their approach to moral problems is different from that of men, using different criteria and a different set of priorities. Theirs is the 'voice of care', and it is contrasted with the 'justice' voice, typical of males. To this extent, an 'ethics of caring' derived from Gilligan's work would presumably target men, together with those women who do not adopt a 'caring' voice (two-thirds of Gilligan's original sample). It would not necessarily claim that the 'voice of care' is superior to the 'voice of justice' (Gilligan herself does not make this claim). However, it would certainly suggest that justice should be complemented by caring, on the grounds that this 'voice' represents a significant proportion of humanity, who should not be marginalized. Interestingly, this justification of 'caring ethics' is itself ethical, and appears to hang on an appeal to justice.

Gilligan's studies are regularly cited in discussions of the 'ethics of caring' (Liaschenko & Peter 2003, Råholm 2003, van Hooft 2003, Watson & Smith 2002). Unlike Heidegger's philosophy, it is rooted in empirical findings, so any attempt to derive a 'caring ethics' from Gilligan's work would be seriously compromised if these studies proved unreliable. Unfortunately, there is persuasive evidence suggesting that they are. A review of over 100 psychological studies by Lawrence Walker notes: 'sex differences in moral reasoning in late adolescence and youth are rare' (Walker 1984 p 681). Another review observes that there is 'very little support in the psychological literature for the notion that girls are more aware of others' feelings . . . than boys. Sex differences in empathy are rarely found and are generally very small when they are reported' (Colby & Damon 1983 p 475). It would appear that Gilligan's findings are not typical. Moreover, even feminist writers have expressed a degree of scepticism about her methods: 'Gilligan . . . never quantified anything. The reader never learns anything about 136 of the 144 people from [one of her studies], as only 8 are quoted in the book. One probably does not have to be a trained researcher to worry about this tactic' (Crosby 1991 p 124).

There is nothing to prevent writers promoting an 'ethics of caring', even if there is no robust evidence that anyone actually adopts the 'caring voice' in their approach to moral issues and dilemmas. However, a good reason for recommending it will have disappeared, and the arguments for claiming that a 'caring ethics' can be given analytical support will have to take a different form. The possibilities boil down to: (1) an alternative meta-ethical grounding; and (2) further attempts to make the normative claims of 'caring ethics' look plausible (it would help to explain, specifically, what these claims are). However, I do not believe that either of these strategies has any chance of succeeding.

CONCLUSION

I have argued that there are at least two ambiguities that make an evaluation of the 'ethics of caring' difficult. One poses the question: is 'caring' one moral value among others, or the dominant value, or possibly an exclusive value? The other concerns the fact that the 'emergent' sense of 'care' is three distinct senses run together: the affective, the cognitive and the motivational. Despite these ambiguities, I have commented on two versions of the 'caring ethic': a strong version, which proposes that nurses form personal relationships with their patients, and a weak version, which, although its specific claims have never been spelled out, can be identified in a series of characteristics constantly alluded to in the literature. The strong version is a failure. The weaker version is profoundly inadequate as a public-service ethic because it ignores the most significant moral questions associated with providing healthcare services to large numbers of people. Finally, I have considered two meta-ethical arguments that have been used in an effort to establish the viability of an 'ethics of caring'; neither works.

Putting it succinctly, the 'caring ethic' is hopelessly *incomplete*, at best, and cannot be the *foundation* for an ethics of nursing. Surprisingly, however, this gloss suggests an alternative line of thought. Can care ethicists get part of what they want from some other moral theory? A theory in which caring, in some form, would have a role? Might that be acceptable, even if 'caring' was subordinate to some other set of concepts? Even if those other concepts set limits to caring, and made it subject to rationality? The answer to these questions, with one exception, might well be 'yes'.

One possibility is to explore the place of 'caring' in Kantian ethics. Although the 'ethics of caring' is regarded as the antithesis of a Kantian 'ethics of principle' (Benner et al 1994), the hostility to Kant is based on a reading of him long since superseded in philosophy (Paley 2002b). According to several writers, we no longer have reason to think that 'the care perspective and the perspective of the moral law are, in fact, mutually exclusive' (Nagl-Docekal 1997 p 106). Of course, there are some major differences between 'caring ethics' and Kantian theory; and the Kantian view holds all the advantages. It is still possible, however, to suggest that Kantian ethics 'qualifies the care ethic by locating it within a fuller account of moral conduct and moral character' (Paley 2002b p 141). In particular, by placing reason, not emotion, at the centre of moral thinking, Kantian theory makes possible an ethics of the one–many and the many–many, and therefore an ethics of equity and justice in health care. It also provides a necessary check on unrestrained, unevidenced and unanalysed 'moral knowing'.

The other possibility is that the 'caring ethic' might be incorporated into utilitarianism. This is the line taken by Kuhse in a book that should be compulsory reading (Kuhse 1997). She introduces the idea of 'dispositional care', which is 'an openness to apprehend the health-related reality of the other', and which she regards as 'a proper and necessary part of a two-level utilitarian approach' (p 150–151). This incorporation, however, comes at a price – the same price as that exacted by the Kantian view: reason rules. In the case of utilitarianism, there would be much greater emphasis on evidence. In order to maximize well-being, we need to know what interventions will lead to what outcomes. A utilitarian 'ethics of care', whatever its other characteristics, would primarily be an 'ethics of evidence'.

Both Kantian and utilitarian theories embody one–many and many–many relations, as well as one–one relations; so they are not limited to individual-to-individual concerns. They can certainly find a space for 'caring', but only at a price that care ethicists might find unacceptable. That price is rationality. What rationality provides is scepticism, equity, evidence. There can be no reasonable ethics, and certainly no professional ethics, which does not satisfy all three of these requirements.

References

Allmark P 1995 Can there be an ethics of care? Journal of Medical Ethics 21, 19–24.

Appleby J, Harrison A, Devlin N 2003 What is the real cost of more patient choice? King's Fund, London.

Benhabib S 1986 The generalized and the concrete other: the Kohlberg–Gilligan controversy and feminist theory. Praxis International 5:402–424.

Benner P 2000 The roles of embodiment, emotion and lifeworld for rationality and agency in nursing practice. Nursing Philosophy 1:5–19.

Benner P, Janson-Bjerklie S, Ferketich S, Becker G 1994 Moral dimensions of living with a chronic illness: autonomy, responsibility, and the limits of control. In: Benner P (ed) Interpretive phenomenology: embodiment, caring and ethics in health and illness. Sage, Thousand Oaks, CA, p 225–254.

Bevis EO 1981 Caring: a life force. In: Leininger M (ed) Caring: an essential human need. Charles B. Slack, Thorofare, NJ, p 49–59.

Bishop AH, Scudder JR 1990 The practical, moral and personal sense of nursing: a phenomenological philosophy of practice. State University of New York Press, New York.

Bowden P 1997 Caring: gender sensitive ethics. Routledge, London.

Campbell AV 1984 Moderated love: a theology of professional care. SPCK, London.

Cheung J 1998 Caring as the ontological and epistemological foundations of nursing: a view of caring from the perspectives of Australian nurses. International Journal of Nursing Practice 4:225–233.

Colby A, Damon W 1983 Listening to a different voice: a review of Gilligan's In A Different Voice. Merrill-Palmer Quarterly 29:473–481.

Crosby FJ 1991 Juggling: the unexpected advantages of balancing career and home for women and their families. Free Press, New York.

Curzer HJ 1993 Is care a virtue for health care professionals? The Journal of Medicine and Philosophy 18:51–69.

Downie R, Telfer E 1980 Caring and curing. Methuen, London.

Dunlop M 1994 Is a science of caring possible? In: Benner P (ed) Interpretive phenomenology: embodiment, caring, and ethics in health and illness. Sage, Thousand Oaks, CA, p 27–42.

Dyson L 1997 An ethic of caring: conceptual and practical issues. Nursing Inquiry 4:196–201.

Farias V 1989 Heidegger and Nazism. Temple University Press, Philadelphia.

Fawcett J, Watson J, Neuman B, Walker PH, Fitzpatrick JJ 2001 On nursing theories and evidence. Journal of Nursing Scholarship 33:115–119.

Fritsche J 1999 Historical destiny and national socialism in Heidegger's Being and Time. University of California Press, Berkeley, CA.

Fry S 1989 Toward a theory of nursing ethics. Advances in Nursing Science 11:9–21.

Fry S 1991 A theory of caring: pitfalls and promises. In: Gaut DA and Leininger M (eds) Caring: the compassionate heder. National League for Nursing, New York.

Gadow S 1995 Narrative and exploration: toward a poetics of knowledge in nursing. Nursing Inquiry 2:211–214.

Gilligan C 1982 In a different voice: psychological theory and women's development. Harvard University Press, Cambridge, MA.

Gottman JM, Murray JD, Swanson CC, Tyson R, Swanson KR 2002 The mathematics of marriage: dynamic nonlinear models. The MIT Press, Cambridge, MA.

Greenhalgh J, Vanhanen L, Kungäs H 1998 Nursing caring behaviours. Journal of Advanced Nursing 27:927–932.

Griffin AP 1983 A philosophical analysis of caring in nursing. Journal of Advanced Nursing 8:289–295.

Grimshaw J 1986 Philosophy and feminist thinking. University of Minnesota Press, Minneapolis.

Hall C 2002 'We can't pull the plug on a conscious patient we have known for a year'. Daily Telegraph, 7 March 2002, London.

Heidegger M 1962 Being and time. Blackwell, Oxford.

Heidegger M 1993 Letter on humanism. In: Krell DF (ed) Martin Heidegger: basic writings, revised and expanded edition. Routledge, Kegan and Paul, London, p 213–265.

Hoagland SL 1991 Some thoughts on 'Caring'. In: Card C (ed) Feminist ethics. University of Kansas Press, Lawrence, p 246–263.

Holmes S 1989 The permanent structure of antiliberal thought. In: Rosenblum NL (ed) Liberalism and the moral life. Harvard University Press, Cambridge, MA, p 227–253.

Jacono BJ 1993 Caring is loving. Journal of Advanced Nursing 18:192–194.

Kapborg I, Bertero C 2003 The phenomenon of caring from the novice student nurse's perspective: a qualitative content analysis. International Nursing Review 50:183.

Koehn D 1998 Rethinking feminist ethics: care, trust and empathy. Routledge, London.

Kuhse H 1997 Caring: nurses, women and ethics. Blackwell, Oxford.

Kyle TV 1995 The concept of caring: a review of the literature. Journal of Advanced Nursing 21:506–514.

Lea A, Watson R 1996 Caring research and concepts: a selected review of the literature. Journal of Advanced Nursing 5:71–77.

Lea A, Watson R, Deary IJ 1998 Caring in nursing: a multivariate analysis. Journal of Advanced Nursing 28:662–671.

Leininger M, Watson J 1990 The caring imperative in education. National League for Nursing, New York.

Liaschenko J, Peter E 2003 Feminist ethics. In: Tschudin V (ed) Approaches to ethics: nursing beyond boundaries. Butterworth Heinemann, Edinburgh, p 33–43.

McCance TV, McKenna HP, Boore JRP 1997 Caring: dealing with a difficult concept. International Journal of Nursing Studies 34:241–248.

McCance TV, McKenna HP, Boore JRP 2001 Exploring caring using narrative methodology: an analysis of the approach. Journal of Advanced Nursing 33:350–356.

Mackintosh C 2000 Is there a place for 'care' within nursing? International Journal of Nursing Studies 37:321–327.

Manning R 1992 Speaking from the heart: a feminist perspective on ethics. Rowman & Littlefield, Lanham, MD.

Maslach C 1982 Burnout: the cost of caring. Prentice-Hall, Englewood Cliffs, NJ.

Mayeroff M 1971 On caring. Harper and Row, New York.

Morse J, Solber SM, Neander WL, Bottorff JL, Johnson JL 1990 Concepts of caring and caring as a concept. Advances in Nursing Science 13:1–14.

Mossialos E, Thomson S 2003 Access to health care in the European Union. In: Morgan M (ed) Access to health care. Routledge, London, p 143–173.

Mulhall S, Swift A 1996 Liberals and communitarians, 2nd edn. Blackwell, Oxford.

Nagl-Docekal H 1997 Feminist ethics: how it could benefit from Kant's moral philosophy. In: Schott RM (ed) Feminist interpretations of Immanuel Kant. Pennsylvania State University Press, University Park, PA, p 101–124.

Noddings N 1984 Caring: a feminine approach to ethics and moral education. University of California Press, Berkeley.

O'Neill O (1996) Towards justice and virtue: a constructive account of practical reasoning. Cambridge University Press, Cambridge.

Oppenheimer H 2003 Mattering. In: Tschudin V (ed) Approaches to ethics: nursing beyond boundaries. Butterworth Heinemann, Edinburgh, p 73–82.

Paley J 2000 Heidegger and the ethics of care. Nursing Philosophy 1:64–75.

Paley J 2002a Caring as a slave morality: Nietzschean themes in nursing ethics. Journal of Advanced Nursing 40:25–35.

Paley J 2002b Virtues of autonomy: the Kantian ethics of care. Nursing Philosophy 3:133–143.

Paley J 2004a Commentary on Wiman and Wikblad: 'Caring and uncaring encounters in an emergency department'. Journal of Clinical Nursing 13:122–123.

Paley J 2004b Commentary: the discourse of moral suffering. Journal of Advanced Nursing 47:364–365.

Peacock JW, Nolan PW 2000 Care under threat in the modern world. Journal of Advanced Nursing 32:1066–1070.

Philipse H 1998 Heidegger's philosophy of being: a critical interpretation. Princeton University Press, Princeton, NJ.

Råholm M-B 2003 Caritative caring ethics: a description reflected through the Aristotelian terms phronesis, techne and episteme. In: Tschudin V (ed) Approaches to ethics: nursing beyond boundaries. Butterworth Heinemann, Edinburgh, p 13–23.

Ray MA 1981 A philosophical analysis of caring within nursing. In: Leininger M (ed) Caring; an essential human need. Charles B. Slack, Thorofare, NJ, p 25–36.

Roach MS 1984 Caring, the human mode of being: implications for nursing. Faculty of Nursing, University of Toronto, Toronto.

Stockdale M, Warelow PJ 2000 Is the complexity of care a paradox? Journal of Advanced Nursing 31:1258–1264.

Swanson KM 1999 What is known about caring in nursing science. In: Shaver JJF (ed) Handbook of clinical nursing research. Sage, Thousand Oaks, CA, p 31–60.

van Hooft S 1987 Caring and professional commitment. Australian Journal of Advanced Nursing 4:29–38.

van Hooft S 2003 Caring and ethics in nursing. In: Tschudin V (ed) Approaches to ethics: nursing beyond boundaries. Butterworth Heinemann, Edinburgh, p 1–12.

Walker LJ 1984 Sex differences in the development of moral reasoning: a critical review. Child Development 55:67–691.

Warelow PJ 1996 Is caring the ethical ideal? Journal of Advanced Nursing 24:655–661.

Watson J 1985 Nursing, human science and human care: a theory of nursing. Appleton-Century-Crofts, Norwalk, CT.

Watson J 1988 Nursing: human science and human care. National League for Nursing, New York.

Watson J, Smith MC 2002 Caring science and the science of unitary human beings: a trans-theoretical discourse for nursing knowledge development. Journal of Advanced Nursing 37:452–461.

Wilson TD 2002 Strangers to ourselves: discovering the adaptive unconscious. The Belknap Press of Harvard University Press, Cambridge, MA.

Chapter 15

Caring and caring ethics depicted in selected literature: what we know and what we need to ask

Anne J. Davis and Marsha Fowler

CHAPTER CONTENTS

INTRODUCTION

Everyone wants a competent nurse and we recognize such nurses when in their presence, but what does competent mean in this context? Some people would include as a main characteristic of competence the notion of caring. The literature asks what characteristics these nurses demonstrate that permit us to say they are caring. Generally, nurses view themselves as members of a caring profession, although the profession has striven to be more scientific and professional. Caring is vital to life and not limited to nursing. Caring is central in numerous relationships; however, caring remains difficult to conceptualize and especially in western ethics where historically it has not been a dominant value.

Why did Western philosophy mostly overlook the construct, caring? Many societies have historically been patriarchal in character: male-dominated, male-identified, and male-centered (Johnson 1997). In such societies caring was, and in many places remains, women's work and was therefore defined as socially and economically not important. Caring for children, elderly, sick and poor people usually fell to women.

Another potential reason for the lack of caring in literature is the dominance of natural sciences in the west. It is not possible to describe human capacities in context-free features and abstracted from their everyday context as the natural sciences have done (Dreyfus 1986). The nurse anthropologist, Madeleine Leininger, points out that caring is highly context-dependent and that this creates certain difficulties in developing a science of caring (Leininger 1978).

Caring has been written about by several philosophers and Milton Mayeroff has written one of the clearest philosophical statements available (Mayeroff 1971).

This chapter traces the development of caring and caring ethics in selected nursing literature, limited mainly to major authors who forwarded this construct and selected contributions from non-nurses. Space does not allow us to include the entire literature that either promotes caring as central to nursing, or questions the adequacy of caring as a basis for nursing ethics. We have included some literature that supports caring and some literature that questions it because we believe that teachers should know something of both sides of the debate. In addition, we provide some general ideas and questions that teachers can use in the classroom and make general suggestions for the teaching of caring ethics. The terms caring ethics, care ethics, and an ethics of care are found in the literature and are used interchangeably here.

The word 'care' has been central in the nursing literature for many years and is used in two distinct ways that differ from one another but also interact: (1) taking care of or giving care to and (2) caring about.

THE FIRST MEANING OF CARING: GIVING CARE TO

The first definition means performing activities for, to, and with another person thought beneficial for that person. Most people think of this when they say, nursing care. This nursing care usually involves two people whose connection is mainly governed by the responsibility of one person to respond to and serve the needs of the other. Unlike relationships of family members or friends, these relationships are usually between strangers who often lack a shared history and they occur within the professional norms and sanctions (Bowen 1997).

THE SECOND MEANING OF CARING: EMOTIONAL RESPONSE TO THE PATIENT

The second meaning of caring reflects how one person feels about or feels committed to and responds to another person. Generally speaking, this caring is an emotional response that includes a concern for the other, places emphasis on relationship, attachment, openness, and attentiveness to the needs of the one cared for. This is not about the various tasks that nurses perform, but about their attitude towards the other person – the one receiving care – and their engagement with that other person. This meaning depicts the psychosocial dimensions of the nurse–patient relationship and has become a value with moral connotations that believes that nurses should be caring, empathic and attentive to patients. The good nurse gives competent nursing care and cares about the patient in an empathic manner. This meaning of caring has attained a special place in the nursing discourse since the 1980s.

Regardless of the approach to the study of caring in nursing, two common themes emerge in the literature:

- Caring is not one single entity and in the strictest sense it cannot be measured
- Caring spans the instrumental (first meaning) and existential or expressive (second meaning) aspects of nursing (Lea et al 1998)

THE NURSE–PATIENT RELATIONSHIP AND CARING

Jean Watson sees care as a foundational value in nursing and views the ideal caring nurse–patient relationship as total encounter (Watson 1985, 1994, 1999, 2004). This relationship should be deep, meaningful and intimate and akin to what the philosopher Martin Buber calls the I–Thou relationship as opposed to the I–It relationship in which the other becomes an object of attention or an It rather than a person (Buber 1970).

Watson writes that in true transpersonal caring the nurse forms a union with the other person that transcends the physical so that both persons are freed from their separation and isolation. The nurse enters the life space of each patient (Watson 1985). The nurse–patient relationship differs from many other types of relationships between people. Many relationships are fleeting because of the social norms dictating appropriate behaviour combined with the realities of time and energy. While we are respectful and polite, we invest little of ourselves in these relationships. This can be true with our co-workers, neighbours, and even with some friends. Usually people come together to achieve a specific goal, to solve a specific problem, or to enjoy each other's company. Many adults have limited intimate caring relationships, except with some family members and friends.

Caring and caring ethics emphasizes the nurse–patient relationship and assumes a relationship between these two people. Patients can interact with numerous nurses but do they have a relationship with each one? That depends on how we define relationship. It also depends on how the patient and the nurse define what is important in their interpersonal contacts. One study reported that nurse educators consider comfort and trusting factors more important, whereas patients said behaviour associated with physical care are more important (Komorita et al 1991). In this study, nurse educators think the second meaning of emotional caring is more important while patients think the first meaning, giving care to, is more important.

In preparing to teach caring and caring ethics, an examination of the nurse–patient relationship literature to determine what we know about that dyad may be enlightening. Some questions for classroom discussion are:

- How does the literature inform us as to the nature of the nurse–patient relationship?
- Do all patients have a patient–nurse relationship?

- If so, how is this relationship developed and maintained?
- Can numerous nurses collectively be considered to have one relationship with a patient?
- Can each encounter, including fleeting ones, between a nurse and a patient be considered a relationship with a patient?
- Do all patients want or need a caring nurse–patient relationship (Davis 2001)?

Since concerned caring for the other occurs within the context of a nurse–patient relationship, this context needs examination not only as an ideal but as a reality factor in the clinical nursing world.

Nursing places high value on relationship but can leave it unexamined. To understand 'relationship' more fully, we must make it problematic and not take it for granted as a given good. An examination does not imply that the nurse–patient relationship lacks importance, but opens this ideal of relationship to scrutiny. This helps us to understand caring relationships and caring ethics better. In recent explorations of this long held nursing value of caring empathically, an attempt at a more systematically articulated meaning has been made in order to understand what we mean when we say a nurse cares about a patient.

PROBLEMS OF DEFINITION AND THEORETICAL GROUNDING

One problem in this attempt has been that different basic definitions are given by authors to the phrase 'caring about', therefore it is unclear exactly what is under discussion. Such words as disposition, feeling, sentiment, virtue and commitment have been used in the definition of caring (McCance et al 1997). These differences are important because they have implications for how we proceed to develop theory. Some nurses writing in the 1980s about caring are now attempting to develop a theory of care ethics. A basic and as yet not entirely clear or agreed upon definition of caring will provide the foundation for the development of a care ethics.

In 1990 authors concluded that knowledge development related to caring in nursing was limited by several factors:

- The lack of refinement of caring theory
- The lack of definitions of caring attributes
- The neglect in examining caring from the dialectic perspective
- The focus of the theorists and researchers on the nurse to the exclusion of the patient (Morse et al 1990)

In 1991, a slightly different team of nurses published a comparative analysis of conceptualizations and theories of caring. They used five major conceptualizations of caring:

- A human trait
- A moral imperative
- An affect

- An interpersonal interaction
- As intervention

They concluded that caring as a construct, was relatively undeveloped, had not been clearly explicated and often lacked relevance for nursing practice (Morse et al 1991).

Some years later, authors conducted a content analysis on caring and identified four critical attributes of caring:

- Serious attention
- Concern
- Providing for
- Getting to know the patient

They also found that amount of time, respect for persons and an intention to care were identified as antecedents of caring (McCance et al 1997).

When teaching care ethics, this issue of definition can provide an early focus for the teacher and can raise the following questions:

- How do the nursing literature and other sources inform us on this question of definition?
- Do students or teachers agree that nursing lacks a coherent definition of caring?
- Is a care ethics possible if nursing has not defined the key concept of care in a coherent fashion?
- Is the nursing profession any closer to developing a coherent care definition and theory than in the 1980s when the nursing literature began more specifically to focus on these ideas?
- If the nursing profession remains unclear on what constitutes caring, so fundamental to a care ethics, how do we proceed with the development of this ethics?
- How best can we deal with these questions in our preparation as teachers of nursing ethics and in the classroom with students?

This is not to say that people examining this issue of definition are anti-caring but it does mean they think a solid foundation seems necessary for the development of any ethical theory.

Another issue in the development of the central value of caring goes beyond the problem of definition. Caring is a large construct that could include a set of behaviours based on concern, compassion, worry, fondness, affection, a commitment to a person, being careful and attentive to details, responding in a sensitive way to the other's situation, listening to the other, or all of the above and more. In examining these non-mutually exclusive caring behaviours, one question becomes: is caring a virtue? Stan van Hooft, a philosopher, says that caring can be understood as a holistic virtue. Although courage is also a virtue, courage is a trait that lies dormant and comes to expression only as specific occasions demand it. Caring is a framework or form given to all aspects of our existence insofar as that existence expresses our caring for others. In caring there is also a concern for oneself (van Hooft 2003).

Virtues, or aspects of character, and virtue ethics have been part of nursing since Nightingale's time and then reflected what Victorian society considered morally right behaviour for middle- and upper-class women. If caring is a virtue, then caring ethics belongs in virtue ethics because caring is an additional virtue (see Chapters 10, 11 and 12 on virtue ethics).

Is caring a duty like the duties of truth-telling, promise keeping and non-infliction of harm? Or is caring an end, a telos something we seek, such as health, well-being, human dignity and respect?

Should we conceptually place caring and caring behaviour in the theories of philosophy, psychology, theology or some other knowledge base such as feminist ethics? (See Chapters 16, 17 and 18 for a discussion on feminist ethics.) Recently, scientists have said that genes determine altruistic behaviour but more studies are needed to support this (Singer et al 2004, Wilson 2003). If this is true or not:

- Can altruistic behaviour, so akin to caring, be taught and – importantly – can students learn and apply this knowledge to their interactions with patients?
- Is there a difference between knowing about caring and developing caring behaviour?
- Is caring a set of communication techniques called the therapeutic use of self, as taught to psychiatric nurses in the 1950s–1960s?

How best to explore and examine caring as a construct and what knowledge base to use remain important questions because the way we answer them will determine the form that caring will take. Various fields of knowledge have different frames for definitions, questions, answers and what counts as important. Even within one field of knowledge, different concepts arise to create various theoretical foundations. For example, Bandman and Bandman (1990) indicate that an ethics of caring gains appeal from several philosophical sources:

- The early Greek philosopher Aristotle's emphasis on natural virtues such as wisdom, prudence and temperance
- The thirteenth-century Italian philosophical theologian Aquinas' altruism or love-based ethics
- The eighteenth-century Scottish philosopher David Hume's utilitarianism, which bases ethics on people's wants and likes and the avoidance of people's dislikes and aversions

Nursing's focus on this second sense of caring (the emotional response to the patient) has led to the development of care ethics also being referred to as an ethics 'in a different voice' that attempts to challenge the dominant principle-based ethical theory of justice (see Chapter 7).

Some take the position that nurses feel fulfilment in their professional role when the two meanings of care – to give care and to care about – converge so that articulation of the professional sense of practice discloses the moral sense. Caring and care ethics can create this convergence (Bishop & Scudder 1990).

ETHICS IN A DIFFERENT VOICE: THE BEGINNING

Many consider two non-nurses, Carol Gilligan and Nel Noddings, to have given birth to care ethics. Gilligan's first book (1982) and Noddings' book on feminine caring (1984) received great attention and critique. Gilligan said that people use two different moral voices: a language of justice or impartiality that is male, and a relational language of self and social relationships or a voice of care that is female.

Noddings' book on feminine ethics and moral education discusses the two roots of caring: (1) the universal memory of being cared for and (2) the natural sympathy human beings feel for each other that enables them to feel the pain and joy of others (Noddings 1984).

Both authors detail the importance in ethics of personal histories and context and criticize principle-based ethics for overlooking these factors. These works had a major impact that included the development of caring as a major construct in feminist ethics and nursing ethics.

Some authors think of care ethics as an embryonic form of feminist ethics and a new ethics theory. For example, Rosemarie Tong (1993) finds the distinction between feminine and feminist ethics useful. She makes a contrast between care-focused feminine ethics and power-focused feminist ethics and says that feminine ethics needs to rehabilitate culturally associated feminine values such as empathy and kindness whereas a power-focused feminist approach has the duty to eliminate or modify any system, social structure, or set of norms that contribute to women's oppression. This statement has implications for nursing and an ethics of care.

One feminist author has argued for a necessary connection between care and justice and details their compatibility (Friedman 1987). Notions of compatibility also have implications for nursing's development of a care ethics.

Aristotle believed that women and men differ morally and wrote:

Moral virtues belong to all but the temperance of a man and a woman, or the courage and justice of a man and of a woman, are not as Socrates maintained, the same; the courage of a man is shown in commanding, of a woman in obeying. (Aristotle 1986)

Other recent western philosophers believed that women could not or should not be sufficiently rational to be moral. Sigmund Freud embraced this idea and used these social constructs of the female in the development of psychoanalysis. Throughout his theory, developed in the nineteenth century, he did not state directly but assumed that the male is the norm and the female is a deviation of the norm (Freud 1923/1990). The nineteenth-century Victorians believed that women had certain virtues different from men that limited women to caring work such as nursing and teaching. These beliefs in the lack of female rationality and specific female virtues helped to keep women from participating in the wider world. They could not vote, work outside the home, own or inherit property, or enrol in colleges and universities. Dominant religions helped to create and supported the social definitions of the good woman. Women should be passive, submissive, loyal and caring. This history reveals the fact that people do not live in a social vacuum, but rather that they live in a complex social world and this in large part influences how they see and act in that world. This has major ramifications for nursing as it attempts to define its boundaries and essence (Bowen 1997, Chambliss 1996, Kuhse 1997).

The legacy of these social, philosophical, and religious beliefs remains in some form today, although changes have occurred internationally but in an uneven fashion. One could argue that these beliefs about womanly virtues became a major factor that helped Nightingale to develop modern nursing as a female occupation.

An important potential issue that needs addressing is the danger of invoking the concept, gender essentialism, that assumes that women and men have unique characteristics and dispositions determined by their biological differences (Volbrecht 2002). Gender essentialism allowed the discrimination of women to occur. As early as 1792 the English feminist writer, Mary Wollstonecraft, viewed such ideas as a double-edged sword more capable of hurting than helping women (Wollstonecraft 1792/1996). Some writers believe it is not gender but class and education that make the difference in the way people view and try to solve ethical problems (Walker et al 1984).

Some authors viewed caring as the essence and central focus of nursing before Gilligan and Noddings published. For example, Leininger published that idea in 1977 and continued with this topic into the 1990s (Leininger 1977, 1980, 1981, 1990). Nursing journals published articles on caring but not until the 1980s and 1990s did a critical mass of literature begin to develop on caring and caring ethics in a renewed examination and extension of an old central value in nursing. During these years Patricia Benner (Benner 1984, 1994, Benner & Wrubel 1989, Benner et al 1994) and Watson (1985, 1994, 1999) published works that added considerably to the literature on caring. These contributions have implications for the development of caring ethics. Other North American and British nurses made major contributions to the development of caring ethics. Some of these contributions will be noted below. We are less familiar with nurses from other parts of the world who may also have contributed to the development of caring ethics; this is a major limitation of this chapter.

CARE AND CARING ETHICS IN THE NURSING LITERATURE

Anyone teaching a nursing ethics course that includes care ethics should be familiar with these nursing pioneers and others who developed caring and caring ethics. To agree or disagree with them, teachers need an understanding of what they have written and their contributions to the nursing dialogue.

Principle-based ethics asks 'what should I do to be ethical?', while caring ethics asks 'how should the carer interact with the one being cared for?' Watson reacts to principle-based ethics by pointing out that in nursing and caring we are not concerned primarily with ethical principles and laws that indicate an act is right or wrong. Caring, as a moral ideal, entails a commitment to the protection and enhancement of human dignity and preservation of humanity. An ethics of moral caring and curing needs a nursing ethics that favours subjective thinking, not objective principles (Watson 1985). This is a reaction against rational principle-based ethics that also has limitations. Helga Kuhse, a philosopher, raises the question: 'can an ethics of care be spelled out adequately without reliance on some principles, rules, or norms, that is, without a prior defence of the values or principles we should be caring about?' (Kuhse 1997 p147).

Benner's research of nursing competencies represents one of the most extensive and thorough articulations of nursing practice available. She focuses on the knowledge embedded in actual practice and believes that nurses have not explored this knowledge in actual nursing practice because they have not understood the difference between theoretical knowledge and practical knowledge (Benner 1984). Aristotle defined practical wisdom as one of the chief intellectual virtues that includes knowledge of how to secure the aims of human life. Patricia Benner and Judith Wrubel considered the facets of personhood that influence and are influenced by the stress of disruption to the usual smooth functioning of a person's existence (Benner & Wrubel 1989). They say that the experience of illness depends on its personal meanings to the patient and an understanding of each patient's own personal involvement and commitment allows nurses a healing entrance into patients' disrupted world.

Benner argues in her discussion of individual practice that nurses do care by displaying clinical competence and caring attitudes in the nurse–patient relationship. To some extent she also deals with the tension between personal caring and the impersonal context in which it occurs. Disillusionment with institutional nursing and the belief that the organization and social constraints in hospitals render nurses impotent remain widespread in the professional culture. Nursing care can be determined by its institutional demands rather than by the patients' personal needs. Schedules, resources, efficiency requirements, physicians' orders, routines, and shift work combine to structure relationships with patients (Chambliss 1996).

Sally Gadow, a nurse philosopher, began writing in the 1970s and has influenced a generation of nurses and other caregivers. In 2003, the journal *Nursing Philosophy* devoted an entire issue to her work, noting her major contribution in nursing practice, education and research. Gadow's recurring themes include the demand for objectivity in science and the subjectivity of both patient and nurse; the sick person as object of scientific knowledge and the sick person as the subject of a lived life; the importance of the body and embodiment to living with these contradictions; the significance of meaning in the experience of illness and the significance of that experience to healing; relational narratives as a way of moral engagement that resists the dangers that beneficence poses for the sick person; and the importance of interpretive inquiry. Gadow's work, pertinent to an understanding of caring and caring ethics, includes articles that specifically address the nurse and patient in a caring relationship (Gadow 1980, 1985, 1990).

Sara Fry, another nurse philosopher, also contributed to the caring literature. In 1989 she published two articles on caring, challenging the presumption of medical ethics and its principle-based and moral justification ethics as an appropriate model for nursing ethics (Fry 1989a). She maintained that the development of nursing ethics, as a field of inquiry, largely paralleled developments within bioethical ethics. She pointed to growing evidence that the future development of a nursing ethics theory might not follow a similar pattern because the value foundations of nursing ethics are derived from the nature of the nurse–patient relationship rather than from ideas of patient good, rights-based autonomy or the social contract of professional practice found in medical ethics. Fry maintained that the value of caring ought to hold a central place in any theory of nursing ethics (Fry 1989b) and later (in 1996) makes the point that:

> *The context of nursing practice requires a moral view of persons rather than a theory of moral action or behavior or a system of moral justification. Present theories of medical ethics . . . do not fit in with the practical realities of nurses' decision making in patient care and that, as results, tends to deplete the moral agency of nursing practice rather than enhance it.* (Fry et al 1996)

Fry says that some contemporary moral theorists have criticized traditional moral theory for its inadequacies in accommodating the demands of special relationships in that past moral theorists did not envision today's moral challenges. She views care-based reasoning, caring, and the ethics of care as contemporary responses to the need for new moral theories adequate for today's moral questions (Fry 1989a).

Sister M Simone Roach, a Canadian, was an early and major force in the development of the contemporary Canadian code for nurses. She has published several books among her many activities in Canadian nursing ethics (Roach 1992, 1997, 1998). Another Canadian, Janet Storch, has been active nationally and internationally in nursing ethics for some years and recently published an important book that discussed caring ethics among a wide array of topics (Storch et al 2004).

Verena Tschudin, editor of the international journal, *Nursing Ethics*, has focused her writing on ethics, including caring ethics. As the editor of the only nursing journal given over entirely to ethics, her contribution continues as both a facilitator and a scholar. She has authored or edited several books that have a wide international circulation (Tschudin 2003). Megan-Jane Johnstone, an Australian, has also been active in national and international nursing ethics and has authored several important publications, including a book on ethics in nursing (Johnstone 1989).

Katie Eriksson has written extensively on caring and suffering since 1990; however, her contributions are published only in Swedish. With a colleague she wrote an article in English focused on the caring conversation (Fredriksson & Eriksson 2003).

This attempt at theoretically developing caring and caring ethics is very new when compared with virtue ethics and principle-based ethics and, like them, did not arrive fully grown and mature. The growing pains that caring ethics experiences are not unique but represent the usual progression towards refining knowledge.

A topic has come of age when extensively critiqued. While some might not like such critique because they view caring above these debates, nevertheless, such critique and dialogue remain vital to the development of knowledge. We arrive at faith in one way and at knowledge by quite another method.

Nursing ethics teachers should be familiar with the caring literature and with two important journals, *Nursing Philosophy* published since July 2000 and *Nursing Ethics* published since March 1994. In addition, many other journals publish this literature.

TEACHING CARING AND CARING ETHICS

No longer can teachers of nursing ethics completely avoid caring ethics. The latest edition of the well known book by Thomas Beauchamp and James Childress has a chapter entitled *Ethics of care: relationship-based accounts* (Beauchamp & Childress 2001).

An important question for all nursing teachers is: Can caring be taught? One answer is: Yes, caring can be taught, but there is a difference between teaching people about caring as a construct and teaching people to be caring. The first type of teaching should be easy while the second may be more difficult. Some people might say that authentic caring cannot be taught to young adult students. This depends on how one defines caring and where it fits into the larger body of knowledge. Watson maintains that caring can be taught. She lists carative factors that include the formation of a humanistic–altruistic value system that begins developmentally at an early age with values shared with parents. Several authors suggest that caring based on humanistic values and altruistic behaviour develops through examination of one's own views, beliefs, and interactions with various cultures and personal growth experiences, and can be taught and learned (Bevis & Watson 2000, Leininger & Watson 1990, Watson 2002). People, and that means mostly women, enter nursing for many reasons. Some may be caring people on arrival but others may not be especially caring. If so, what happens to these students? Do they learn caring and, if so, what is the nature of that caring? Benner and Wrubel found numerous examples of caring nurses in their study of specific nurse–patient relationships (Benner & Wrubel 1989). Have they always been caring; did they learn to be caring in nursing school; did they learn this behaviour as a practising nurse? The answer may be yes to all three of these possibilities.

Pioneers such as Watson and Benner made their contribution in caring and caring ethics because they thought nurses lacked adequate moral voice and agency in their work, and the reasons for this situation may be a combination of using biomedical ethical theory that some say does not fit nursing, plus the nature of the work setting. In 1978, Anne Davis and

Mila Aroskar raised questions about the possible social and institutional constraints that can inhibit the ethical practice of nursing (Davis & Aroskar 1978). Although both Watson and Benner discuss the importance of the nurse–patient relationship, they pay scant attention to the context that led them to undertake their work. In any classroom discussion on caring ethics, as with any ethics theory, it is useful to discuss this larger context within which nursing ethics occurs. In the clinical world of nurses and patients, ethics is not lofty abstractions but a set of behaviours based on ethical thinking and acting that occurs in the context of healthcare facility norms and demands.

Most of us and most of the time want a clinically competent and sensitive-to-others nurse when we are patients in the healthcare system. Can nursing ethics teachers help to prepare such nurses? One way might be to focus on the developments made in caring and see them not as ideology and a given good but as important topics in need of further critique, research, and development.

SUMMARY OF QUESTIONS FOR TEACHERS OF NURSING ETHICS

This chapter listed questions for nursing ethics teachers to ask themselves and students so as to become more aware. We grouped these and additional questions by subtopics in the chapter.

1. **Caring and relationship: concepts basic to caring ethics:**

a. Why did Western philosophy mostly overlook caring?

b. What is the nature of the nurse–patient relationship?
    - How does the nursing literature inform us on this relationship?
    - Do all patients have, need or want a nurse–patient relationship?
    - How is a relationship developed and maintained?
    - Can each encounter be a relationship between nurse and patient?
    - Can a nurse be caring even in fleeting encounters with patients?
    - Can a patient have one relationship with a collective of nurses?

c. What is the definition of caring?
    - Does nursing have an adequate definition of caring for clinical work, teaching, research?
    - Where does caring as a construct fit into the organization of knowledge in psychology, philosophy, theology, and genetics?
    - Is caring a virtue?
    - Is caring one of several concepts in feminist ethics?
    - Is caring a duty or is it an end that we want to achieve?

2. **Caring ethics:**

a. Can nursing have an ethics of care without an adequate definition of caring?

b. Can an ethics of caring be fully developed without reliance on some principles, rules, or norms?

c.   What values should nurses be caring about?

d.   Can nurses use caring ethics in their relationships with patients and principle-based ethics to cope with ethical questions outside that relationship?

We wonder if conceptualizing principle-based ethics and caring ethics as opposing and mutually exclusive theories helps nurses in dealing with ethical issues. Both theories have limitations but both may be helpful in understanding the complex world where nurses practice. How can this tension best be taught to students?

SOME FINAL WORDS ON TEACHING

When teaching undergraduates, teachers often provide the knowledge base of a subject but then do not invite students to question too much because they think the students know too little. Ethics may not entirely fit this mould. While students need some basic understanding of ethical theories before they critique them, the question before teachers is: what do we want to accomplish in an ethics class? Certainly the students' further development of ethical awareness and sensitivity is a basic goal. This seems best achieved in a seminar with dialogue where students are actively engaged in the discussion. If the class is large then a combination of lecture, case studies and small group work is possible. One important objective is not only reaching some ethically right action but to think carefully about the process of arriving at that action. Students begin to see various ethical theories at work. They may discuss relationships and context (caring ethics), or rights and duties (principle-based ethics) or the good nurse (virtue ethics) or some combination of these and other theories.

Students' prior experiences with ethical issues in general can be used. As some of the literature indicates that caring ethics needs more development and all ethical theories have limitations, the ethics class can become a wonderful opportunity to enhance students' critical thinking while examining ethical problems. Ethics as education and not indoctrination is assumed in all of these comments.

References

Aristotle 1986 Nichomachean ethics (trans. Irwin T). Hackett, Indianapolis, IN.

Bandman EL, Bandman B 1990 Nursing ethics through the life span, 4th edn. Prentice Hall, Englewood Cliffs, NJ.

Beauchamp TL, Childress JF 2001 Principles of biomedical ethics, 5th edn. Oxford University Press, New York.

Benner P 1984 From novice to expert: excellence and power in clinical nursing practice. Addison-Wesley, Reading, MA.

Benner P (ed) 1994 Interpretive phenomenology: embodiment, caring, and ethics in health and illness. Sage, Thousand Oaks, CA.

Benner P, Wrubel J 1989 Primacy of caring: stress and coping in health and illness. Addison-Wesley, Reading, MA.

Benner P, Hooper-Kyriakidis PL, Stannard D 1994 Clinical wisdom and interventions in critical care: a thinking-in-action approach. Saunders, Philadelphia.

Bevis EO, Watson J 2000 Towards a caring curriculum: a new pedagogy for nursing. Jones and Bartlett, Sudbury, MA.

Bishop AH, Scudder JR Jr 1990 The practical, moral, and personal sense of nursing. State University of New York Press, Albany.

Bowen P 1997 Caring: gender-sensitive ethics. Routledge, London.

Buber M 1970 I and thou, 3rd edn. T&T Clark, Edinburgh.

Chambliss D 1996 Beyond caring: hospital nurses, and the social organization of ethics. University of Chicago Press, Chicago.

Davis AJ 2001 Labelled encounters and experiences: ways of seeing, thinking about and responding to uniqueness. Nursing Philosophy 2:101–111.

Davis AJ, Aroskar MA 1978 Ethical dilemmas and nursing practice. Appleton Lang, Stanford, CT.

Dreyfus HL 1986 Why studies of human capacities modeled on ideal natural science can never achieve their goal. In: Margolis M, Krausy M, Burain RM (eds) Rationality, relativism, and the human sciences. Martinus Nijhoff, Dordrecht, p 3–22.

Fredriksson L, Eriksson K 2003 The ethics of the caring conversation. Nursing Ethics 10:138–148.

Freud S 1990 The ego and the id: the standard edition of the complete psychological works of Sigmund Freud. Norton, New York.

Friedman M 1987 Beyond caring: the de-moralization of gender. In: Hanen M, Nielsen K (eds) Science, morality, and feminist theory. University of Calgary Press, Calgary, BC, p 87–110.

Fry ST 1989a The role of caring in a theory of nursing ethics. Hypathia 4(2):88–103.

Fry ST 1989b Toward a theory of nursing ethics. Advances in Nursing Science 11(4):9–21.

Fry ST, Killen AR, Robinson EM 1996 Care-based reasoning, caring and ethics of care: a need for clarity. Journal of Clinical Ethics 7(1):41–47.

Gadow S 1980 Existential advocacy: philosophical foundation of nursing In: Spicker SF, Gadow S (eds) Nursing: images and ideals – dialogue with the humanities. Springer, New York, p 79–101.

Gadow S 1985 Nurse and patient: the caring relationship. In: Bishop A, Scudder J (eds) Caring, curing, coping: nurse, physician, patient relationship. University of Alabama Press, Tuscaloosa, AL, p 34–37.

Gadow S 1990 The advocacy covenant: care as clinical subjectivity. In: Stevenson JS, Tripp-Reimer (eds) Knowledge about care, and caring: state of the art and future developments, proceedings of a Wingspread conference. 1–3 February, ANA Publications, Washington, DC.

Gilligan C 1982 In a different voice: psychological theory and women's development. Harvard University Press, Cambridge, MA.

Johnson AG 1997 The gender knot: unraveling our patriarchal legacy. Temple University Press, Philadelphia.

Johnstone MJ 1989 Bioethics: a nursing perspective. Saunders, Sydney.

Komorita NJ, Doehring KM, Hirchert PW 1991 Perceptions of caring by nurse educators. Journal of Nursing Education 30: 23–29

Kuhse H 1997 Caring: nurses, women, and ethics. Blackwell, Oxford.

Lea A, Watson R, Deary I 1998 Caring in nursing: a multivariate analysis. Journal of Advanced Nursing 28:662–671.

Leininger M 1977 Caring: the essence and central focus of nursing. In: The phenomenon of caring, Part V, American Nurses' Foundation. Nursing Research Report 12:2–14.

Leininger M 1978 Transcultural nursing: concepts, theories, and practices. John Wiley, New York.

Leininger M 1980 Caring: a central focus in nursing: understanding the meaning, importance, and issues. In: Leininger M (ed) Care: the essence of nursing and health. Wayne State University Press, Detroit, MI, p 45–59.

Leininger M 1981 Caring: an essential human need: proceedings of three national caring conferences. Slack, Thorofare, NJ.

Leininger M 1990 Ethical and moral dimensions of care. Wayne State University Press, Detroit, MI.

Leininger M, Watson J (eds) 1990 Caring imperative in education. National League of Nursing, New York.

McCance T, McKenna H, Boone J 1997 Caring: dealing with a difficult concept. International Journal of Nursing Studies 34:241–248.

Mayeroff M 1971 On caring. Harper and Row, New York.

Morse J, Solberg S, Neander W et al 1990 Concepts of caring and caring as a concept. Advanced Nursing Science 13:1–14.

Morse J, Bottoroff J, Neander W Solberg S 1991 Comparative analysis of conceptualizations and theories of caring. Image 23(2):119–126.

Noddings N 1984 Caring: a feminine approach to ethics and moral education. University of California Press, Berkeley.

Nursing Philosophy 2003 Special issue on Sally Gadow's work. 4(2).

Roach MS 1992 The human act of caring. Canadian Hospital Association, Ottawa.

Roach MS (ed) 1997 Caring from the heart. Paulist Press, New York.

Roach MS 1998 Caring ontology: ethics and the call of suffering. International J for Human Caring 2:30–34.

Singer T, Seymour B, O'Doherty J et al 2004 Empathy for pain involves the affective but not sensory components of pain. Science 303:1157–1162.

Storch JI, Rodney P, Starzomski R 2004 Toward a moral horizon: nursing ethics for leadership and practice. Pearson-Prentice Hall, Toronto.

Tong R 1993 Feminine and feminist ethics. Wadsworth, Belmont, CA.

Tschudin V 2003 Ethics in nursing: the caring relationship. Heinemann, Edinburgh.

Tschudin V (ed) 2003 Approaches to ethics: nursing beyond boundaries. Butterworth Heinemann, Edinburgh.

van Hooft S 2003 Caring and ethics in nursing. In: Tschudin V (ed) Approaches to ethics: nursing beyond boundaries. Butterworth-Heinemann, Edinburgh, p 1–12.

Volbrecht RM 2002 Nursing ethics: communities in dialogue. Prentice Hall, Upper Saddle River, NJ.

Walker LJ, deVries B, Trevethan SD 1984 Sex differences in the development of moral reasoning. Child Development 55:677–691.

Watson J 1985 Nursing: the philosophy and science of caring. University of Colorado Press, Denver.

Watson J (ed) 1994 Applying the art and science of health care. National League of Nursing, New York.

Watson J 1999 Nursing: human science and human caring: a theory of nursing. Jones and Bartlett, Sudbury, MA.

Watson J 2002 Assessing and measuring caring in nursing and health science. Springer, New York.

Watson J 2004 Caring science: a core science for health professions. FA Davis, Phildelphia.

Wilson EO 2003 The future of life. Vintage, New York.

Wollstonecraft M 1792 The vindication of the rights of women. Reprinted 1996 Dover Publications, New York.

Further reading

Bishop AH, Scudder JR Jr 1996 Nursing ethics: therapeutic caring presence. Jones and Bartlett, Sudbury, MA.

Brabeck MM (ed) 1989 Who cares? Theory, research and educational implications of the ethics of care. Praeger, New York.

Brown JM, Kitson AL, McKnight TJ 1992 Caring: explorations in nursing and ethics. Chapman & Hall, London.

Hothchild AR 2003 The managed heart: commericalization of human feelings. University of California Press, Berkeley.

Jameton A 1984 Nursing practice: the ethical issues. Prentice Hall, Englewood Cliffs, NJ.

Reich WT 2003 History of the notion of care. In: Post SG (ed) Encyclopedia of bioethics. Macmillan, Basingstoke, UK, p 345–374.

Reverby S 1987 Ordered to care: the dilemma of American nursing, 1850–1945. Cambridge University Press, Cambridge.

Tronto JC 1993 Moral boundaries: a political argument for an ethic of care. Routledge, New York.

Chapter **16**

Feminist ethics: a way of doing ethics

Joan Liaschenko and Elizabeth Peter

Many misconceptions about feminist ethics abound among those not familiar with its major tenets. There is, for example, the belief that feminist ethics solely concerns women or that feminist ethics is equivalent to care ethics. While it is the case that feminist ethics is an intellectual project done mostly by women and is indisputably for women, one need not be a woman to be a feminist. To quote Alison Jaggar: 'it is worth reemphasizing that all women are not feminists and that some men are' (Jaggar 1991 p 94). However, all feminist ethicists believe that there is male bias in moral theories and they are committed to correcting that bias. Such bias is revealed, for example, in the view of women as incomplete or inadequate moral agents who cannot reason morally because they are considered too emotional. This view is explicit in the work of Plato and Aristotle and continues through the work of the major philosophers in western thought, including Thomas Aquinas, Thomas Hobbes, Immanuel Kant, Friedrich Nietzsche and John Rawls (Okin 1988).

To be a feminist is to recognize that women, at intersections with class, race, age, ethnicity and religion, occupy a social and moral space different from that of the privileged few who define the terms of moral discourse and structure forms of living by assigning divisions of labour and moral status accordingly. Feminist ethicists do not merely observe these differences from afar but, like other women, live their lives in some version of such a space. They know firsthand that the moral experience of women in everyday life, which is concerned with the responsibilities for paid and unpaid caring of children and people who are sick or disabled, does not fit with the representation of morality and moral agents in moral theory. Therefore feminist moral philosophers are rethinking the very project of ethics and morality.

Feminist ethics and feminist healthcare ethics are broad and ever-evolving approaches to ethics and bioethics. We have chosen to characterize feminist ethics as Margaret Urban Walker (2003) has, as a way of doing ethics as opposed to a static subject matter. Feminist ethics is committed to a process of emancipatory politics related to everyday moral life in such a way that it can be viewed as critical scholarship possessing some fundamental similarities with post-structuralism and post-colonialism. In this regard, feminist ethics can be described as a critique of mainstream ethical theory and a critique of life and its inequities. Walker (2003) aptly states:

> Feminist ethics insists we look at the impact of intersections and distributions of social authority, privilege, and power both on morality as an aspect of moral life and on ethics as the reflective and systematic representation of morality. What is crucial to feminist ethics and its importance for ethics is the link between these two dimensions of its inquiry, the impact of power on morality, and its effects on ethics. A premise of feminist ethics is that both in theory and in life unequal distributions of power and privilege will tend to reproduce themselves, and each will tend to reinforce and legitimate the other. (Walker 2003 p 207)

In this chapter we explore three overarching, but interrelated, dimensions of feminist ethics or healthcare ethics that represent this critique. First, we examine how feminist ethics blurs the boundaries between ethics and morality and politics. In doing so, it critiques the impact of power on how both everyday morality and ethical theory are shaped. Second, we examine how feminist ethics critiques aspects of mainstream ethical theory, in particular, the dominant conceptualization of persons as autonomous, equal and rational. Third, we explore the naturalistic basis of ethics and morality that has been proposed by feminist ethicists, such as Walker (defined in Glossary, p 360). Naturalism is a critique because mainstream ethical theorizing has generally depicted moral knowledge as pure and idyllic and derived from reason, not real life experiences. We show how the naturalistic approach is already the way in which nurses make moral sense of their work and how it helps nurses to articulate their moral understandings in a language that counters the neglect of nurses' experience by mainstream bioethics.

BLURRING THE BOUNDARY BETWEEN ETHICS AND POLITICS

The boundary between ethics and politics in philosophical thought has often been unbending. Feminists, however, have questioned this boundary and have articulated well the interrelationships between ethics and power. Fundamentally, feminist ethics is a discourse about morality and power. First, feminists describe how moral and social practices are inextricable. In other words, moral identities and practices are constituted through people's sociopolitical positioning. How we define our range of accountability and moral positions is an outcome of how we are situated in society. For instance, nurses' definitions of their moral responsibilities for health care are inherent in their moral positioning within healthcare systems. Nurses often act in-between the values of others to deliver the healthcare services for which they are accountable and consequently view their moral identity as evolving and emerging (Rodney et al 2002).

Second, feminists examine the morality of specific practices and distributions of power. Although there are variations of feminist ethical thought, one common thread is that feminist ethicists regard oppression as morally and politically wrong and endeavour to bring about social change to eliminate oppression in all its forms (Baier 1994, Brennan 1999, Sherwin 1992, Tong 1996, Walker 2003). Traditionally, feminists have addressed the domination of men over women, but feminists must also oppose oppression that is the result of hierarchies and exclusions based in class, race, sexual orientation, age and ability, not only because these are morally problematic in themselves, but also because they intersect with gender oppression (Liaschenko & Peter 2003, Walker 2003). For example, nurses need to examine how race, class and gender impact on an individual's access to needed health services.

Power itself is morally neutral, i.e. to exercise power is not in itself good or evil; however, how power is used is of moral significance. Therefore, it is necessary to ascertain the power differences that are legitimate and unavoidable and those that are not. For example, the power of the nurse in relation to sick and vulnerable patients can be legitimate if this power helps to restore the health and well-being, and ultimately the power, of patients. In contrast, this power is not legitimate if it is used to dominate and silence patients into becoming passive objects of care. When teaching nursing ethics it is essential for nurses, both students and instructors, to understand and reflect on their own use of power and to avoid the tendency of viewing themselves as powerless. Like those who have relative power over us, we sometimes have the freedom to choose to exercise power in such a way that it can promote human flourishing or we can choose to exercise power in such a way that we oppress others. More commonly, nurses have examined how the power of others has been oppressive to them to the extent that nurses' moral agency is constrained. The use of feminist ethics in the classroom can facilitate discussion with respect to nurses' oppression also. This type of discussion often helps students to find the words they need to express the moral distress they so frequently experience in their work lives.

How power is used to form what constitutes 'legitimate' moral and other knowledge is another focal point of feminist ethics for moral and epistemic privilege to be appraised and diminished. For example, those who possess medical knowledge, especially those considered experts, can be viewed as possessing epistemic privilege because of the vast power and esteem that is given to medical knowledge in society. Feminist ethics is deeply reflective and directs its attention to examining the social impact and usefulness of moral, medical and other theorizing (Held 1984, Walker 2003). Feminist ethics emphasizes the need to challenge ethics and bioethics. Without this challenge, ethics and bioethics have the potential simply to reproduce existing structures of power and privilege. For example, the lack of attention paid to nursing perspectives in bioethics perpetuates the invisibility of nurses' contribution to health care and diminishes an appreciation of nurses' moral agency. Uncovering nurses' moral knowledge of issues concerning overall quality of life, not just disease and treatment, the importance of relationship building in healthcare contexts, and also the impact of health policy and law on the individual lives of people could begin to shift the current moral and epistemic privilege of medicine.

KEY POINTS: **Blurring the boundary between ethics and politics**

- Moral and social practices are inseparable.
- Feminist ethicists regard oppression as morally and politically wrong.
- Power is morally neutral, but requires us to reflect on how we use it.
- Feminist ethics critiques epistemic and moral privilege.

THE CRITIQUE OF RATIONAL AND AUTONOMOUS PERSONHOOD

Feminist ethics rests on a definition of personhood that is largely consistent with the conception of persons inherent in the ethic of care. Seyla Benhabib (1987) has named this conception the 'concrete' other, versus the 'generalized' other underlying the ethic of justice. The concrete other requires us to view others as individuals with a concrete history and a unique identity, including motives, needs, desires, and emotions. The conception of persons underlying the ethic of justice and much of mainstream philosophy emphasizes what people have in common, as opposed to their differences. Consequently, the characteristics given to persons are abstract and general in nature, leading to Benhabib's (1987) label of the generalized other. People assume that the other is like us with broadly similar needs, desires, and affects. By virtue of the common humanity of others, they are worthy of respect.

Some of the attributes assumed to describe all people, in a generalized sense, are included in the following definition. Persons are equal, rational, autonomous, independent, self-realizing, self-interested, or at least mutually disinterested. This portrayal of persons reflects the self-conceptions likely to be held by the theorists who constructed theories that assumed this definition. It comes as no surprise that this conception of persons has been widely criticized by feminist theorists (Baier 1986, Code 1987, Walker 2003, Young 1990). Specifically, Annette Baier (1985a), Virginia Held (1987) and Will Kymlicka (1990) argue that persons are not primarily autonomous because their lives are filled with many largely unchosen relationships, such as children, family, fellow workers, superiors, etc. These are often relationships of dependency, resulting in a restriction of personal goals and activities.

The claim that persons are autonomous in the sense that they are self-realizing has also been criticized. Baier (1985b) states, 'A person, perhaps, is best seen as one who was long enough dependent upon other persons to acquire the essential arts of personhood. Persons essentially are second persons, who grow up with other persons' (p 84). Children grow up highly influenced by their caregivers and within a cultural heritage that directly affects the persons they come to be. Personhood is never fixed even in adulthood because we always influence and are influenced by those people with whom we have relationships (Code 1987). Definitions of persons that deny the influence of culture and personal history, in their attempt to be universal, often have the shortcoming of also denying relevant differences between persons such as gender, class, and race. Feminist ethics, through its challenge to the traditional person or moral subject, has resulted in new models of persons that are more open-textured. The models allow for important differences between individuals, which have much of their basis in culture and history, and which need to be acknowledged. In short, feminist ethics tends to view persons as interdependent, vulnerable, unequal in power, unique, gendered, racialized, embodied and historically, economically, culturally and politically located.

KEY POINTS: **The critique of rational and autonomous personhood**

- A feminist conception of persons critiques the notion that persons are purely rational and autonomous.

- Feminist ethics views persons as unique, gendered, connected to others, and interdependent, i.e. vulnerable and unequal in power. It focuses on how persons are positioned in society, including culture, race, history, politics, and socioeconomic status.

- A feminist conception of persons acknowledges difference.

FEMINIST NATURALISM

Feminist ethics does not separate ethics from politics and holds a different view of moral agents. Because feminist ethics, in contrast to traditional philosophical ethics, holds that the everyday moral experience of people is highly relevant to what is defined as a moral issue, how people think about the issue, and what solutions are possible, feminist moral philosophers are rethinking the very project of ethics and morality. Underlying assumptions and the exclusion of real life experiences are being re-examined along with the ways in which traditional theory, despite its affirmation of disinterested moral agents, actually serves to construct privilege for an elite few. This was accomplished by determining the 'norms' of morality and justifying them through the representations of ethical theory, which is characterized by universals, abstractness, and detachment. This representation of morality functions to obscure or rationalize the subordination of women and other marginalized groups by ignoring their moral experiences, concerns, and ways of approaching moral solutions (Jaggar 2000; Walker 1998). As Jaggar (2000) states, 'Relatively few persons have ever been sanctioned to define moral knowledge and so conceals the fact that western ethics has functioned as a practice of authority that has often rationalized masculine privilege' (p 462). The corrective for this problem is to look at the moral understandings of actual moral agents in real time and space.

Moral knowledge is concerned with the following questions: What is moral knowledge? Where do we look for it? How do we know we have it? Ethics is commonly understood as the philosophical justification of what ought to be done; the behaviours in keeping with the justification are then moral, or right or good. Justifications of actions involve claims of moral knowledge that include determinations of relevant facts, nature of evidence, limits of the problem or question at hand, correct ways of thinking about the problem, and acceptable solutions. Claims of moral knowledge also entail assumptions of moral agency and who counts as a moral agent under what circumstance. These issues are worked out and represented in moral theories. According to the claims of traditional moral theories, the 'oughts' hold for all moral agents of reason in similar situations. In this way, the moral knowledge represented in the theory is thought to be objective. Objectivity implies being freed from the contingencies of everyday life that actually render moral agents, what they know, and what they can do, quite different from the ideal, pure, objective idea of moral theories. Feminists question the structure and politics of 'oughts' by asking 'who gets to say and why?' This question is not straightforward in societies highly stratified by gender, race, class, age, sexual orientation, and so forth (Walker 1998).

Feminist moral philosophers want to know whose interests are being served as well as the social, political, material, and moral costs to those whose interests are not so served. As Jaggar (2000) pointedly indicates at the beginning of this section, those privileged to define moral knowledge have been staggeringly few. The moral experience of most people has been ignored, dismissed, or negated under the guise of universal truths understood only by a select few. As a corrective, feminist moral philosophers use a naturalized moral epistemology in rethinking the very notion of morality itself. In what follows, we discuss briefly a feminist alternative view of morality, specifically that of Walker in *Moral understandings* (1998).

Walker's concern with the representative claims of traditional moral theory has led her to reconceptualize morality itself. Examples of how morality is represented in the following two descriptions are worth considering. The first is found in an introductory philosophy text:

> *Ethics, as a reflective philosophical endeavor, attempts to make theoretical sense out of our classification of actions into the basic categories of the morally permissible, the morally impermissible, and the morally obligatory.* (Earle 1992 p 177)

From this description, ethics is only concerned with actions of a certain kind. The task of philosophers is to sort this out, which means specifying which actions under what conditions count as morally permissible, impermissible, and obligatory, and to formulate the justification for each. The point Richard Taylor (1985) makes so masterfully, however, is that the notion of right or wrong, or permissible or impermissible requires a lawgiver or rule maker. In the history of western ethics, the ancient Greeks took these ideas as products of human beings, albeit those of the elite male citizens of Greek city states. With the advent of Christianity, the lawgiver or rule maker became God. This remained in effect until the Enlightenment, and Kant, who did not like the idea of God, nonetheless kept the question of the lawgiver. Kant's answer was reason: universal, abstract, and detached. Even though the lawgiver had changed, women were still denied the status of moral agents and their concerns were negated.

Just who is the stand-in for this universal reason? Who is the 'our' in 'our classifications'? What views of moral agency are represented in this view? What counts as a moral issue and who is authorized to label it as such? What solutions are possible? These are precisely the questions that occupied Walker in her critique of moral theory, and led to her rejection of not only traditional moral theory, but also the traditional understanding of morality itself.

Within traditional moral philosophy, morality is represented 'as a compact, propositionally codifiable, impersonally action-guiding code within an agent' (Walker 1998 p 7). Morality is limited to evaluative judgements of morally permissible, impermissible, or obligatory actions by moral agents who are represented as impartial judges. Walker calls this view the theoretical–juridical (TJ) model, which 'shrinks morality "proper" down to a kind of purified core of purely moral knowledge' (Walker 1998 p 8). Such a view lends itself to the conviction held by moral philosophers that morality is attainable by 'mostly or entirely non-empirical reflection on conceptual and logical relations' (Walker 1998 p 8). In this way, morality becomes the province of those trained for particular styles of reasoning and the TJ model is 'the template for "serious" or "important" moral theorizing' (Walker 1998 p 7).

Walker rejects this representation of morality, arguing that morality is not fundamentally about moral theories or thought in individuals. It is also about what is 'perceived, felt, and acted out' and not only in individuals but between people (Walker 1998 p 8). This cannot be emphasized too strongly. While this may make sense to some, such an understanding is a marked difference from the TJ model. If morality cannot be found in the heads of individuals, where is it to be found? Walker locates morality in *practices of responsibility* that implement commonly shared understandings about who gets to do what to whom and who is supposed to do what for whom' (Walker 1998 p 16). She defends a view of morality that she calls the expressive–collaborative (EC) model. This view conceives of 'morality as a socially embodied medium of understandings and adjustments in which people account to each other for the identities, relationships, and values that define their responsibilities' (Walker 1998 p 61). In the EC model, morality is fundamentally interpersonal and negotiated. Feminist ethics, however, holds that individuals are not all equal in opportunities, social and material resources, social standing, status, and power. Many live their lives in poverty, have limited education, are marked by stigma, suffer disabilities and illness, and are confined by gender stereotypes. Thus morality happens in a real world marked by profound social differentiation.

For feminist ethics, these realities are of the utmost significance. For Walker, they are inseparable from how people come to understand their responsibilities and are held accountable for them. The moral understandings of our agency, identity, the responsibilities we take ourselves to have, how we will be judged, and by whom, are inseparable from our social location. Our social location is critical to morality because 'in the ways we assign, accept, or deflect responsibilities, we express our understandings of our own and others' identities, relationships, and values' (Walker 1998 p 16). It is precisely our own and others' identities, relationships and values that are at stake in morality. There are costs, risks and privileges associated with who gets to assign, who must accept and who can deflect what sorts of responsibilities. The idea that there are costs and risks to morality associated with people's social location is a morally important insight from feminist naturalism.

KEY POINTS: **The place of naturalism in feminist ethics and moral theory**

- Feminists endorse naturalism as an approach to the generation of knowledge to ensure that more than a privileged few can define moral knowledge.

- Walker has critiqued mainstream moral theory, what she has called the theoretical–juridical model, and has offered in its place the expressive–collaborative model.

- Morality in the expressive–collaborative model is naturalistic because it draws on the everyday lives of people reflecting the situated, interpersonal and negotiated character of actual morality.

CONCLUSION

The core idea of feminist naturalism is quite simple: it is that philosophers must attend to the insights obtained from empirical methods, that is, science. For feminist ethics, it means attending to what is actually occurring in the everyday lives of people in real time and space. Feminist moral philosophers use this knowledge to support several claims that weaken the claims of the standard TJ model. Significantly, such knowledge shows that morality is not static but ongoing and constantly negotiated by people engaged in practices who are not afforded the luxury of armchair detachment. The EC model is important because it argues for a view of morality, not as an ideal, but as deeply embedded in forms of life and everyday practices. Feminist naturalism shows that the traditional model of morality represents moral agents in a way that favours those who construct such accounts. Under the guise of there being pure, ideal, and objective moral knowledge and disinterested, impartial but equal moral agents, those who construct and control moral discourse can in fact be blind to how responsibilities are assigned, accepted, or deflected and the costs and risks associated with them. Feminist naturalism is a corrective because it challenges assumptions about what morality and ethics are within the standard account.

Finally, feminist naturalism provides a method for comparing and thereby evaluating different moral understandings and their justifications. This is unlikely to provide either confidence or comfort to those who believe that there exist absolute and universal moral truths, be they God or reason, to which we can appeal. These are issues that one of us (EP) addresses in the next chapter. In this chapter, our goal was to present what we understand as the main features of feminist ethics with a particular focus on the work of Walker.

References

Baier A 1985a What do women want in a moral theory? Nous 19:53–65.

Baier A 1985b Postures of the mind: essays on mind and morals. University of Minnesota Press, Minneapolis, MN.

Baier A 1986 Trust and antitrust. Ethics 96:231–260.

Baier A 1994 Moral prejudices: essays on ethics. Harvard University Press, Cambridge, MA.

Benhabib S 1987 The generalized and the concrete other: the Kohlberg–Gilligan controversy and moral theory. In: Kittay EF, Meyers DT (eds) Women and moral theory. Rowman & Littlefield, Lanham, MD, p 154–177.

Brennan S 1999 Recent works in feminist ethics. Ethics 109:858–893.

Code L 1987 Second persons. In: Hanen M, Nelson K (eds) Science, morality and feminist theory. University of Calgary Press, Calgary, BC, p 357–373.

Earle WJ 1992 Introduction to philosophy. McGraw-Hill, New York, NY.

Held V 1984 Rights and goods. Free Press, New York.

Held V 1987 Non-contractual society: a feminist view. In: Hanen M, Nelson K (eds) Science, morality and feminist theory. University of Calgary Press, Calgary, BC, p 111–137.

Jaggar AM 1991 Feminist ethics: projects, problems, prospects. In: Card C (ed) Feminist ethics. University Press of Kansas, Lawrence, KS, p 78–106.

Jaggar AM 2000 Ethics naturalized: feminism's contribution to moral epistemology. Metaphilosophy 31:452–468.

Kymlicka W 1990 Contemporary political philosophy: an introduction. Clarendon Press, Oxford.

Liaschenko J, Peter E 2003 Feminist ethics. In: Tschudin V (ed) Approaches to ethics: nursing beyond boundaries. Butterworth Heinemann, Edinburgh, p 33–43.

Okin S 1988 The subjection of women. Hackett Publishing, Indianapolis, IN.

Rodney P, Varcoe C, Storch JL et al 2002 Navigating towards a moral horizon: a multisite qualitative study of ethical practice in nursing. Canadian Journal of Nursing Research 34(3):75–102.

Sherwin S 1992 No longer patient: feminist ethics and healthcare. Temple University Press, Philadelphia.

Taylor R 1985 Ethics, faith and reason. Prentice Hall, Englewood Cliffs, NJ.

Tong R 1996 An introduction to feminist approaches to bioethics: unity in diversity. Journal of Clinical Ethics 7(1):13–19.

Walker MU 1998 Moral understandings: a feminist study in ethics. Routledge, New York.

Walker M U 2003 Moral contexts. Rowman & Littlefield, Lanham, MD

Young IM 1990 Justice and the politics of difference. Princeton University Press, Princeton, NJ.

Further reading

Benner P 1984 From novice to expert. Addison Wesley, Menlo Park, CA.

Benner P, Wrubel J 1989 The primacy of caring. Addison Wesley, Menlo Park, CA.

Code L 1991 What can she know? Feminist theory and the construction of knowledge. Cornell University Press, Ithaca, NY.

Gilligan C 1982 In a different voice: psychological theory and women's development. Harvard University Press, Cambridge, MA.

Lloyd G 1984 The man of reason: 'male' and 'female' in western philosophy. University of Minnesota Press, Minneapolis, MN.

Schott R 1990 From cognition to eros: a critique of the Kantian paradigm. Beacon Press, Boston, MA.

Williams B 1985 Ethics and the limits of philosophy. Harvard University Press, Cambridge, MA.

Chapter 17

Feminist ethics: a critique

Elizabeth Peter

Feminist ethical theories have been described as sharing two central aims: (a) 'to achieve a theoretical understanding of women's oppression with the purpose of providing a route to ending women's oppression and (b) to develop an account of morality which is based on women's moral experiences)' (Brennan 1999 p 860). This concise articulation of feminist ethics encapsulates the core elements of feminist ethics. Although these core elements are highly valued by feminists who regard these aims as necessary correctives to much of traditional ethical theory, they are also at the centre of debate and critique.

Two common charges against feminist ethics have been that of moral relativism and the privileging of gender oppression. The concern of moral relativism arises from the naturalistic basis of feminist ethics. Moral knowledge from this perspective is grounded in the experience of embodied, socially situated knowers, not abstract reasoning alone. Normative evaluation regarding moral practices and understandings, however, remains possible even though it is always partial and subject to revision. Both within and between cultures, norms must be continually redeveloped in ways that make mutual recognition and cooperation possible. In this regard, feminist ethics is not so much morally relativistic as it is morally pluralistic.

The critique of the privileging of gender oppression is related to the first concern of moral relativism in that the emphasis upon gender is rooted in tenets of feminist moral epistemology. The criticism stems from the tendency of feminist ethics to emphasize the moral experience and oppression of women as opposed to other forms of oppression that are related to race, class, and disability. I argue that an intersectional analysis that views various forms of oppression as interlocking can mitigate this problem.

Throughout, I provide examples of how these criticisms can have great ethical significance to nurses and nursing students and offer strategies to work with them in a way that promotes the teaching of feminist ethics as both content and process.

FEMINIST MORAL EPISTEMOLOGY: NATURALISM

Moral epistemology investigates sources of moral knowledge. Existing at the interface of ethics and epistemology, moral epistemology has been described as a neglected area of philosophy (Dancy 1992). Its questions can include: What kinds of knowledge does morality depend on? How do we discover what is right and wrong? Do any of our moral views count as knowledge? How do we ground or justify such knowledge? (Dancy 1992, Walker 1998a). Feminist moral epistemology attends to how power and oppression have influenced how these questions have traditionally been answered and how they could be answered in a way that better promotes human flourishing for all.

Mainstream ethical theorizing, such as principle-based ethics, has produced a representation of morality in which moral judgement and justification are depicted as the application of a set of law-like and impersonal principles and codes that direct moral agents or explain moral behaviour. Moral philosophers have regarded this model of moral inquiry, which Margaret Urban Walker (1998b) has called the 'theoretical–juridical' model, as serious and important. Such a status is granted because the model presumes that moral philosophers can gain access to a pure core of moral knowledge through conceptual and logical reflection, which is independent of the contexts of human practices and empirical inquiry (Walker 1998b). The belief that moral knowledge is pure and therefore transcends the boundaries of a social world divided by gender, race, class, ethnicity and religion, rather conveniently shields moral theorists from viewing moral knowledge as culturally situated. Failing to see that moral theory is shaped by a theorist's social positioning results in the negation of the moral lives of nearly all of us (Peter & Liaschenko 2003).

This theorizing also presupposes that moral agents are independent, self-interested, autonomous and equal persons who seek relationships with others that are based on non-interference. Women, children, economically disadvantaged people, people of visible minority groups and people with disabilities typically do not live lives that are characterized by the degree of autonomy inherent in dominant perspectives of moral agency. For example, the autonomy of most women has been curtailed because they have been expected to care for others who are often vulnerable and dependent, such as children and old, sick and injured people (Walker 1998a). Dominant moral perspectives do not capture the complexities of the moral judgements required to perform such work, nor do they adequately recognize the interdependencies and power differential among persons. Because nurses' work tends to typify women's caring labour, bioethical theory when rooted in the theoretical–juridical model does not anchor nurses' identities, responsibilities, and moral experiences well at all. Nursing concerns can be discounted as truly 'ethical' problems or can be considered merely practical problems. This dismissal or redefinition is a major way in which the legitimacy of nurses' concerns and moral knowledge can be questioned and nurses' concerns can become invisible, leading to nurses' moral self-doubt. It can also result in nurses becoming morally paralyzed when attempting to embrace theoretical ideas far removed from their world (Peter & Liaschenko 2003).

To counter the theoretical–juridical model's tendency to ground moral knowledge in the abstract and conceptual, feminist ethicists have required that moral theory be based on experience. Ethical theorizing begins with racialized and gendered subjects who come from particular communities, have particular histories, and have particular visions and ideals of what constitutes human flourishing (Morgan 1991). Although an emphasis has been placed on women's moral experiences, feminists recognize the significance of drawing on all persons' moral experiences. Since feminists recognize that oppression is a fundamental moral wrong, they address this wrong in all of its manifestations, including oppression resulting from race, class, disability, sexual orientation and so forth (Liaschenko & Peter 2003). Because the experiences of oppressed persons have been so frequently marginalized, listening to the moral voices of all persons is one way of transforming society.

The teaching of feminist ethics similarly involves listening to and drawing on the moral experiences of all students, thereby bringing together both feminist content and process. Ann Manicom (1992) reminds us that teaching from a feminist perspective is political: 'to develop feminist analyses that inform/reform teachers' and students' ways of acting in and on the world' (p 365). An atmosphere of mutual respect, trust and community must be established in the classroom so that students' experiences are valued and heard. Students' own experiences should form the basis of in-class discussions and assignments. In addition, as much as is possible in academic settings, the power differences among teachers and students must be acknowledged and minimized for students' perspectives to be legitimized (Kimmel & Worell 1997, Manicom 1992).

The experiences of patients must also find a central role in the teaching of feminist ethics. Their stories of illness can be brought forward through various narrative approaches such as film, poetry, literature and in some instances, qualitative research findings. Hearing patients' perspectives can cultivate our moral sensibilities and perceptions and can enhance our compassion when we are engaged in healthcare decision making (Nelson 2001). Patients' voices can too easily be neglected in the teaching of nursing ethics because of the attention that must be given to the moral constraints nurses experience in their workplaces. Ultimately, gathering patient moral knowledge adds to the fullness of our own moral understandings.

KEY POINTS: **Feminist moral epistemology**

- Feminist moral knowledge is not derived from reason alone, but also draws on people's experiences as they live their lives.

- Moral knowledge is influenced by how persons are situated. Class, race, gender, sexual orientation and so on are relevant.

- Uncovering the moral experiences of oppressed people is necessary to overcome the biases in current mainstream moral theory.

- It is necessary when teaching feminist ethics to draw upon the experiences of students and patients.

THE PROBLEM OF MORAL RELATIVISM

The process of drawing on a diversity of moral experiences and perspectives, however, is not unproblematic. It raises concerns regarding moral relativism. Moral knowledge from feminist moral theorists, such as Walker, is founded not in something 'higher' such as God, the natural law, science or pure practical reason, but in the moral practices and experiences of persons that can be variable and seemingly incommensurable. The western philosophical tradition, in contrast, has valourized the universal and abstract and has deeply distrusted and despised the embodied and the particular that represents the starting point for feminist ethical theorizing (Morgan 1991). Questions regarding moral relativism arise especially when various moral experiences and judgements conflict. For instance, should all perspectives be given equal weight? Are all equally valid? What if one group morally disagrees with the cultural practices of another group? Ultimately, particularist accounts of morality make it difficult to decide which particulars matter, or matter most (Brennan 1999).

In a classroom setting in which students are from diverse backgrounds and have experienced variable and sometimes intersecting or interlocking forms of oppression, it is inevitable that moral disagreement will develop. Multiple narratives of both patient and personal experiences are often shared from differing vantage points. I have found it challenging to value and respect all perspectives simultaneously, while attempting not to endorse a relativistic stance. A disquieting encounter with moral relativism is common in students studying nursing ethics or moral philosophy who, perhaps for the first time, may be subject to an array of different moral perspectives. While this breadth of particular perspectives is both enriching and engaging, it can be anxiety provoking for students when a common ground is not readily achieved.

It is important to recognize that moral relativism has its variations. Drawing on the work of Bimal Matilal (1989), Kathryn Morgan (1991) differentiates 'hard' moral relativism from 'soft' moral relativism and also differentiates moral relativism from moral pluralism. Hard relativism is the view that culture-bound norms are both mutually incomprehensible and incommensurable. In other words, a hard moral relativist would argue that particular moral beliefs cannot be brought together by a common norm of any kind, nor can those with conflicting beliefs truly understand the other's position. On the other hand, soft relativism holds that there are many particular moral norms that vary from culture to culture and from person to person. While these norms may be comprehensible across people and cultures, they are incommensurable because there is no way to judge their merit from any objective basis.

Using these definitions of hard and soft relativism, I argue that feminist ethics does not support either form of relativism despite its reliance on particular experiences. Feminists have endorsed several related norms that limit the possibility of relativism in feminist ethical theory. For example, Alison Jaggar (1991) writes that feminist ethics is 'incompatible with any form of moral relativism that condones the subordination of women or the devaluation of their moral experience' (p 95). In my own work, I have held to the values and beliefs of care, social justice and interdependence within a political perspective to counter both relativism (Peter 2000) and the values inherent in neoliberalism (Peter 2004). Walker (1998b) has likewise spoken of the possibility of moral justification through coherent social arrangements that are based on the centrality of mutual recognition and cooperation as opposed to deception, oppression, and violence. A community of people must be able to have a set of social arrangements and a kind of shareable and stable sense of themselves within a community for coherence to exist. Therefore feminist ethics is not so much a relativistic approach or set of approaches, as an example of an approach that is morally pluralistic. Moral pluralism refers to the plurality of norms that can exist interculturally or intraculturally that require continual ordering and reordering of priorities depending on the context and other variables (Morgan 1991). This iterative process of creating norms relies on a naturalistic process in feminist ethics, whereby those carrying out particular responsibilities are in the best position to declare whether the norms operating within a particular social arrangement are intelligible and coherent (Walker 1998b).

With respect to the teaching of nursing ethics, moral disagreement can be mitigated by explicitly examining what norms are operating within a particular debate. Norms that foster oppression and silence the voices of oppressed people cannot be endorsed. These norms are often deeply embedded within a debate and require some effort to uncover. Within the classroom it can be difficult, however, to attain sound knowledge of the experiences of others, if research regarding, or student exposure to, the experiences of a particular group is lacking. We sometimes do not know how oppressed people experience an aspect of their lives that is related to debates within healthcare ethics. For example, we may not have full knowledge of how single and poor women experience their lives when their technology-dependent children are discharged from hospital with minimal home supports. Understanding the perspectives of all people, such as these women, can enable us to have better knowledge of what constitutes adequate informed consent and what kinds of supports strengthen the capacity of patients to make decisions.

KEY POINTS: The problem of moral relativism

- Moral relativism is a potential problem for feminist ethics because of its reliance on a diversity of moral experiences and perspectives.

- Feminist ethics can best be described as morally pluralistic in character, as opposed to morally relativistic.

- Norms that counter oppression limit the moral relativism of feminist ethics.

LIVING AND TEACHING WITH MORAL PLURALISM

Susan Sherwin (1996) and Margaret Walker (1998b, 2003) have reworked John Rawls' (1971) conception of a reflective equilibrium in ways that offer guidance on how we can live and teach with the moral pluralism that feminist ethics entails. From Rawls' perspective, a reflective equilibrium exists when our theoretical principles or norms coincide with our considered moral judgements. It entails a dialectical process in which theoretical considerations, i.e. principles and norms, are developed and tested against considered moral judgements and similarly, moral judgements are developed and tested against theoretical considerations. This process is one in which individuals deliberate within themselves to examine how their moral judgements correspond with their theoretical principles and norms and the reverse, to examine how their theoretical principles and norms correspond with their moral judgements. It is primarily an intellectual exercise that can result in the modification of theoretical principles or moral judgements.

In a modified version of Rawls' reflective equilibrium, Sherwin (1996) proposes that attention should not only be given to developing and testing conceptual and theoretical propositions against considered moral judgements, but it also should be given to the practical world of actual moral life. Questions of domination and power are highly relevant moral concerns and need to be raised when issues in healthcare ethics are explored. Sherwin's modification is important because it brings Rawls' reflective equilibrium into the realm of actual moral life with all of its political and social nuances.

Walker (1998b, 2003) also transforms Rawls' (1971) conception of moral norms from that of abstract action guides that direct individuals to communally created achievements. She broadens the conception of a reflective equilibrium by going beyond the idea that individuals, as autonomous and self-realizing subjects, must strive to find equilibrium and coherence between their individual practices and their moral beliefs to include the notion that equilibriums can be achieved *between* individuals, not just within them. Social arrangements must cohere for those who participate in them and communities of people must be able to create a lasting sense of themselves and their moral responsibilities and knowledge that they can communicate to others. Moral knowledge, from this point of view, is a communal product that is constructed through interactions among people, rather than a set of theoretical action-guiding principles within individual people.

Under critical reflection, mutual equilibriums between individuals or groups may become unstable or may be revealed as merely apparent. This type of reflection, or transparency testing, is necessary so that it can become clear who has responsibility for what and what provisions are available to distribute and evaluate these responsibilities. This type of analysis makes it possible to examine the extent to which differently situated people experience their responsibilities as intelligible and coherent and how the costs and burdens of these responsibilities are distributed. Mutual intelligibility is sustainable when people's understandings and responsibilities are placed in rough equilibrium. This equilibrium becomes evident when we can make its conditions and consequences explicit among us. Although this transparency testing sometimes results in disequilibrium, disorientation and conflict, it can also open opportunities for critique and change (Walker 1998b, 2003).

The moral authority of morality, or the normativity of ethics, does not emanate from a believed-to-be ideal or pure source of moral knowledge, as it would in mainstream ethical theorizing. Normative evaluation, or the capacity to make justified moral claims, regarding moral practices and understandings, however, remains possible, but not in the absolute sense. Although normative evaluation is always partial and subject to revision, we can critically examine whether the moral understandings that hold communities together sustain practices of responsibility and whether they make sense to differently positioned persons within those particular communities. Walker states:

> The 'normativity' of morality – the specifically moral authority of morality, whatever powers hold its practices in place – does not descend from someplace outside all human judgement; it inheres in the durability of our understandings and the trust they support under the right kind of tests.
> (Walker 2003 p 109)

While these moral understandings will always be incomplete, tentative and subject to revision, Walker maintains that this is the nature of morality. In this regard, Walker represents an account of morality that is consistent with moral pluralism because she gives support to a process that is iterative in nature. A plurality of possible norms is reflected on and reprioritized as needed by those who must make their moral responsibilities and understandings intelligible and coherent. Even though moral certainty cannot be attained, we can be reassured that when transparency testing results in the reinforcement of our moral understandings, we can at least temporarily have confidence in our moral knowledge (Walker 1998b, 2003).

For example, a teacher can foster discussion in the classroom that brings out the plurality of nursing students' values in a fashion that instils confidence. Graduate students, in particular, often express values that are distinct from those of the healthcare systems in which they practise. It is common for these nurses to express that their values – caring for patients' unique needs and providing socially just care – are incompatible with the corporate values that are embedded in many healthcare systems. The process of drawing out the plurality of values expressed by these students is a type of transparency testing because it reveals the incoherence of students' values and responsibilities in relation to those of the broader system. The elicitation of the plurality of values, which often results in the exposure of incoherence, can produce anxiety and uncertainty. Nevertheless, it provides students the opportunity to gain confidence in their moral understandings as a representation of valid moral knowledge instead of diminishing their own experiences and judgements.

Thus, we can live and teach in a morally pluralistic world that a feminist perspective opens up to us, not by having a false confidence in absolute moral norms, but instead by having confidence in the norms we possess, even if they are potentially subject to revision. In theory, the norms that feminists have advanced, such as social justice, are not absolute either. Nevertheless, because the development of these norms has been empirically informed, at least in part, by oppressed groups, it is unlikely that they would ever be rejected entirely. For example, it is difficult to imagine that oppressed people would ever find their responsibilities under examination coherent and intelligible in a way that would render norms supporting social justice as somehow morally unjustified. Social justice is necessary for humans to thrive because it ensures that people have the necessary goods, such as food, clean water, safety and employment, to live a life. These goods are in themselves naturalistic because they fulfil basic human needs.

KEY POINTS: **Living and teaching with moral pluralism**

- Equilibriums need to be achieved between individuals, not just within them.

- Transparency testing is necessary to determine whether the responsibilities of differentially situated people are coherent and intelligible to them.

- Norms are not transcendent in nature, but instead are always subject to revision.

THE PRIVILEGING OF GENDER

The term 'feminist ethics' implies that close attention is paid to women's oppression and moral experiences, as Samantha Brennan's (1999) characterization of feminist ethics at the beginning of this chapter suggests. Indeed, feminist ethics has some of its beginnings in the work of Carol Gilligan (1982) who examined the moral orientation of women empirically and concluded that women's orientation differed from men's in that it reflected an ethic of care as opposed to an ethic of justice. In the succeeding decades the ethic of care has been criticized by feminists as perpetuating women's invisible and exploited caregiving and as ignoring the moral concerns of distant and unknown others. Because the ethic of care only describes the moral experiences of women, it has been considered to be an example of 'feminine' ethics, but not 'feminist' ethics. In order for an ethic to be considered feminist, it must not only account for women's moral experiences, it also requires a political perspective (Sherwin 1992). Nevertheless, an ethic of care, although not sufficient on its own, has remained an important and necessary aspect of feminist ethics because it reveals the value of women's moral experiences.

This focus on women, however, raises concerns that feminist ethics privileges the experiences of women over other groups and that it considers gender oppression to be the most significant and serious form of oppression. While there is some validity in this criticism of feminist ethics, it is inconsistent for feminists not to be concerned with other forms of oppression, especially because many women simultaneously experience several related forms of oppression. Other critical perspectives, for instance post-colonialism, have well described other forms of oppression and can further enhance how feminist ethicists address what has been called intersecting or interlocking forms of oppression.

Post-colonialism holds race as an overarching theme, yet it does not necessarily consider race to be more significant than all other forms of oppression. Sheryl Reimer Kirkham and Joan Anderson (2002), who draw on the work of Patricia Hill Collins (1990), describe how an intersectional analysis that views various types of oppression, such as sexism, classism and racism as interlocking categories, can help us to understand how each form of oppression is embedded in the contexts of the other types. In this way, a fuller analysis of oppression is possible. In my own teaching, as a white, middle-class, able-bodied, heterosexual woman, I need to be continually aware that my position of relative privilege and my life experiences may not mirror those of my students. Because I live and work in Toronto, Canada, which is a highly diverse city, the student body is also very diverse. Understanding the experiences of students can be severely limited if it is confined to a gender analysis exclusively. Students often come with a complex array of concerns that calls for an intersectional analysis. To embrace the teaching of feminist ethics as both content and process, therefore, it is imperative to acknowledge openly any differences in power, privilege, and oppression regardless of the forms they may take (Kimmel & Worell 1997). Similarly, it is most important that the health issues of patients, who have also often experienced multiple forms of oppression, be understood fully so that our healthcare systems can be examined in the pursuit of furthering social justice.

Thus, while feminist ethics has emphasized gender, it has not done so at the expense of not allowing for the potential analyses of other forms of oppression. Nevertheless, more active engagement across critical perspectives by feminist ethicists and others would enhance this theoretical perspective's capacity to avoid any tendency, even if merely perceived, to privilege gender.

KEY POINTS: The privileging of gender

- The ethic of care, which has been described as representing the moral orientation of women, is necessary but not sufficient for feminist ethics.

- Feminist ethics must address multiple types of oppression, not merely gender oppression.

CONCLUSION

In summary, the related requirements of feminist ethics both to bring attention to women's oppression and also to develop an account of morality based on women's moral experiences open up both potential problems and possibilities when teaching. For example, teachers need to emphasize with students that while gender may be a starting point for feminists it is not necessarily the most salient form of oppression. Without this recognition, students can too easily exclude feminist ethics as a workable perspective. In addition, because feminist ethics as a way of doing ethics is dynamic and critical in nature, it may lead to a sense of uneasiness in students and teachers when definitive answers cannot be readily found. Yet students can begin to experience the validation of their moral knowledge in classrooms where their judgements are not merely put aside as practical or trivial in nature. The morally pluralistic character of feminist ethics is what makes it possible for students' moral experiences to be given credibility, even when they conflict with dominant perspectives. Their moral voices can contribute to revealing the mere appearance of current reflective equilibriums that exist at the level of healthcare systems.

References

Brennan S 1999 Recent works in feminist ethics. Ethics 109:858–893.

Collins PH 1990 Black feminist thought: knowledge, consciousness, and the politics of empowerment. Routledge, New York.

Dancy J 1992 Moral epistemology. In: Dancy J, Sosa E (eds) A companion to epistemology. Blackwell, Oxford, p 286–291.

Gilligan C 1982 In a different voice: psychological theory and women's development. Harvard University Press, Cambridge, MA.

Jaggar AM 1991 Feminist ethics: projects, problems, prospects. In: Card C (ed) Feminist ethics. University Press of Kansas, Lawrence, p 78–106.

Kimmel E, Worell J 1997 Preaching what we practice: principles and strategies of feminist pedagogy. In: Worell J, Johnson N (eds) Shaping the future of feminist psychology: education, research, and practice. American Psychological Association, Washington, p 121–153.

Kirkham SR, Anderson J 2002 Postcolonial nursing scholarship: from epistemology to method. Advances in Nursing Science 25(1):1–17.

Liaschenko J, Peter E 2003 Feminist ethics. In: Tschudin V (ed) Approaches to ethics: nursing beyond boundaries. Butterworth Heinemann, Edinburgh, p 33–43.

Manicom A 1992 Feminist pedagogy: transformations, standpoints and politics. Canadian Journal of Education 17(3):365–389.

Matilal BK 1989 Moral dilemmas in the Mah-abh-arata. Shimla: Indian Institute of Advanced Study in association with Motilal Banarsidass, Delhi.

Morgan K 1991 Strangers in a strange land. In: Stewart C (ed) Perspectives on moral relativism. Agathon Books, Lander, WO, p 33–62.

Nelson HL 2001 Damaged identities: narrative repair. Cornell University Press, New York.

Peter E 2000 The politicization of ethical knowledge: feminist ethics as basis for home care nursing research. Canadian Journal of Nursing Research 32(2):103–118.

Peter E 2004 Home health care and ethics. In: Storch J, Rodney P, Starzomski R (eds) Toward a moral horizon: nursing ethics in leadership and practice. Pearson-Prentice Hall, Toronto, p 248–261.

Peter E, Liaschenko J 2003 Whose morality is it anyway? Thoughts on the work of Margaret Urban Walker. Nursing Philosophy 4:259–262.

Rawls J 1971 A theory of justice. Harvard University Press, Cambridge, MA.

Sherwin S 1992 No longer patient: feminist ethics and health care. Temple University Press, Philadelphia.

Sherwin S 1996 Theory versus practice in ethics: a feminist perspective on justice in health care. In: Sumner LW, Boyle J (eds) Philosophical perspectives on bioethics. University of Toronto Press, Toronto, p 187–209.

Walker MU 1998a Moral epistemology. In: Jaggar AM, Young IM (eds) A companion to feminist philosophy. Blackwell, Oxford, p 363–371.

Walker MU 1998b Moral understandings: a feminist study in ethics. Routledge, New York.

Walker MU 2003 Moral contexts. Rowman & Littlefield Publishers, Lanham, MD.

Chapter 18

Teaching feminist ethics

Joan Liaschenko

Feminist ethics is grounded in feminist epistemology, which is making different claims on knowledge than traditional philosophical views. Feminist epistemologists argue that all knowers are situated in historical and social contexts, that emotions are relevant to the acquisition of knowledge, and that power dynamics figure in claims to knowledge. In terms of ethics, these epistemological assumptions challenge traditional understandings in ethics about what counts as moral knowledge, who can be a knower, what is important to consider in moral inquiry, and what counts as adequate and acceptable moral reasoning. Margaret Urban Walker claims that 'feminist ethics isn't a subject matter, but a way of doing ethics' (Walker 2003 p 207). Therefore, how does one do it? Where does one begin? In this chapter, I describe my current teaching of graduate students in nursing.

Since my first research and writing in nursing ethics, I have believed that traditional bioethical theory did not serve the interests of nurses (Liaschenko 1993). Rather, I believe that traditional bioethical theory actually silences nurses in disallowing their moral concerns by relabelling, ignoring, denigrating, and dismissing them. My teaching of nursing ethics to masters and doctoral students over several years has confirmed these earlier beliefs and in fact, my position is even stronger now. By silencing nurses, they are denied recognition as moral agents, their moral competence is negated, and their actual contributions to the moral well-being of communities are denied (Liaschenko & Peter 2003, Peter et al 2004, Storch et al 2004). For their part, nurses have generally accepted this failure to acknowledge their moral concerns as an indication that they are, in fact, less knowledgeable than others in bioethical theory. Some have struck bargains such that they thought they might be able to make their case if they did not challenge this view.

In keeping with my experience and beliefs, I have always taught feminist ethics. My approach was to use a variety of literature and approaches to explore the moral concerns of nurses through narratives written by students about an experience of moral concern. Recently, I have used *Moral understandings: a feminist study in ethics* by Margaret Urban Walker (1998). Her expressive collaborative (EC) model of morality (see Chapter 16) accommodates the empirical findings and theoretical articulations of my own work. Specifically, as one of the first researchers in nursing ethics to use narratives as sources of data, I articulated the concept of 'moral geographies' (Liaschenko 1994, 1996, 1997, 2001) that, although novel to nursing, is similar to that of Walker. The EC model of morality can account for the moral experience of nurses as actual moral agents in real time and space and, importantly, it provides concepts and language that can serve as an intellectual resource for nurses and indeed, everyone involved in clinical care. I find Walker's conception of morality a powerful resource in helping me with my two goals for the course. One of these is that students will own their moral concerns and not let anyone convince them that their concern is not a moral or ethical matter. Indeed, it is the case that nurses, and not only students, are told that their concerns are not an ethical issue but simply a practical matter, a communication problem, a 'boundary' problem, an overemotional response, or some other definition that negates and thereby justifies ignoring both the issue and the nurse as a moral agent. This goal requires a second: that nurses articulate their concerns in moral terms that both insist on their recognition as full moral agents with knowledge and concerns relevant to the community of carers involved; and that they demand accountability from that community.

In working towards these ends, I use readings from *Moral understandings* and the history and sociology of nursing, narratives of students' practice about which they experienced some moral concern, and discussion of these narratives in class. Final assignments have included a paper in which students rewrote their narrative of moral concern in the light of some aspect of the literature read during the semester. I have used final presentations in which students worked in groups and, using a select narrative or group of narratives, explored a specific concept from Walker's (1998) *Moral understandings*.

Space limitations do not permit even an outline of the EC model that would do justice to Walker's articulation. For that, readers must turn to the work itself (Walker 1998). To see a brief discussion of the four hypotheses underlying *Moral understandings*, readers are referred to Peter and Liaschenko (2003). In the next three sections, I restate Walker's central point of differentiation between two models of morality, introduce basic ideas regarding her understanding of moral justification, and briefly discuss her idea of moral ethnography. Following this, I use a narrative written by a student for class to illustrate, as best as possible, the ways in which I teach feminist ethics using *Moral understandings*.

MODELS OF MORALITY

Although Walker uses both 'ethics' and 'morality' in her 1998 title, *Moral understandings: a feminist study in ethics*, she challenges the basis of traditional ethics through her comparative descriptions of the 'theoretical–juridical' (TJ) and 'expressive–collaborative' (EC) models of morality.

For Walker, morality is 'a socially embodied medium of mutual understandings and negotiation between people over their responsibility for things open to human care and response' (1998 p 9). These understandings of responsibilities cannot be extricated from other social roles and practices; morality is not something transcendent but part and parcel of everyday social life. She calls this view, the 'expressive–collaborative' model of morality, contrasting it with the prevailing view of morality as theories, which she calls the 'theoretical–juridical' model. The latter 'prescribes the representation of morality as a compact, propositionally codifiable, impersonally action-guiding code within an agent, or as a set of law-like propositions that "explain" the moral behaviour of a well-formed moral agent . . . by "explaining" what should happen' (p 7–8). Walker emphasizes activities, not merely codes of behaviour, demonstrating that morality is about how people live every day. Morality is not about specified codes but about the practices we enact, specifically practices of responsibility for what is open to human care. Through these practices, we learn to whom we are accountable and for what. 'Morality tells us something deep and central about how to live' and 'ethics . . . . is a reflective and normative study of morality' (p 3).

Walker's EC model of morality locates morality in 'practices of responsibility that implement commonly shared understandings about who gets to do what to whom and who is supposed to do what for whom' (p 16). In other words, moral accountability is determined through divisions of labour that establish how responsibilities are to be shared, define the scope of our agency, affirm who we are and what we care about, and designate who has the authority to judge and blame us. We comprehend and sustain these moral responsibilities through narrative understandings that constitute our sense of relationships, moral identity, and moral values. Morality from this perspective is embodied and lived out by people in real time and space.

KEY POINTS: Models of morality

- The theoretical–juridical (TJ) model represents morality as a code or a set of propositional guides that explain and direct moral behaviour within individuals.

- The expressive–collaborative (EC) model does not locate morality in codes and theories but in actual human practices of responsibility and accountability.

MORAL JUSTIFICATION

For Walker (1998, 2003), moral justification or the 'normativity' of morality does not come from some essential core of pure moral knowledge outside of everyday human experience but inheres in the durability of our shared moral understandings and the practices of responsibility they sustain. These understandings and practices, however, must be put under the right kinds of scrutiny. Moral arrangements in social orders must be made transparent so that it can become clear who has responsibility for what and what terms are available to distribute and evaluate these responsibilities. This type of analysis makes it possible to examine whether differently situated people experience their responsibilities as intelligible and coherent and how the costs of these responsibilities are distributed. Walker states:

> If our way of life in reality betrays our shared understandings, or if these understandings turn out to be driven by deception, manipulation, coercion, or violence directed at some of us by others, where all are nonetheless supposed to 'share' in the purported vision of the good, then our trust is not sustained and our practices lose their moral authority, whatever other powers continue to hold them in place. They become then nothing more than habits or customs. (1998 p 109–110)

We live in stratified societies in which divisions of labour and responsibility are deeply marked by race, gender, class, occupation and income level. Not everyone has the same opportunities, resources and responsibilities. Rather, these responsibilities are assigned, accepted or deflected on the basis of these forms of social positioning. Some of us are able to demand accountability of others, but do not have to provide it to those of whom we demand it, whereas others are called to be accountable but cannot demand it. When considerable differentials in power exist in social moral orders, transparency testing can result in significant disequilibrium and conflict. This disequilibrium, however, can result in the development of critical spaces to open up opportunities for change. We can begin to consider whether our ways of life are better or worse than others we know of, or can imagine, and we can also begin to embrace the moral knowledge of those previously denied any moral or epistemic authority (Walker 1998, 2003).

KEY POINTS: Moral justification

- Moral justification is the result of the durability of our shared moral understandings and the practices of responsibility they sustain.

- Moral arrangements in social orders must be made transparent and scrutinized to examine whether differently situated people experience their responsibilities as intelligible and coherent and how the costs of these responsibilities are distributed.

■ The disequilibrium and conflict that transparency testing can produce can also result in the development of critical spaces to open up opportunities for change.

MORAL ETHNOGRAPHY

Walker's (1998) interpretive moral ethnography is the process through which social–moral orders are made transparent, reflected upon and critiqued. In short, moral justification is made possible through moral ethnography. It is a form of moral inquiry and, like ethnography as a method of social science, moral ethnography takes into account multiple kinds of data. For example, Walker speaks of the importance of including 'documentary, historical, psychological, ethnographic, and sociological' (p 11) data in moral inquiry. This range of 'data' sources extends the inquiry of moral concerns beyond the usual range of what is considered relevant within the TJ model. Yet it is only through such data that the moral understandings of particular social–moral orders can be made transparent. Many of the contemporary practices of responsibility and accountability experienced by nurses, for example, have their origins in the long history of gendered and hierarchical relationships between nurses, as primarily women, and physicians, as primarily men. Psychological data are important because they provide insights into how people see themselves and others as moral agents and how they appraise situations. Documentary data reveal practices of representation and so forth. Like the ethnography of social science, the data of moral ethnography are given in narratives.

Narratives illustrate a naturalized epistemology in that they reveal the knowledge nurses have access to and produce by virtue of their engagement with the work that constitutes nursing. This knowledge is a combination of several things including, but not limited to:

- Skill in multiple domains
- A general discourse about nursing and what is obtained through formal nursing education
- Knowledge of people in general
- Knowledge of how other patients with similar situations have responded
- Local knowledge of the actors and practices of a particular unit or institution
- Knowledge of the recipient of care

Nurses in academia have known the value of narratives in revealing nursing knowledge since the early work of Patricia Benner (1984).

Narratives also reveal nurses' moral understandings of the situation in question. Narrative ethics is now a recognized approach to ethics. For Walker, however, narrative is more than an approach to ethics, it is itself part of morality and of how people understand themselves and the world. Moral knowledge is not primarily developed, made visible, and communicated in the limited context of formal philosophical discourse, but in ordinary interpersonal contexts. Indeed, for Walker, *'we' are the members of some actual moral community, motivated by the aim of going on together, preserving or building self and mutual understanding in moral terms. We will try not only to harmonize our individual practices of moral judgement with the standing moral beliefs we each avow but to harmonize judgement and actions among us. We need equilibrium between people as well as within them.* (Walker 1998, p 64–65, emphasis in original).

Equilibrium is made possible through narratives because narratives show how a situation came to be and how it might be changed. For Walker, 'A *story* is the basic form of representation for moral problems' (p 110) and the basic forms of moral reasoning are analogy and narrative.

KEY POINTS: Moral ethnography

- Moral ethnography is the process through which social-moral orders are made transparent and critiqued, making moral justification possible.

- Narrative is more than an approach to ethics. It is how people understand themselves and their moral responsibilities in ordinary interpersonal contexts.

THE STORY OF G

Nurses are storytellers. I use their stories of moral concern to show the kinds of questions that can be asked. In the following narrative, I convey, as well as I am able, a classroom discussion. I am grateful to Terryann Clark, of New Zealand, for her willingness to share her narrative and the discussion publicly. Ms Clark is currently a doctoral student in nursing at the University of Minnesota.

The story of G

'G' is a 16-year-old Maori male with insulin-dependent diabetes mellitus (IDDM) who was referred to me at the youth centre by a staff nurse on a medical ward. He was being discharged, after having been admitted in diabetic ketoacidosis (DKA) three days earlier. The staff nurse said that he was 'non-compliant', 'obstructive' and had been aggressive toward the hospital staff. He had refused to see the dietitian and said that she was stupid. The hospital had discharged him but G was reluctant to leave. They were sending him to me by taxi and wanted me to 'sort him out'.

As G arrived, I could see by his body language that he was really not pleased to be here. He walked in, looked at me and said, 'I bet you're just another bloody nurse, who's going to tell me what to do...' I realized that I needed to approach this in a really different way. I said, 'Shall we go and get something to eat?' He said, 'okay', and so we went and had something to eat and drink. I asked him about his tattoo, which was a Maori design. He talked about the tattoo and how it was his family's tattoo design. He got quiet, and then said. 'I don't know where my family is.' This young man had stayed with a friend about a month ago, and when he came home his family was gone. His family had been in trouble with the law and had left the city without him. He had no money, no food and had been staying at friends' places. He had been stealing food and money to survive and had run out of insulin. He became very sick and landed in hospital. I was horrified that the staff had not noticed that his family had not come to visit him and had not called welfare services.

In Maori culture, family is central to well-being and this young man clearly felt abandoned, alone and angry. I asked him if he had any other family, like aunties, uncles or cousins. He said that he knew he had cousins, but was unsure where they lived. I asked him if he wanted help to find his cousins; he said yes and was very excited about this. Then he said, 'but they don't have a lot of money, and have lots of kids. They wouldn't be able to afford to let me stay with them.' I thought about the 'independent youth benefit', a New Zealand benefit programme for children who live away from their parents and told him that I might be able to help him apply for a benefit. That might help financially with his cousins, until he found his family or found somewhere else to live.

I started to check out other issues. He had a girlfriend; she was 13 years old and he had been sneaking into her house and staying with her when he couldn't find anywhere to live. He told me that she thought that she might be pregnant and that he was feeling really bad because he had threatened her to 'get rid of the baby' and now she wouldn't talk to him. His mood was justifiably low and angry.

He told me that he was really into Kapa Haka, Maori performing arts, and used to play the guitar and lead his performance group when he used to go to school. I knew that he must be very talented and have a wonderful voice because leaders are only chosen for their expertise in singing, performance and instrument playing. He clearly missed this part of his life.

Finally, I asked him about his diabetes care. He was clever, articulate and had a high level of knowledge about diabetes. He showed me the prescription that he had been given on discharge from the hospital. He obviously had no way of paying for the prescription, even if it was only $3. He laughed and said this is the first time that a nurse hadn't lectured him about testing and not taking his insulin. I told him that, considering the circumstances, I thought he was doing a great job of caring for himself. I was angry about how he had been treated by the health professionals who had missed all of this important information. We were not going to make any difference to his health if we didn't sort out all these other issues.

I talked to the diabetes consultant who had cared for G while in hospital. The consultant told me that G really needed to start taking his medication or 'next time he won't be so lucky'. He then went on to say that G needed to take this particularly complicated insulin regime, based on testing his sugar levels. I knew that G wasn't testing his sugar levels because he didn't have a meter. I tried to advocate for a much simpler regime, but was told that I was giving him suboptimal care. The consultant then said that 'this was a social worker's job', i.e. trying to sort out his social issues, accommodation and benefits. I was even angrier now, and called a community endocrinologist whom I know to be a youth friendly doctor. He agreed that the insulin regime was completely inappropriate and agreed to see G. We came up with a very simple plan that G felt that he could manage and the community physician gave G the insulin so he didn't have to pay for it. I knew that the consultant was not going to be pleased that I had undermined his decision about diabetes care.

I also knew that I needed to find a safe place for G to stay. I called a Maori social worker and asked her if she knew anywhere that G could stay for the night. I also asked her if she by any chance knew G's cousins' family. She said the name sounded really familiar and that she would think about this for a while. She found an emergency youth home for him where he stayed temporarily. My social worker colleagues found his cousins and a week later found his family. The family signed the forms so that G could access a welfare benefit to stay with his cousins. His cousins provided him with good support and a loving and stable home.

I went back and talked to my team about this case. I felt that I had been ethical and safe and acted in the best interests of G, but it had meant undermining a consultant's decision. My team was completely supportive of my decision. There had been previous 'tensions' between the community health teams and inpatient teams. The community physician who had prescribed the insulin offered to talk to the consultant. I was pleased that I had the support of my team but was disappointed that my nursing decisions and assessment weren't valued as much as a physician's decision. In the end, I talked to the consultant with my team leader and community physician present and the consultant agreed that 'it was probably the right decision at the time'. However, the relationship between this ward and our community health team remained strained and we noticed a reduction in the referrals that our service received from this consultant.

Two months later G asked me if I would come to his powhiri, a cultural formal welcoming, because he had gotten a part-time job working for a kohanga reo, a Maori total immersion preschool. He was teaching little children to speak Maori, to sing Maori songs and to participate in Maori performing arts. I agreed excitedly and felt very privileged that he had invited me. His diabetes control is still 'less than optimal', but I feel that it is much better for him to be happy than to have perfect diabetes control at this time in his life.

Like the majority of the narratives that I have seen in my teaching and research there is no explicit statement of moral concern. After the student finished reading the story, I asked what the moral concern was. The narrator (N) said that she wondered if she had done the right thing in going over the consultant's head by seeking out the endocrinologist in the community. She indicated that she felt fine with the rest of what she did. Another student suggested that the concern was more to do with justice in the allocation of nursing resources. If N was spending so much time with this patient, then other patients might not be receiving services. These labels of moral concern suggest schooling in traditional representations of morality in healthcare contexts. To voice the moral concern as one of challenging medical authority indicates an acceptance of a representation of morality that gives epistemological privilege to organized medicine in all contexts, even when it is not reasonable to do so. Likewise, to see the concern with justice as the acceptance of a traditional view of morality negates the moral agency and understanding of the narrator.

Yet, the written story of N's moral concern illustrates a variety of moral understandings about responsibilities and how people negotiate and adjust to them. Walker uses the term, 'geographies of responsibility' as a metaphor for making responsibilities transparent by 'mapping the structure of standing assumptions that guides the distributions of responsibilities' (p 99). Interestingly, Walker notes, that 'much of it may hardly be visible to us from within because of its apparent "naturalness"' (p 99). In the class discussion, I challenged the students to view the narrative through Walker's expressive–collaborative model.

In this model, there is no separation between the understandings of N's work and the morally central issues – there is no ethical issue outside of the concerns of day-to-day work. Identities and responsibilities are introduced in the first paragraph. The young man is a troublemaker disrupting the hospital ward by ignoring rules and because he does not take responsibility for himself – he is 'non-compliant'. He is also Maori. He no longer requires hospitalization and therefore there is a shift in responsibility from the hospital nurses to community centre nurses who are charged to 'sort him out.' There are differences in the moral understandings of each place.

In the geography of care that he has experienced, G's moral understanding is that nurses 'tell him what to do'. N recognizes that more typical approaches will not work so she makes the nearly subversive suggestion (given the diagnosis) that they go to get something to eat. This interaction is highly skilled with the result that N now knows how to gain understanding of his world and concerns and how to respond. She is 'horrified' that the hospital nurses were blind to those circumstances that make it possible for one to care for oneself as a person with diabetes: he lacks insulin, the money to obtain it, the means to store it, the equipment to test blood glucose levels, the availability of proper food, and a stable enough life so that the care of his diabetes can assume its necessary space in his life. N responds because she understands her responsibilities to help make it possible for G to have what he needs to live with diabetes. She helps him in the broader sense to live. She responds because she can. By this I mean that she is a highly skilled community nurse, working in a structure in which the problems of this young man are not unique. She responds because she is Maori and because she knows what cultural strengths can be enlisted to help him. Her actions reveal integrity. Walker's view of integrity is relational, which makes 'it interpersonally, and not just intrapersonally, indispensable' (p 116). For Walker, integrity is 'a kind of reliability' whose point is 'to maintain – or re-establish – our reliability in matters involving important commitments and goods' (p 106). The nurse necessarily takes multiple

actions to make the best of this situation, importantly asking the consultant to change the insulin regimen. She recognizes that the young man's
situation will require leeway if he is to achieve any measure of control.

The consultant, on the other hand, sees himself as responsible for
charting a course of optimal care in terms of the strictly medical management of diabetes. This involves fine-tuning insulin requirements in
response to specific physiological measures. To do anything else would
be 'suboptimal' he tells N, even though she has told him that his proposed management is impossible given the circumstances. Here the
physician makes a clear division of labour, separating the nurse from the
social worker and himself from both. In his view, the social realities of
this young man's life are viewed as either irrelevant to optimal care or
not his responsibility. Neither, he tells N, are they her responsibility. To
the social worker go the 'social issues' and to N goes the mandate to
make G compliant. In refusing to alter the complicated regimen of
insulin because it is suboptimal, the consultant protects himself from
possible charges of racism. While this may be understandable, there is
the odd fact that the consultant's insistence on optimal treatment is far
more likely to have a negative, even fatal outcome.

How are we to make sense of this? Assignments or deflection of
responsibilities are usually associated with certain forms of privilege. As
Walker indicates, 'assignments of responsibility are a form of moral
address, but some are addressed as peers, others as superiors or subor-
dinates' (p 99). The consultant's assignment of responsibility to maintain
compliance is a mix of serving the consultant's interest in achieving good
outcomes supposedly in response to strictly medical knowledge and his
interest in deflecting his own responsibility for acknowledging and
working within the limitations of what was actually possible for G to do.
There is no collaboration here; no willingness to address what is needed
and how best to adjust responsibilities. What is at stake in these moral
understandings? Walker argues that identity and integrity, sustainable
responsibilities, valued relationships and values in general, in the sense
of what people think worth being accountable for, are at stake. Here the
social location of the moral actors is important, but not simply as individual moral actors appealing to some abstract moral theory. The well-
being of this young man does not depend solely on any one of the moral
agents involved, not the nurse, not the social worker, not the consultant.
Yet the consultant's moral understandings would have us believe otherwise. Moral judgements are made not by some purely 'autonomous'
moral agent but by human beings engaged in ongoing activities that
share moral understandings that intersect from various embodied practices. That the consultant refuses to alter the insulin regimen is relevant
for many reasons, but most importantly because if the optimal course of
treatment is not followed, 'next time, G won't be so lucky'.

Morality 'consists in a family of practices that show what's valued by
making people accountable to each other for it' (p 10). In this situation,
N is unable to make the consultant accountable for seeing and understanding the conditions of the young man's world that markedly
increase the risk of the optimal course of treatment failing. From the

situated knowledge of N this is a ludicrous position, but from the consultant's perspective it is not. He has divided the labour and deflected responsibility for the patient's compliance onto the nurse and the social worker, to the extent that the latter is seen to make a contribution at all. The consultant can stand in this position because he is from a group privileged to claim epistemic authority on matters of disease and treatment. Furthermore, as a consultant, he is of a higher status than is the community endocrinologist. While at least etiquette requires that he respond to the community physician, most representations of moral understandings between nurses and physicians are not predicated on any requirement to listening to nurses on matters that involve courses of treatment.

The consultant cannot sustain his responsibility for optimal treatment given G's social situation, so his claim on that becomes suspect. Other moral understandings reveal themselves in the history and practices of the gendered relationships between nurses and physicians and the evolution of status regarding medical knowledge. For the consultant, there is no value attached either to listening to the nurse's account of why treatment should be altered or to taking any responsibility for altering the social world that G inhabits. If he were to take responsibility it would not involve his going into the community and doing something directly. Rather it would come in the form of *genuine* collaboration with N and the social worker. It would involve working with them and would disallow appeals to traditional divisions of labour that permit physicians to assign and deflect responsibilities when, in fact, the young man is vulnerable to the actions of all involved with him. As it stands, for a nurse to suggest that a consultant alter his treatment is, to the consultant, unthinkable. Depending on the moral understandings of readers, one could say something like: 'well it turned out OK so why is the nurse so upset?' I believe that those who raise such a question mean it rhetorically because there can be no question but that N's integrity and identity are at stake. N's knowledge as a Maori and as a community nurse specializing in working with adolescents is negated and, with it, her knowledge and moral understandings that offer more workable and life-sustaining courses of action.

There is much more that the class discussed than can be presented here. For example, the class reflected on the social space of the hospital nurses and what that might mean in terms of their responsibilities and accountability. We discussed the consequences for the relationship between the community clinic, which depended on referrals from the hospital unit, and the hospital. This relationship was clearly strained and referrals were down. I want to conclude the discussion of this narrative by commenting briefly on moral justification. N takes this situation back to the community health team and submits herself and her course of action for review of her moral justification. I would suggest N's language that, 'did she do the right thing?' is a limited view of moral justification. Walker claims: 'we learn progressively from our moral resolutions and their intelligibility and acceptability to ourselves and others who and how we are and what our moral concepts and standards mean' (p 113). Walker's expressive–collaborative model of morality provides concepts and a language robust enough to examine the way people in real time and space enact their daily lives.

TOWARDS A PEDAGOGY OF FEMINIST ETHICS FOR NURSES

In this chapter I have tried to demonstrate both the content and the process of my teaching of nursing ethics. I deliberately say nursing ethics rather than feminist ethics because, like Walker, I believe that feminist ethics is about ethics. I focus on *Moral understandings* because I am absolutely convinced that Walker's EC model of morality is a more accurate reflection of how people understand their day-to-day moral experience than is the TJ model. Because the EC model views morality not as formal moral knowledge but embodied practices of responsibility, moral agents and their understandings of themselves, of each other and of situations are central. The EC model admits to a wide range of data relevant to moral agents and the issues they see as problematic and, very importantly, the EC model of morality is concerned as much with those who do not have a voice as with those who do. This view of morality articulates identity, sustainable relationships, valued relationships and certain values themselves as what is at stake in morality and, in so doing, provides a language and the conceptual resources to all moral agents; one need not be a philosopher or bioethicist to name a moral issue, share in the articulation of moral understandings, and participate in the negotiations for resolution.

I believe that the discussion of narratives in class and working to connect students' understandings of situations with the concepts and language of Walker is invaluable but there are also trade offs. Even in a 3-hour class, there is little time for discussion of other readings. Although there is little on feminist ethics in the nursing literature, some of it is excellent, for example, the sections on nursing ethics in Megan-Jane Johnstone's *Bioethics: a nursing perspective* (1999) and Rose Mary Volbrecht's, *Nursing ethics: communities in dialogue* (2002). The new book edited by Janet Storch, Patricia Rodney and Rosalie Starzomski, *Toward a moral horizon: nursing ethics for leadership and practice* (2004), is noteworthy in two respects. While there are sections on feminist ethics, the entire text addresses many of Walker's ideas even though the authors are not writing from Walker's theoretical perspective. A faculty looking to teach feminist ethics might want to start with these texts, and in particular with *Toward a moral horizon*.

References

Benner P 1984 From novice to expert. Addison-Wesley, Menlo Park, CA.

Johnstone M-J 1999 Bioethics: a nursing perspective, 3rd edn. Harcourt Saunders, Marrickville, NSW.

Liaschenko J 1993 Faithful to the good: morality and philosophy in nursing practice. Unpublished doctoral dissertation. University of California, San Francisco.

Liaschenko J 1994 The moral geography of home care. Advances in Nursing Science 17(2):16–26.

Liaschenko J 1996 Home is different: on place and ethics. Home Care Provider 1(1):49–50.

Liaschenko J 1997 Ethics and the geography of the nurse-patient relationship: spatial vulnerabilities and gendered space. Scholarly Inquiry for Nursing Practice 11(1):45–59.

Liaschenko J 2001 Nursing work, housekeeping issues, and the moral geography of home care. In: Weisstub DN, Thomasma DC, Gauthier S, Tomossy GF (eds) Aging: caring for our elders. Kluwer Academic Press, Dordrecht, p 123–137.

Liaschenko J, Peter E 2003 Feminist ethics. In: Tschudin V (ed) Approaches to ethics: nursing beyond boundaries. Butterworth-Heinemann, Edinburgh, p 33–43.

Peter E, Liaschenko J 2003 The conception catches you and you fall silent: an analytic strategy for empirical ethics research in nursing. October Paper presented at the Nursing Ethics Pre-conference, American Society of Bioethics and Humanities and Canadian Bioethics Society 22 October 2003, Montreal, Canada

Peter E, Macfarlane A, O'Brien-Pallas L 2004 An analysis of the moral habitability of the nursing work environment. Journal of Advanced Nursing 47(4):356–364.

Storch JL, Rodney P, Starzomski R (eds) 2004 Toward a moral horizon: nursing ethics for leadership and practice. Pearson-Prentice Hall, Toronto.

Volbrecht RM 2002 Nursing ethics: communities in dialogue. Prentice Hall, Upper Saddle River, NJ.

Walker MU 1998 Moral understandings: a feminist study in ethics. Routledge, New York.

Walker MU 2003 Moral contexts. Rowman & Littlefield, Lanham, MD, p 207.

PART 3

Teaching ethics

PART CONTENTS

Chapter 19

Introduction to the teaching and different country chapters

Verena Tschudin

The step from theory to practice, from knowing to doing, is always the hardest. This is true in every aspect of life, but in health care it often seems to present particular problems. When ethics first appeared as a subject on the nursing and midwifery curricula, it tended to be taught in lectures; it was thought that if health practitioners know about the basic principles, they can and will apply them in practice. It was only with time that research was conducted with nurses who had been taught the principles of biomedical ethics. Prompted by something I had read, I asked a class of students which of the principles they tended to use most often in decision making. Their answers surprised me because they admitted that actually, when they make a decision, they do so on the basis of their conscience or experience and not on any formal principles or theories. After that, my methods of teaching changed.

There are relatively few situations within health care where nurses and midwives have to make ethical decisions entirely on their own. For it to be an ethical decision, it will probably involve more than just one person, or just one health professional. That is the point of ethics: it is always concerned about how to live and work together for the good of all.

Teaching and learning ethics takes place within a context, and this Part highlights this, with contributions from colleagues in various countries and cultures. Ann Gallagher gives a wide-ranging overview of teaching ethics in her opening chapter. Ann is concerned not only with the knowing and doing of ethics, but with many aspects in between: ethical seeing, reflecting and being are also addressed. These must surely be part of the role of any professional who is concerned for the health and well-being of any patient or client.

In our multi-cultural world, all health carers find themselves working with people from very many different backgrounds, beliefs, traditions and practices. It is no longer enough to know the dietary habits of certain groups of people to claim that good care was given. The migration of people, and especially healthcare professionals, is a major problem as well as a wonderful opportunity and challenge to learn from each other.

The chapters in this part of the book give some indications of the various historical developments of nursing and ethics teaching in the different countries represented. This in turn gives an insight into the possible competencies of the nurses concerned, but also the culture and development of the country. A rich and diverse pattern of practice is visible, but underlying this is often also a background of a culture and practices that may shock and challenge readers. The chapter written by Elizabeth Rozsos from Hungary is an example of this in particular and it is to her credit that she is willing to share some of it.

In her chapter, Elizabeth describes how she had to start her ethics teaching by making nurses aware of right and wrong. Most of the chapters in earlier parts of the book take it for granted that nurses work within codes of practice, are completely familiar with professional values, have had a sound moral education, and can make professional decisions of the highest calibre. Reading this chapter can make one wonder if all this is simply idealism when faced with the reality as it presented itself when Communism collapsed not so long ago. Yet there is no hint of bitterness in the chapter; rather, it is an account of what can happen when a system becomes so powerful that it pervades every aspect of life. Despite working in systems and institutions that condone cruelty, such acts are done by individuals. We may all have to have our ethical antennae well functioning because the power over others, especially dependent patients, can be forceful and seductive.

In their own way, each chapter highlights the inequities that most nurses and health carers still work with, be this with displaced people in Colombia, as described by Nelly Garzón, or immigrant Pakistani men in Norway, who are the concern of Eli Haugen Bunch. Ancient traditions and beliefs, such as those described by Nili Tabak in Israel, Adamson Muula in Malawi and Emiko Konishi and Anne Davis in Japan, are being challenged by modern technology and healthcare situations that can very easily turn received wisdom into questionable practices. The resulting turmoil can be devastating, not only medically but in terms of family coherence and the meaning of life generally. In stark contrast, as Leyla Dinç's chapter from Turkey shows, political movements can also bring a reversal of lifestyles and systems that were in their day considered to be enlightened and modern.

Taking these various strands into consideration, Miriam Hirschfeld sums up in a very global way what the future of health care generally will be. Her wide experience with WHO gives her a unique overview that gives a legitimacy to the country-specific chapters that they would not have otherwise.

Nursing generally is heading in a direction that becomes clearer when a global view is taken. The profession as a whole has increasingly to address itself to global issues and to working together with other agencies. This gives nursing and midwifery a professional autonomy that they never had before, but it is also a different autonomy from that envisaged in earlier decades. It is not a going-it-alone autonomy but one that is capable of bringing together the other health professions and enables all of them to work together for the benefit of patients and clients. Maria

Gasull addresses this specifically in her chapter. Professional autonomy is a clear call to all health carers. Interestingly, Maria does not favour a 'going alone' strategy. Rather, she considers professional autonomy to be necessary as the basis for patient advocacy. Ethical action is increasingly needed when caring for vulnerable people who may find themselves in situations that professionals would not tolerate for themselves. Perhaps that is when their consciences and their instincts play a particularly large role.

Chapter 20

The teaching of nursing ethics: content and method.
Promoting ethical competence

Ann Gallagher

Ethical nursing practice can be viewed variously: as nurses possessing and demonstrating moral qualities or virtues in practice; as nurses understanding and adhering to principles in practice; as nurses demonstrating qualities and actions of care; and as nurses considering ethics from a more political and gendered perspective. This chapter signals the beginning of the discussion of the more applied or practical aspects of teaching nursing ethics. No one theoretical approach is sufficient and a more eclectic approach to nursing ethics is necessary that involves more than understanding theory and which accommodates more than one theoretical perspective.

The stance taken here is that the purpose of ethics education is the promotion of 'ethical competence'. I will argue that the goals or aims of ethics education and the components of ethical competence are: ethical 'knowing'; ethical 'seeing' or perception; ethical 'reflecting'; ethical 'doing'; and ethical 'being'. Each component will be elucidated and I will suggest how each component might be promoted. Formal 'teaching' is only one part of ethics education. Other strategies include: self and other scrutiny, habituation, role modelling, coaching and engagement with the humanities.

INTRODUCTION

- How do the theoretical perspectives of nursing ethics square with the meaning, aims and purposes of teaching them?
- Is an understanding of ethical theory sufficient in nurse education?
- What should teachers of ethics aim for and what is their purpose?
- Should we even talk in terms of 'teaching' ethics at all? Perhaps another term would be more appropriate?
- It seems obvious that those labelled 'teachers of ethics' should be concerned with these issues but what about other people – nurses and managers, for example?

The promotion of ethics in practice is everybody's business and not just the domain of those perceived to be ethics experts.

The challenges of teaching nursing ethics relate to individuals, institutions and to the ideas surrounding teaching ethics. I propose an eclectic approach to ethics teaching based on a model of ethical competence. Ethical practice requires that nurses not only 'do', but also 'know', 'see', 'reflect' and aspire to 'be' a certain kind of nurse.

First, something about the challenges that may confront those engaged in the promotion of ethics in education or in practice.

CHALLENGES TO TEACHING NURSING ETHICS

The first challenge relates to definition; should it be 'teaching ethics' or 'ethics education'? One definition of teaching is that it is:

> ...a system of activities intended to induce learning, comprising the deliberate and methodical creation and control of those conditions in which learning does occur. (Curzon 1990 p 18)

The two concepts of teaching and learning are inextricably linked. It is very possible that much that is labelled 'teaching' may lead to little or no learning at all. However, those who take teaching seriously, in particular the teaching of ethics, need to appreciate how learning can occur and that much professional learning takes place without formal teaching. One of the limitations of focusing on 'teaching' in relation to ethics is that it may arise from or lead to the assumption that learning needs to be orchestrated and controlled by someone else and that learners are passive recipients or vessels to be filled. This is a false assumption. With encouragement, learners can take control of their own learning, engage with practice in an ethically knowing and reflective way, demonstrate that they can see the ethical implications of their everyday practice and come to understand the implications of their professional actions or omissions on patients, families and colleagues.

Three main types of challenge arise for teachers/educators in relation to nursing ethics teaching/education:

- Those the teacher/educator may encounter in the individual nurse: student – moral blindness, moral complacency and moral distress

- Institutional challenges or attitudinal obstacles
- Philosophical challenges, which inevitably arise when ethics is on the curriculum, such as indoctrination and relativism

A range of individual challenges arise in relation to nursing ethics and some of these are introduced here.

Moral blindness is a familiar problem and is apparent when nurses deny that there is an ethical problem or say 'I don't think of that as a moral/ethical problem'. If practice situations are not viewed in ethical terms then it seems unlikely that nurses will respond ethically. If, for example, resuscitation is thought of purely in clinical, technical or research terms (focusing on the use of the defibrillator or success rates) with the nurse being 'blind' to the ethical considerations, then the patient will be worse off. Moral blindness can have tragic consequences as professionals might not respond appropriately in moral situations. According to Megan-Jane Johnstone (1999 p 169), professionals can be 'conditioned' to 'see' the moral aspects of a situation. Ethical 'seeing' necessarily precedes ethical doing and being.

A second type of problem, *moral complacency*, is characterized as 'a general unwillingness to accept that one's moral opinions may be mistaken' (Unwin 1985 p 205). Johnstone (1999 p 174) is hopeful that this problem can be overcome by moral education and 'moral consciousness raising'. She states that the objective is 'to produce in the morally complacent person the attitude that nobody can afford to be complacent in the way they ordinarily view the world – least of all the moral world'. Reflective strategies discussed below are relevant here.

A third, and significant, moral problem is that of *moral distress*, which is discussed by Andrew Jameton (1984) and described as 'the conflict between the nurse's knowledge of the ethically appropriate action and institutional constraints that prevent or make that action difficult'. It is important that a concern with ethics education considers also the nature of the institution as these have the capacity to contribute to or alleviate the moral distress of conscientious nurses.

One challenge in relation to institutions relates to the 'hidden curriculum'. The conventional nurse education curriculum makes the knowledge, values and attitudes explicit, as well as the means to put them into practice in a transparent and organized way. The 'hidden curriculum' is not so organized and is quite subtle. This concerns the knowledge, values and attitudes that students are actually exposed to in practice or in the university, and which may challenge or contradict learning on the explicit curriculum. Students are likely, for example, to learn about the significance of enhancing an individual's dignity as part of scheduled classes, but they may find via the 'hidden curriculum' that in practice individual dignity is not promoted. If ethics is to be taken seriously then the character of the institution must also be considered. An additional institutional obstacle is the crowded curriculum. This raises problems of time for ethics sessions. While cost-effective, the lecture format is clearly an inadequate strategy to promote ethics if it is meant to contribute to betterment and non-deterioration.

At least two potentially serious philosophical challenges can be levied at anyone who claims to be interested in teaching ethics: indoctrination and relativism. If only one view of ethics is promoted, then the charge is indoctrination; if none or many are proposed, then the charge is relativism – a case, perhaps, of 'damned if you do and damned if you don't'. Daniel Callahan discusses this in relation to doubtful goals in ethics teaching. He states:

I do not want to endorse an easy ethical relativism. That no teacher can have a full grasp of final moral truth does not imply that there is no final moral truth. (Callahan 1980 p 69)

In relation to indoctrination, which is 'wholly out of place', Callahan accepts that students may come to share the teachers' convictions but the important question is whether their convictions have emerged from their own process of analysis or whether they have been unduly influenced by the teacher. If a particular perspective is promoted, even if this is a more eclectic ethics, does this amount to indoctrination? It seems not. What is important is that students are made to reflect for themselves on the nature of professional practice, on the requirement of professional obligations and, most significantly, on what is worth aspiring to in terms of their ethical 'being'.

Moral relativism or subjectivism is commonly presented as a way of explaining differences in values between cultures or individuals. It denies that there is any one universal moral code. Those who teach ethics may have encountered this in practice or in the classroom. Students may argue that ethics is relative to culture or is just a matter of individual opinion. This is undoubtedly a challenge to nursing ethics, but not an insurmountable one. One strategy to counter such views in the classroom that may be suggested to students is outlined by Joan Callahan:

Suppose at the end of the semester – everyone, no matter what his or her performance on the course – is given a D. The subjectivist is not free to complain that this would be unfair because he or she is committed to the view that there are no objective standards for moral evaluation of behaviour. (Callahan 1988 p14)

Callahan concludes that 'the students quickly see that they do not really believe that morality is reducible to the arbitraries of taste or mere opinion' (1988 p 14).

Despite this discussion, the question of how to justify ethics as a subject on the professional curriculum remains open.

THE AIMS AND PURPOSES OF TEACHING NURSING ETHICS – PRELIMINARIES

There are narrower and broader views of the aims and purposes of teaching nursing ethics. Judith Cassels and Barbara Redman (1989), for example, focus on skills in ethical decision making; Tziporah Kasachkoff (1989) focuses on reflection, decision making and articulation; Sara Fry (1989) focuses on commitment, reflection, moral reasoning and judgement, and ethical decision making. Ursula Gallagher and Kenneth Boyd (1991) focus on professionalism, understanding value systems, reasoning and the humanitarian nature of nursing. Win Tadd (1994) focuses on the development of moral consciousness, on seeing with 'a moral eye', on the acceptance of dissension and clarification of meaning, on an awareness of moral responsibility, and on the promotion of moral behaviour. This is similarly echoed in the broader healthcare ethics context (see, for example, Boyd 1987, Hope & Fulford 1994, Spiecker & Straughan 1988).

Five goals or aims of ethics education are discernable: knowledge aims, perceptual aims, cognitive aims, behavioural aims and character aims. These can be articulated as: ethical 'knowing', ethical 'seeing' or perception, ethical 'reflecting', ethical 'doing' and ethical 'being'. The next section relates these goals to a model of ethical competence. Developing ethical competence is arguably the purpose of teaching ethics or ethics education.

ETHICAL COMPETENCE IN NURSING

The drive to competence-based education is very much evident in health professional education and in recent writing on ethics education. This development is traced to the 'new managerialism in the public sector' in the 1980s and 1990s (Hodkinson & Issitt 1995 p 1), which requires 'that the quality of service can be demonstrably measured as can the competence of those employed as service providers'. The Nursing and Midwifery Council (NMC) in the United Kingdom, for example, requires that nurses demonstrate a wide range of specified competencies or proficiencies before they can be admitted to the professional register.

Competence-based approaches to learning have been criticized for their 'narrow, behaviourist conceptions of learning, and on a functional analysis of current jobs, which risks atomizing the job, so that the whole becomes less than the sum of its parts' (Hodkinson & Issitt, 1995 p 5). Competence need not, however, focus purely on behavioural outputs, nor is it the case that the individual is necessarily fragmented or reduced to parts. Competence can be defined much more broadly in a way that is amenable to being 'filled in' so that it is appropriate for professional practice and education. Wolfgang Brezinka writes:

'Competence' means a relatively permanent quality of personality, which is valued positively by the community to which the person belongs. It is the ability of an individual to meet specific demands which are placed upon him to their full extent. This ability is acquired as a result of personal effort. The quality of competence is attributed to a person who shows himself to be up to the tasks which life presents to him. 'To be competent' means to be able to do what is required . . . A person is competent by being able to perform a certain kind of task. If a person possesses the disposition for certain kinds of achievement then he is described as competent in relation to this task: 'competent to work', 'professionally competent', 'a com-

petent sportsman', 'morally competent', and so forth. There are as many kinds of competence as there are requirements and corresponding dispositions. (Breziaka 1988 p 76)

As the concern of professional ethics is with conduct and character, ethics is inseparable from professional competence and competencies. Where professionals are engaged with patients and colleagues, the competencies demonstrated will have an ethical dimension.

It makes sense, then, to talk of moral or ethical competence as something distinct from general professional competence because it cannot be assumed that ethical competence will inevitably emerge during the development of general professional competence. Nurses might be technically competent but morally or ethically incompetent. Ethical competence is a fundamental part of, and inextricably linked with, general professional competence. Extricating ethical competence from other kinds of competence, however, enables educators, students and practitioners to appreciate more fully the complexities, subtleties and skilfulness of ethics in professional practice.

As with more general competence, ethical competence should be understood not just as a minimal set of standards, but as a continuum that indicates a development process. David Leach (2002) has suggested that competence develops over time and that the stages of novice, advanced beginner, competent, proficient, expert and master can be attached to this development. He also points to the possibility of professionals being competent in some areas but not in others. These insights are applicable to a view of ethical competence that facilitates a more eclectic view of ethics.

ETHICAL 'KNOWING' – PROMOTING THE KNOWLEDGE COMPONENT OF ETHICAL COMPETENCE

The idea of knowledge or knowing in relation to ethics raises some contentious questions about the possibility and nature of knowledge in ethics:

- What does such knowledge consist of?
- What does it mean to be 'knowing' ethically?
- What knowledge is required for a more eclectic approach to ethics that incorporates a range of ethical perspectives?

Below I suggest learning objectives, curriculum content, teaching and learning strategies and methods of evaluation in relation to the development of a syllabus for ethical competence.

In 1994, Ian Thompson, Kath Melia and Kenneth Boyd proposed the following areas of knowledge that continue to be applicable to nurses in 2004:

- Relations between personal, public and professional ethics
- Ethics in health care and in specific nursing applications
- Ethics in theory and in practical moral decision making

The first area focuses on roles, rules, power and authority (Thompson et al 1994 p 179). Nurses need to understand particularly the nature of and relationship between personal and professional values. Students therefore need to be introduced to and begin to appreciate what commitment to a professional code requires and how this relates to their pre-professional values. A more eclectic approach to ethics requires that students know about professional obligations to be adhered to and virtues to be aspired to.

Second, nurses need also to consider the nature of professional–patient and professional–professional relationships. Health care is not value free and students should be enabled to consider the kind and range of everyday ethical issues that arise in health care more than the dramatic quandary. Some of these issues will arise from studying the professional codes.

The third area identified by Thompson et al (1994 p 180) relates to 'theory and practical moral decision making'. The process of decision making in the context of reflection on practice will be discussed below. Students should be introduced to distinctions and common ground between the range of ethical approaches (e.g. virtues, principle-based, caring and feminist approaches) and should be enabled to distinguish between theoretical and applied ethics and to consider the foundation of ethics in relation to nursing.

Learning objectives in relation to the 'ethical knowing' component of ethical competence should then include the following:

- An appreciation of the nature of a health professional role
- Knowledge of the historical and ethical foundations of nursing and medicine
- An ability to distinguish among personal, professional and theoretical ethics
- An understanding of empirical ethics (Hope 1999) and the contribution this can make to professional ethics
- An ability to describe the nature of everyday ethical issues in health care
- An acceptance of uncertainty and ambiguity in health care

Curriculum content is potentially wide-ranging and must be linked to the learning objectives above. There will be limits to what can be covered in an already crowded curriculum. However, there may be opportunities to incorporate aspects of this ethical knowledge within sessions other than those labelled 'ethics'. The health professional role is appropriate in sociology and history sessions, and empirical ethics can be addressed in research sessions. To avoid the danger of ethics being 'integrated out' of the curriculum, some sessions need to be protected as purely 'ethics'.

Strategies to facilitate the students' acquisition of theoretical and empirical knowledge necessary for ethical competence are many and various. Lectures, although a more passive pedagogical strategy, can be used to sketch the ethical territory. Students may also be more engaged in smaller seminar groups to share practice experience and to analyse cases (such as those in the following chapters) that invite them to identify the ethical issues that arise and consider how they may arise.

The acquisition of knowledge, however wide-ranging, is only one component of ethical competence. The evaluation of such knowledge is less problematic than in relation to other aspects of ethical competence. Conventional written assessments and examinations are also indicated. Yet, however much students 'know' about ethics it does not necessarily follow that they will practise ethically. They may fail because of moral blindness. Ethical 'seeing' or perception is therefore the next component of ethical competence.

ETHICAL 'SEEING' – PROMOTING THE PERCEPTUAL COMPONENT OF ETHICAL COMPETENCE

Tadd (1994) emphasized seeing with 'a moral eye' as a key outcome of ethics education. Two key components of moral perception and ethical practice are paying attention to particularities and drawing on the moral imagination. This was developed in relation to virtue ethics in earlier chapters. Perception is an important part of ethical competence. If nurses do not know how to draw on their moral imagination to perceive or see what a situation presents, they are unlikely to act well.

An educational strategy to develop this kind of perception or seeing is to incorporate the medical humanities, particularly literature, into nursing programmes. One of the claims made about literature is that it enhances the professional's ability to see or perceive. Attention to stories or narratives in fiction may help to develop the student nurses' ability to appreciate the patient's perspective. This is suggested by Kathryn Montgomery Hunter, Rita Charon and John Coulehan:

> *More specifically, literature has been included in the medical curriculum to develop students' narrative competencies, for example, the capacity to adopt others' perspectives, to follow the narrative thread of complex and chaotic stories, to tolerate ambiguity, and to recognize the multiple, often contradictory, meanings of events that befall human beings.*
>
> (Montgomery et al 1995)

Anne Scott (2000) points to the strengths of developments in nursing research where a movement can be traced from the traditional scientific methods, common in medicine and social science, to more 'narrative-based methodologies' that take seriously the experience of individual patients. In addition to the arts or humanities, particularly literature, making a contribution in terms of providing insight into 'individual differences or uniqueness', as argued by Robin Downie (1991; see also Downie 1994), narrative-based research methodologies also provide insight into 'common patterns of response' (common or shared human experience) and also in enriching language and thought. Scott cites Gordon Allport (1955; that:

Each person is like every other person, like some other people, like no other person. Each of us contains within us both general patterns and the particular, that which is peculiar to me and my context. (Scott 2000 p 5)

One trend that complements the learning that can be gained from literature is the incorporation of the patients' perspectives into professional education. There is now in health professional education a movement towards patient (or 'service user') involvement in the development and presentation of education programmes for all healthcare professionals. This may consist of consultation before and during curriculum development and by incorporating written and audio recordings of patient narratives into teaching materials. Students may be encouraged to speak with, listen carefully to and record in writing the experiences of people (preserving anonymity and gaining consent) who have experienced mental and/or physical health problems. These strategies form part of work-based learning preregistration nursing programmes at the Open University in the UK. This does not mean that there is no place for literature or other humanities, but rather that there are also other ways of developing the students' perceptual abilities, enabling them to pay attention and to exercise their moral imagination in a bid to understand the experience of patients better. There is also much to be gained from a consideration of qualitative research that places patient experiences at the centre.

Learning objectives in relation to ethical perception therefore include the following:

- An appreciation of a whole person perspective
- An understanding of common patterns of response
- The development of the moral imagination
- Enrichment of the student's language in relation to the experience of illness, disease or distress
- The development of the ability to see and hear deeply

Curriculum content relates to the learning objectives and, as with ethical knowing, there is scope for the development of some aspects of moral perception within other subject areas. The development of observation and listening skills may be in the context of learning about communication skills. Schools and faculties may vary in how and where they place the humanities, such as literature.

Apart from the development of ethical perception through literature and patient narratives, learning activities may also be devised to encourage students to listen to the patients' perspectives on their predicament. This can be very effective in distant learning materials but is also possible in face-to-face teaching where students can be given 'homework' prior to their next practice experience.

The evaluation of teaching and learning in relation to ethical perception is more challenging than in relation to ethical knowing. However, verbal and written accounts of what students perceive in literary narratives and in their professional practice would appear to be the most appropriate means of evaluation.

ETHICAL 'REFLECTING' – PROMOTING THE REFLECTIVE COMPONENT OF ETHICAL COMPETENCE

However much student nurses think they know or believe they see of the ethical aspects of care situations, it is how they process and respond to this perception that influences how they act. Students need to be able to think critically about what they know, do and are. Three kinds of reflection seem most relevant to ethical practice and education:

- Reflection on ethical ideas, concepts and theories
- Reflection on professional practice, people and events
- Reflection on self

The first most closely resembles reflection as part of philosophy, the second relates to reflective practice, and the third to self-scrutiny, according to Alasdair MacIntyre (1999). There is overlap between these three areas.

Simon Blackburn (1999 p 5) points out that, in philosophy, thinking skills or engaging in reflection are not just about the acquisition of a body of knowledge: it is a 'knowing how' as much as a 'knowing that'. He points to the example of Socrates who:

> . . . did not pride himself on how much he knew. On the contrary, he prided himself on being the only one who knew how little he knew (reflection, again). What he was good at – supposedly, for estimates of his success differ – was exposing the weaknesses of other peoples' claims to know. To process thoughts well is a matter of being able to avoid confusion, detect ambiguities, keep things in mind one at a time, make reliable arguments, become aware of alternatives, and so on. (Blackburn 1999 p 5)

Whatever professionals do or are is not just related to what or how much they know but is very much influenced by how they think or reflect. Blackburn (1999) describes philosophy as 'conceptual engineering'. Philosophers, he points out, study the structure of thought, seeing how parts function and interconnect, but reflection is not just something that philosophers can engage in. He goes on to say:

> Human beings are relentlessly capable of reflecting on themselves. We might do something out of habit, but then we can begin to reflect on the habit. We can habitually think things, and then reflect on what we are thinking. (Blackburn 1999 p 4)

In 1983 the publication of Donald Schön's *The reflective practitioner: how professionals think in action* signalled the beginning of the professions' acceptance of reflection as a legitimate educational strategy. Schön identified a dichotomy between the 'hard' knowledge of science and scholarship and the 'soft' knowledge of artistry. Professional 'knowing', according to Schön, begins with the assumption that competent practitioners usually know more than they can say. He discusses the 'crisis of confidence' in the professions and points to the 'tangled web' and complexity of healthcare practice. There is now a very large and growing literature relating to reflection and the professions and there continues to be debate as to what reflection really means.

Reflection on self is of much significance in relation to ethics. MacIntyre, for example, writes of the importance of reflection in relation to moral development:

> What each of us has to do, in order to develop our powers as independent reasoners, and so to flourish qua members of our species, is to make the transition from accepting what we are taught by those earliest teachers to making our own independent judgements about goods, judgements that we are able to justify rationally to ourselves and to others as furnishing us with good reasons for acting in this way rather than that. (MacIntyre 1999 p 71)

As well as standing back from and being able to evaluate our desires, MacIntyre also points to the possibility of fallibility regarding self-reflection and highlights the importance of social relationships in affirming and correcting self-knowledge. He writes:

> We may at any point go astray in our practical reasoning because of intellectual error: perhaps we happen to be insufficiently well-informed about the particulars of our situation; or we may have gone beyond the evidence in a way that has misled us; or we have relied too heavily on some unsubstantiated generalization. But we may also go astray because of moral error: we have been over-influenced by our dislike of someone; we have projected on to a situation some phantasy in whose grip we are; we are insufficiently sensitive to someone else's suffering. And our intellectual errors are often, although not always, rooted in our moral errors. From both types of mistake the best protections are friendship and collegiality. (MacIntyre 1991 p 96)

Although MacIntyre (1999 p 97) gives good reasons for the importance of friendship and collegiality, he also points to the possibility that friends and colleagues may lack the virtues necessary to develop and sustain practical reasoning. MacIntyre points to the importance of our not relying completely on others' judgements and of retaining independence in our self-appraisal.

What then should professionals do if they are to reflect and come to a decision about a practice issue?

There are many decision-making frameworks available in the professional literature. I will use Henk Goovaerts' (2003) 'staged plan' as an illustration:

Stage 1: What are the facts?
Stage 2: Whose interests are at stake?
Stage 3: What is the dilemma about? [What is the ethical issue about?]
Stage 4: What are the alternatives?
Stage 5: What is the conclusion?
Stage 6: How to carry out the decision?
Stage 7: Evaluation and reflection.

Learning objectives for moral reflection need to relate to the three types of reflection discussed here: general philosophical reflection in relation to ethical concepts, ideas and theories; reflection in relation to practice situations; and reflection in relation to self. They may be itemized as follows:

- Demonstrate an ability to reflect critically on ethical ideas, concepts and theories relevant to healthcare practice, drawing on the methods of philosophy
- Apply appropriate reflective and decision-making frameworks to practice situations
- Engage honestly in self-scrutiny with a view to moral betterment
- Utilize the moral expertise of friends and colleagues

Curriculum content flows from the learning objectives. Teaching and learning strategies that are likely to promote ethical reflection include Socratic dialogue (Phillippart 2003) and the teaching of frameworks such as the seven stage plan or Thompson, Melia and Boyd's (1994) spiral model of decision-making. The role of friendship and collegiality is important for the development of reflection on self or self-scrutiny. Reflective diaries or journals are also a popular educational strategy in professional education (Banks 2003).

Evaluating reflection is challenging for ethics educators. Coming to a reasoned conclusion as a result of a process of argument can be demonstrated verbally in student debates and in one-to-one discussions with students. Written accounts can be assessed. However, drawing conclusions about how students reflect in and on practice and on themselves is more difficult. It seems therefore important that students understand that professionals and patients are fallible and vulnerable, and therefore honesty is important.

ETHICAL 'DOING' – PROMOTING THE ACTION COMPONENT OF ETHICAL COMPETENCE

Professional actions do not necessarily improve with ethics education. Yet without an aspiration to ethical action, ethics education is futile. However knowing, perceptive or reflective health professionals may be, if they cannot 'do', the components of ethical competence are impotent to bring about ethical practice. Professional actions and omissions have the potential to promote or thwart the well-being of patients. It is the cruel or kind word, the compassionate or indifferent glance, and the gentle or rough touch that impacts for better or for worse on the patient. Ethical action is not just relevant to professional–patient relationships but also to professional relationships with patients' families, with other professionals and with students. There is evidence, for example, that student nurses are not always treated well by qualified professionals. An Australian empirical study reported how student nurses were treated badly when they were gaining practice experience. One student stated:

I'd never seen a resuscitation before. I didn't know that the woman was dead. The charge nurse asked me to wash her. When I asked, 'Is she sleeping?' they both sniggered in this horrible way. I felt desperate – it was as though they really didn't like me or want me to be there. (Alavi & Cattoni 1995 p 344)

Given the subtleties and nuances of action in professional practice, specifying learning objectives in relation to ethical doing raises many questions. An overall learning objective is: to act ethically in relation to patients, families, colleagues and students.

General professional competence should also be apparent in professional action, that is, that professionals can demonstrate profession-specific skills adequately. This goes some way towards identifying what ethical doing implies. but it is unlikely to go far enough in specifying what exactly health professionals do and should do. Professionals also need communication skills. They can and should learn from more experienced or expert colleagues and here role-modelling and coaching emerge as key teaching and learning strategies in relation to action and being.

Having role models in the classroom who are in a position to guide students and share experience is one thing, but looking to role models in professional practice to learn how best to act and be is quite another.

- What is a role model?
- How might students recognize an appropriate role model?
- What might be learnt from a role model?
- Might students not just as easily learn how to act unethically as ethically?

If students were to follow the examples of nurses who appear to extract pleasure from humiliating students, then they are likely to learn how to act unethically.

Being a role model involves being someone who is worthy of emulation for some reason and who can demonstrate the ability to play a role successfully. Role modelling as an educational strategy for professional education has been discussed in relation to teaching how to care generally (Nelms et al 1993); in relation to demonstrating different nursing roles (Wiseman 1994); and in relation to the cultivation of 'a moral sense of nursing' (Pang & Wong 1998).

Role modelling has been described as 'a traditionally accepted method of teaching professional attitudes and behaviours' (Bidwell & Brasler 1989). Ethical approaches leave open the question of how exactly role modelling becomes educational, but social psychology is quite clear. The social learning theory of modelling developed by Bandura is referred to in the three empirical studies mentioned above (Nelms et al 1993, Pang & Wong 1998, Wiseman 1994). Bandura's theory outlines the subprocesses that are involved in role modelling if learning is to occur (Bandura 1965, 1974 and 1977 in Wiseman 1994 p 406). These are:

- Attention to modelled behaviours: students need to observe
  discriminately, as mere exposure will not lead to learning. In the case of

ethical action, for example, students might be asked, as in Pang & Wong's study, to observe for examples of positive and negative nursing practice.

- Retention of observed inputs: students need to retain what they have observed in some symbolic form. It might be that, in an observation of the ethical aspects of health professional practice, students may code what they have observed under headings related to values.
- Production of a motor response: this occurs when what has been observed is put into practice by the student.
- Incentive and motivational processes: the theory proposes that expressions of the modelled behaviour depend on negative and positive sanctions. It seems probable that where students are praised for certain actions, they are likely to repeat them.

Bandura's theory is helpful in advising educators how to guide students regarding role models. Using examples of role models in class (e.g. on video) or sending students to emulate role models in practice is potentially baffling if students are not given guidance as to what it is they are to observe. If nurses are given instruction and have been helped to see and reflect then their observation of role models should reinforce what they consider to be good practice. This should also insulate them from bad practice. Some of the student nurses in Pang & Wong's study (1998), for example, gave quite striking examples of those they had observed modelling good and bad practice. First an example of 'good nursing' and then an example of 'bad nursing':

It was my second day working in the clinical ward. A patient died and the staff nurse asked me whether I would help her take care of the body. I had to say 'yes' because I understood it was part of my duties. During the procedure, the nurse cleansed the body as if it were alive. She took care of the bleeding wound and bodily discharge gently. She told me that the dead had to be treated with respect, as a person, and not as a thing. In that incident, I realized how commendable nursing could be: to treat people with respect even when they are dead. (Pang & Wong 1998 p 438)

There was an elderly patient who had weakness of the upper limbs. It was nearly lunch time. She asked a nurse to peel an orange for her. The nurse did not comply with her request. Instead, she told the patient that she should have the orange after lunch, and then placed the orange at the far end of the table, where the patient could not reach. I found this an example of bad nursing because by her impatient attitude the nurse failed to respect the patient's dignity. (Pang & Wong 1998 p 440)

These student nurses were able to apply ethical concepts, perceive, deliberate and learn from positive and negative role models. To use role modelling as an effective strategy to promote ethical action, educators need to provide a forum where students can reflect on what they have observed and discuss how the practice environment supports or diminishes their own ability to emulate good nursing. Another teaching and learning strategy, which connects with role modelling and has the potential to promote ethical doing, is coaching. This is a strategy promoted by Schön (1987). He writes of the dialogue between coach and student and the stages, which are as follows:

- Telling and listening – in the context of the students' 'doing'
- Demonstrating and imitating
- Combining telling/listening and demonstrating/imitating

This is compatible with the current trend to incorporate mentorship into professional education and acknowledges some strengths of the apprenticeship model whereby students would learn by working and talking with, observing and imitating experienced practitioners. Self-assessment and assessment of professional actions by the student's practice mentor or an experienced colleague also play a role in evaluating ethical 'doing'.

The final component and culmination of ethical competence is 'ethical being'.

ETHICAL 'BEING' – PROMOTING THE CHARACTER COMPONENT OF ETHICAL COMPETENCE

In virtue ethics (see chapters 10, 11 and 12) it is clear that this ethical perspective focuses on the character of the nurse and on her or his 'ethical being'. How one acquires virtue is a question that has challenged moral education for many centuries. On a virtue account it is argued that the character of the agent is improved by the practice of the virtues, by habituation. What needs to be said, however, is that this is not by 'habit' as we normally consider it. It involves practice and repetition. Nancy Sherman (1999 p 247–248) points out that what actually happens when we practise the virtues is more complicated than might seem from using the words 'habit' and 'habituation'. She makes the point that ethical actions are contextual and variable and also engage judgement, emotion and behaviour. She gives the example of justice, but the same also applies to other virtues. In one context courage may involve speaking out about bad practice and in another it may mean standing firm when confronted by an aggressive relative. Sherman's comments are applicable to professional practice where: no two situations are the same; the internal world of the student is as relevant as his or her behaviour; and where there needs to be some aspiration toward betterment in terms of professional action and being.

Habituation can be promoted in professional education by learning about the role and nature of good character in nursing, the nature of professional virtues, and what is required in demonstrating them. Some of the strategies discussed in relation to other components of ethical competence also have a role here, for example, the use of reflective journals and coaching. The evaluation of character is both challenging and contentious. Developing students' reflective abilities to consider their own character and conduct and the possibility of moral progress can only be a step in the right direction.

CONCLUSION

A wide range of learning objectives, teaching and learning strategies and methods of evaluation are necessary to achieve ethical competence. Nursing students need to be prepared as well as possible to respond to the subtleties and nuances of everyday professional practice. The moral life is exceedingly complex and not one of the components of ethical competence is sufficient to equip students to be ethical professionals. Rather, students need all of them.

References

Alavi C, Cattoni J 1995 Good nurse, bad nurse . . . Journal of Advanced Nursing 21:344–349.

Allport G 1955 Becoming: basic considerations for a psychology of personality, Yale University Press, New Haven, CT. Cited in: Scott PA 2000 The relationship between the arts and medicine. Journal of Medical Ethics: Medical Humanities 26(1):3–8.

Bandura A 1965 Influence of models' reinforcement contingencies on the acquisition of imitative responses. Journal of Personality and Social Psychology 1:589–595.

Bandura A 1974 Psychological modeling. Lieber-Atherton, New York.

Bandura A 1977 Social learning theory. Prentice-Hall, Englewood Cliffs, NJ.

Banks S 2003 The use of learning journals to encourage ethical reflection during fieldwork practice. In: Banks S, Nohr K (eds) Teaching practical ethics in the social professions. FESET (Formation d'Educateurs Sociaux Européens/European Social Educator Training). Online. Available: http://www.feset.org

Bidwell AS, Brasler ML 1989 Role modelling versus mentoring in nursing image. The Journal of Nursing Scholarship 21(1):23–25. Cited in: Nelms TP, Jones JM, Gray DP 1993 Role modelling: a method for teaching caring in nursing education. Journal of Nursing Education 32(1):18–23.

Blackburn S 1999 Think. Oxford University Press, Oxford.

Boyd KM (ed) 1987 Report of a working party on the teaching of medical ethics. IME Publications, London.

Brezinka W 1988 Competence as an aim of education. In: Spiecker B, Straughan R (eds) Philosophical issues in moral education and development. Open University Press, Buckingham, UK.

Callahan D 1980 Goals in the teaching of ethics. In: Callahan D, Bok S (eds) Ethics teaching in higher education. Plenum Publishing Corporation, New York.

Callahan JC (ed) 1988 Ethical issues in professional life. Oxford University Press, Oxford.

Cassels JM, Redman BK 1989 Preparing students to be moral agents in clinical nursing practice: report of a national study. Nursing Clinics of North America 24:463–473.

Curzon LB 1990 Teaching in further education: an outline of principles and practice, 4th edn. Cassell Educational, London.

Downie RS 1991 Literature and medicine. Journal of Medical Ethics 17:93–96, 98.

Downie RS (ed) 1994 The healing arts: an Oxford illustrated anthology. Oxford University Press, Oxford.

Fry ST 1989 Teaching ethics in nursing curricula: traditional and contemporary models. Nursing Clinics of North America 24:485–497.

Gallagher U, Boyd KM 1991 Teaching and learning nursing ethics. Scutari Press, London.

Goovaerts H 2003 Working with a staged plan. In: Banks S, Nohr K (eds) Teaching practical ethics in the social professions. FESET (Formation d'Educateurs Sociaux Européens/European Social Educator Training). Online. Available: http://www.feset.org

Hodkinson P, Issitt M 1995 The challenge of competence for the caring professions: an overview. In Hodkinson P, Issitt M (eds) The challenge of competence. Cassell, London.

Hope T 1999 Editorial: Empirical medical ethics. Journal of Medical Ethics 25:219–220.

Hope T, Fulford KWM 1994 The Oxford practice skills project: teaching ethics, law and communication skills to clinical medical students. Journal of Medical Ethics 20:1–6.

Jameton A 1984 Nursing practice: the ethical issues. Prentice Hall, Englewood Cliffs, NJ.

Johnstone M-J 1999 Bioethics: a nursing perspective, 3rd edn. Harcourt Saunders, Marrickville, NSW.

Kasachkoff T 1989 The case for teaching nursing ethics. Medicine and Law 8:593–599.

Leach DC 2002 Competence is a habit. Journal of the American Medical Association 287:243–244.

MacIntyre A 1999 Dependent rational animals: why human beings need the virtues. Gerald Duckworth and Co, London.

Montgomery Hunter K, Charon R, Coulehan JL 1995 The study of literature in medical education. Academic Medicine 70:787–791.

Nelms TP, Jones JM, Gray DP 1993 Role modelling: a method for teaching caring in nursing education. Journal of Nursing Education 32(1):18–23.

Pang MS, Wong T 1998 Cultivating a moral sense of nursing through model emulation. Nursing Ethics 5:424–450.

Philippart F 2003 Using Socratic dialogue, working with a staged plan. In Banks S, Nohr K (eds) Teaching practical ethics in the social professions. FESET (Formation d'Educateurs Sociaux Européens/European Social Educator Training). Online. Available: http://www.feset.org

Schön DA 1983 The reflective practitioner: how professionals think in action. Basic Books, New York.

Schön DA 1987 Educating the reflective practitioner. Jossey-Bass, San Francisco.

Scott PA 2000 The relationship between the arts and medicine. Medical Humanities 26:3–8.

Sherman N (ed) 1999 Aristotle's ethics: critical essays. Rowman & Littlefield, Lanham, MD.

Spiecker B, Straughan R (eds) 1988 Philosophical issues in moral education and development. Open University Press, Buckingham, UK.

Tadd W 1994 Ethics in the curriculum. In: Tschudin V (ed) 1994 Ethics: education and research. Scutari Press, London.

Thompson IE, Melia KH, Boyd KM 1994 Nursing ethics. Churchill Livingstone, Edinburgh.

Unwin N 1985 Relativism and moral complacency. Philosophy 60:205–214. Cited in: Johnstone M-J 1999 Bioethics: a nursing perspective, 3rd edn. Harcourt Saunders, Marrickville, NSW, p 173.

Wiseman RF 1994 Model behaviours in the clinical setting. Journal of Nursing Education 33:405–410.

Further reading

Banks S, Nyboe N-E 2003 Writing and using cases. In: Banks S, Nohr K (eds) Teaching practical ethics in the social professions. FESET (Formation d'Educateur Sociaux Européens/European Social Educator Training). Online. Available: http://www.feset.org

Murdoch I 1970 The sovereignty of good. Routledge, London.

United Kingdom Central Council for Nurses, Midwives and Health Visitors (UKCC) 1999 Fitness for practice. UKCC, London.

Chapter 21

Colombia.
Social justice in nursing ethics

Nelly Garzón

INTRODUCTION

The aim of this chapter is to motivate nurses and nursing students to ethical reflection on the basic elements of social justice and equity and their significance in health services and nursing care. It is important to strengthen the content and extent of this aspect of ethics in the nursing curriculum. Social justice and equity should have an important place in the learning and teaching process of the nursing discipline, together with other elements, such as art and science, aesthetics, philosophy, axiology and epistemology of nursing.

I take an approach that necessitates looking at the ethical aspect of social justice in the specific context where people live. This has to include the cultural characteristics, political organizations, socioeconomic aspects and the main social issues or problems concerning the protection of the rights of the individual considered as a moral person.

Adela Cortina, in her book *Citizens as protagonists* (1999), says that John Rawls is concerned about finding out the minimums of social justice shared by citizens in a pluralistic society. He arrives at the conclusion that the ethical minimums are those described by Kant in his concept of moral person.

Cortina explains that the moral person is a human being who wishes to be happy and does everything possible to be happy. This person also knows that she or he should look for this happiness within a society where she or he must behave justly. This means that the individual must be willing to share with other citizens both the burdens and the benefits.

For this study of social justice it is important to start with some general facts here in the context of Colombia. This will help readers to understand the situations that nurses and health professionals face when trying to apply these ethical components in their professional practice so that a truly humanitarian care based on equity and justice results.

SOME ASPECTS OF THE COLOMBIAN CONTEXT

Colombia is a beautiful country with a privileged location at the upper northwest corner of the South American continent. Three branches of the Andes mountains cover the country from south to north, and west to east. They pose some difficulties for communications within the country but they bring benefits as well. For example, the mountains provide cold and warm weather all year round, depending on the altitude. This in turns accounts for a variety of vegetation and agriculture, which produce many tropical and exotic fruits, high-quality coffee and a wide variety of flowers and vegetables, many of which are now grown for export. The country has thousands of varieties of birds, butterflies and different species of animals, making Colombia one of the leading areas in the world for biodiversity. The subsoil is rich in minerals, oil and precious stones, such as the country's world-famous emeralds. Colombia is a paradox: a rich country with a growing number of people living in poverty.

Colombia is a republic governed by a president and a two-chamber Congress elected by popular vote. There are 33 states, each with decentralized government. The State governors and city mayors are also elected by popular vote; representation of minority groups, such as ethnic and indigenous groups, is guaranteed.

According to the 1993 census, the Colombian population is just over 33 million inhabitants. By now this figure has probably increased to more than 45 million. The rate of urban and rural population growth has reversed in the last 30 years, with now approximately 72% of people living in cities and only 28% in the country. This shift in the population is significant in the sense that we are losing our agricultural tradition in many regions, and young rural people are moving to the cities in search of better opportunities for progress and better living conditions.

This internal migration to the nation's capital and to other important cities has created large belts of misery as a result of the socioeconomic inequities that now exist throughout the country. Almost 50% of the Colombian population lives below the poverty line, facing unemployment, lack of educational opportunities, limited coverage by basic health services, domestic violence, serious problems with drug dealing, the guerrilla and other illegal armed groups, the inhuman and cruel practice of kidnapping by guerrilla groups, the increase in different forms of delinquency, the corruption in public administration and many other factors and situations that are to some extent the origin or consequence of inequity and lack of social justice. What is needed are political decisions and cooperative working on the part of the government and society. The real roots of these social problems and how to solve them have yet to be found, so that a social conscience can be fostered that demands respect and creates dignity and rights for everyone.

According to the nation's political constitution (Constitución Política de Colombia de 1991) Colombia is a democratic, pluralist and participative society. The foundation of its democracy is respect for human dignity, solidarity and a priority to protect the common good and general interests of the people. To fulfil this mandate the authorities must protect the life, beliefs, property, rights and liberty of all people. Human rights of individuals should be safeguarded, as well as cultural and ethnic diversity. All ethnic groups are ensured equal rights.

Health services, social security and environmental sanitation are public services that are the responsibility of the state. The right to decent housing is recognized, as are the right to recreation, to work with a fair wage and safe working conditions. There is freedom of association, the right to education with respect for the specific culture of ethnic groups and religious freedom.

The Constitution also demands respect for the life of all people; for this reason capital punishment is banned, as well as all types of torture, cruel and inhuman treatment, forced disappearance, life imprisonment and exile.

It is urgent that the principles of equity and justice become deeply ingrained in the minds of public servants, people in executive or managerial positions, and in each person individually. If each person in society acts equitably and with social justice in their daily life with family members, with co-workers, and with all types of employees and neighbours, the prospects for living together in peace, with respect and love will be greater.

EQUITY AND SOCIAL JUSTICE IN REAL-LIFE SITUATIONS

Nurses are citizens (and often women), therefore many issues of social injustice and inequity concern us. We are frequently witnesses of inequities in real situations and also get acquainted with many of them reported in the media. Some of them are:

- Scenes of poverty in communities and families
- Homeless children, men and women living on the streets
- Children who have been denied access to a place in school
- A high percentage of school children who are malnourished and hungry
- Children who are mistreated, abused and abandoned
- The rising rate of teenage pregnancy
- Women who head families

- The increasing rate of drugs consumption
- A high percentage of the population with no access to health care
- Difficulties and constraints daily in giving quality nursing care

These and many other situations reflect the existence of inequity and problems with social justice in the health services, which are cause for serious concern among nurses, leading to what Andrew Jameton (1984) calls 'moral distress'.

For an analysis of equity and social justice, I use here the social problem of displaced people in Colombia, as their numbers have grown increasingly in the last two decades for various reasons.

THE EQUITY AND SOCIAL JUSTICE FOR DISPLACED PEOPLE IN COLOMBIA

In 1983, The International Council of Nurses (ICN) discussed and approved a position statement on health services for migrants, refugees and displaced persons, which was revised and ratified in 2000. ICN cites this as a problem of concern for nurses and in this statement condemns the frequent violation of human rights that occur with the migrants, refugees and displaced people and it also promotes strategies that support equity and social justice for these population groups. ICN encourages the National Nurses' Associations to examine the extent of these problems in their countries and to undertake cooperative action to provide adequate health services for the population that suffers the effects of these social problems.

As part of an ethic of care nurses consider the individual person, the family and the groups or collectives in a social, economic, spiritual and psychological context, as opposed to just the narrow context of the pathological problems. Nurses, feel morally and socially responsible to give displaced people and their families humanitarian, integral and comprehensive care, based on a multidisciplinary approach to intervention.

THE DIMENSIONS OF THE PROBLEM OF DISPLACED PEOPLE IN COLOMBIA

Displacement is a social problem known around the world. It has different manifestations but is associated mostly with the cruel context of massacres (the killing of ten or more people) committed in poor communities by guerrilla groups who have also been associated with kidnapping individuals, families and groups of people. This is a very complex situation that requires an interdisciplinary approach, continuing efforts and cooperative work to help people and their families who suffer not only the economic consequences, but the psychological and spiritual repercussions of the social exclusion also associated with displacement.

During the last decade, displacement of the population has increased and caused some very critical social problems. It has become a matter of concern for the government, the Roman Catholic Church, other faiths and many governmental and non-governmental organizations (NGOs), seeking to provide immediate assistance and long-term solutions to the affected population.

Internal displacement in Colombia began many years ago but has intensified year after year. Today the country has the third highest rate of displacement in the world. For example, 40% of the municipalities in Colombia suffered forced expulsions in the years 1996–2000. The human rights research institute CODHES (Consultoria para los derechos humanos y el desplazamiento) reports that in the year 2000, more than two and a half million people were robbed of their properties, expelled from their homes or stigmatized (Hommes 2004). There are no exact statistics, but this represents about 300 000–350 000 families (de Laverde et al 2001).

According to the Interamerican Institute of Human Rights (IIDH), a displaced person is someone who has been forced to migrate within the country and to abandon his or her place of residence and economic activities because his or her life, physical integrity or freedom have been violated or threatened as a result of any of the following situations:

- Internal armed conflict
- Outbreaks of internal tension
- Generalized violence
- Massive violations of human rights
- Any other situation that alters the law and the public order

The main causes of displacement in the first quarter of 2003 were general and specific threat (65%), armed conflict (12%), killing of groups of persons and invasion of municipalities (10%) (Cervellin & Uribe 2000).

Many displaced people are living in very poor conditions. They left behind or lost what little property or possessions they had. They also lost members of their families, friends and relatives. They miss their land and their way of life, and they express their desire and hope to return, but are afraid.

Sante Cervellin and Fanny Uribe (2000) summarize the consequences of displacement as 'the abandonment of crops, the disappearance of small villages, the lack of horizons for the new generations, emigration to other cities in the country or to other nations, and a brain drain'.

A meeting of a Roman Catholic Church group in Cartagena, Colombia, generated attention by saying: 'if we were displaced by violence . . . we should not be further displaced by indifference' (Cervellin & Uribe 2000). This is a call for social justice and is asking for each of us to be concerned, to help people who suffer from displacement and to advocate on their behalf, because it is human dignity, integrity and the rights of individuals that are being violated. This is a matter of equity and social justice that should be of concern to everyone.

As to nursing ethics, the field of study should be broadened to include social situations that are at the root of unresolved human problems, related to equity and social justice in every country. The guerrilla groups in Colombia justify their fighting and violence as being necessary to resolve the inequalities and unjust situations that create huge gaps between a few privileged citizens who have more than enough and the bulk of the population who have little or nothing and live with unsatisfied basic needs and fewer opportunities for progress. However, we should remember the moral principle that 'the end does not justify the means'. We must look for strategies to promote awareness and to encourage every person to be fair and do right by his or her neighbour and harm no one.

ANALYSIS OF SOCIAL JUSTICE AND EQUITY IN SELECTED CASES OF DISPLACEMENT

This section continues the general analysis and adopts a specific approach to the cases presented, focusing on the different generations of human rights. The Episcopal Conference of Colombia (2003) defines human rights as:

> . . . socio-political ideals founded in autonomy, freedom and the common good. These elements are expressed in values of living with others on the basis of respect for human dignity, reason and justice that require material and spiritual conditions that should be guaranteed to all.

The same document lists and describes human rights in three generations (of historical development). The first generation includes individual or fundamental rights, such as:

- Guarantee of respect for a person's identity and dignity
- The value of human life and personal integrity
- Freedom of conscience, religion, opinion, expression and freedom of organization
- The right to have and own property
- The right to a nationality
- The right to political and social participation with no discrimination due to age, sex, race or social class

The second generation of human rights is related to a person's life in the community, to social, economic and cultural aspects, and to the relationship with the natural environment:

- These rights provide the means and instruments to preserve the conditions for meeting the social needs of the population, their economic and social well-being and quality of life. These rights concern equity and justice.
- They are the rights associated with the family, social security, the right to work in proper conditions, with a fair salary, and the right to health care, education, rest and leisure, and decent housing.
- In general, to have equal opportunities for well-being and progress, without any discrimination whatsoever.

The third generation of rights comprises collective and environmental human rights. Their aim is to provide appropriate conditions for a person's development in harmony with the social and physical environment:

- to ensure the protection of people and their surroundings
- to guard against possible abuse or dangers attributed to certain technological advances.

Governmental and non-governmental organizations charged with helping displaced people and their families try to offer equitable protection, taking into consideration every generation of human rights. However, the priority is the protection of the right to life, respect for persons' dignity, their physical, social, spiritual and psychological integrity and satisfaction of their basic needs for food, shelter, health care, education and work. These organizations also help people to use their autonomy and resources for self-development.

The Law 387 (Republic of Colombia 1977) sets out the National Plan on Integral Attention for persons displaced by violence. It defines the term 'displaced person' and establishes the basic principles of integral care for displaced people and interventions to prevent forced displacement. It considers the care, protection, consolidation and socioeconomic stability that should be afforded to internally displaced persons. It ends with the statement: 'It is the government's responsibility to promote conditions that help Colombians to live together and to ensure equity and social justice.'

However, the government and many NGOs lack the resources to meet all the needs of displaced people. Many displaced families and individuals are not receiving the care they need and additional problems have emerged as a result. Some families have taken to begging on the streets and use their children as beggars. This is clearly unjust, as dignity and self-respect are lost often from a very young age.

The expectation is that available resources will be distributed equitably, in equal but small portions to everyone during the first 3 months after displacement. However, this type of help sometimes does not fulfil a family's basic needs. Some needs go unattended, such as the need for privacy in shelters, because the entire family must share the same bedroom and many families have to share space with other families.

The principle of formal justice, that is, equal treatment to equals and unequal treatment to unequals (different treatment for people according to their relevant differences), means giving more to those who have more needs. Yet this is often not possible in the situation under study because resources are scarce. Problems with equity are often beyond the control of nurses.

For instance, in the health services, displaced people receive the same treatment as regular patients but displaced persons might have additional problems, such as stress, anguish, rage, sadness and distress. Some need help to complete the grieving process. Displaced persons need to be listened to; indeed they might need more support, more love and more understanding. We should avoid addressing displaced persons in a demeaning way by referring to them as 'those people', or 'the displaced'. If they are to act with justice, nurses must devote more time and resources to integral care for displaced people. They must become advocates of displaced families so as to promote comprehensive care at the health agencies and the formulation of policies to provide humane and just programmes for care. In some situations, nurses are not in positions of power to influence the political changes that are needed.

Ethical reflection and analysis of situations in the lives of displaced people and families such as those presented below, offer a wealth of in-depth knowledge and help to strengthen ethical, humanitarian and fair attitudes in nursing practice.

Case 1	The film *Little voices* (Caballero 2003) features the testimony of two children, John who is 11 years old and 9-year-old Lilly, who relate their painful experiences with the guerrillas. Lilly describes how she was happy living with her family in a beautiful small country village where they rode horses and played with their little dogs called Puppy and Seagull. 'One day the guerrilla came and told my father he had to leave immediately with his family, because they knew he was helping the other groups. That afternoon, we left our house, leaving behind everything we had. We ran and ran to the road where we took a bus. We were in tears and afraid. Along the way we were attacked by another guerrilla group; they stopped the bus and forced us to get off. They pushed my father in a room with blood on the floor, and my mother and the children were locked in another room. Many days passed; they gave to us one meal of rice, tuna fish and hot water with brown sugar. We could not sleep, and my mother cried all the time. My father pleaded with them to let my mother and children go. Many days later they allowed us to leave. Again we ran for many hours along the road to go to another town. When we got there another group of guerrillas came. They entered the house where we were staying and decided to seize the girls and rape them. My father fought to protect them. In this moment the "paras" (another guerrilla group) came in and started shooting. They killed my father and many of the guerilleros'. After this horrible scene, Lilly said: 'Some people are mean to others because others were mean to them. They want to take revenge on others. We again ran away quickly with my mother, very sad, crying in silence and very fearful. After that terrible day we are always afraid, wherever we are, and feel different from everybody'.

Case 2 *The displaced family* *Perez**	This concerns a young family: Luisa, Ernesto and little David. They had to flee their town, which is a commercial centre that operates as a free port. Ernesto was hired as driver to carry 'merchandise' to different towns and individuals. He knew the merchandise boxes were packed with large amounts of cash that came from cocaine sales or money laundering. Every day he had to drive a different car and contact different people. He never talked about this with anyone but he was afraid of the job. He knew his life was in danger because he knew he had so much information. He did not know how to quit and eliminate the problem. He knew he and his family were in danger. Some days later he was notified that the job was finished. That day one of his relatives told him that he had to leave immediately; if not he would be killed. He left the town with his wife and son. That night they hid at the home of a relative in the capital. Next day they saw some

* NG's interview with the family; names were changed.

suspicious people walking around. He changed his hair cut, and grew a beard and decided to escape to another part of the city. The family changed their location every two or three days. Someone told Ernesto to go to the police and tell them the situation but he did not trust the police and was afraid to ask them for help. He could not work and he was desperate with this way of life. His wife looked to the Church for help. She is a Christian and her faith in God is a source of great strength to her and her husband. Luisa is doing some works for the church, so the family will have some money to live on. They are also connected with an organization that is helping them to gain entrance to Canada as refugees. This is their hope for their future.

Nurses are concerned and understand the realities of social justice. They know that in situations of armed conflict, civilians, families and communities suffer episodes such as those described by Lilly and the Perez family, which make them victims of social injustice. These displaced families must adjust to live in a new social group, with different customs and cultures and with no ties of friendship. They feel alone, afraid and like strangers in their own land. Nurses must learn to understand this situation, and to design strategies to help people in such situations.

Our society is affected by violence from various armed groups, each one with different ideals and world views. They all defend their own reasons for social justice. Some fight for equity in the distribution of land and goods for peasants, others protect the properties of those who own lands and cattle, and the military fight to maintain order and respect for all.

The civilian population is caught in the middle of this fighting and suffers the consequences. This situation can cause confusion. Nurses have to give care to everybody and they have to be prudent in their interpretations and comments. Although nurses might understand the circumstances and thinking of the guerrillas and armed groups, they will not agree with their methods because they go against the nursing philosophy of care and an ethics based on respect for the integrity of the person.

To provide displaced communities with nursing care, we must design interventions to safeguard respect, equity and social justice:

- Children such as Lilly need help and guidance so as not to grow up with feelings of hate and revenge. They must learn that weapons are not the means and way to win justice.
- We must teach children through positive experiences to understand the values of goodness, love and forgiveness in order to be healthy and happy, and be able to live at peace with themselves and each other, as a way to find social justice.
- Besides the effort to design rational models for justice in society, it is necessary to strengthen the sense of belonging in the families and groups of people who are displaced.

- When doing voluntary work with displaced families, nurses need help to meet basic needs, such as shelter, food and clothing, but displaced people also want someone to talk to and to communicate their feelings and concerns. In this sense they require psychological and spiritual support, and they need love and friendship. Nursing policies and care models should include these elements (Morgan de Morillo 2003).
- It is a matter of justice to provide displaced people with ways and means to protect their dignity, to avoid becoming beggars and to strengthen their capacities to be self-sufficient. They should not be treated with pity, and must be oriented to clarify and foster their goals for their future and for life.

All these elements demand that nurses be committed to design new models of nursing care for displaced people, based on equity and social justice, respect for their rights, freedom and autonomy and not on paternalistic interventions.

References

Caballero E (ed) 2003 Little voices [a film]. Directed and produced by Lizeth Santana, Colombia.

Cervellin S, Uribe F 2000 Desplazados. Aproximaciones psicosociales y abordaje terapéutico (Displaced people. Psychosocial and therapeutic interventions). Episcopal Conference of Colombia, Bogotá. May 2000, p 21.

Constitución Política de Colombia de 1991 Edición especial, (Constitution of Colombia 1991, Special edition) ISMAC, Instituto María Cano, Bogotá.

Cortina A 1999 Los ciudadanos como protagonistas (Citizens as protagonists). Galaxia Gutenberg, Barcelona, p 100.

Episcopal Conference of Colombia and other organizations 2003 Una apuesta para la civilización del amor, lineamientos conceptuales y metodológicos para la atención integral del desplazado (A blueprint for the civilization of love, outlines and methods for integral care for displaced people). Editorial Kimpres, Bogotá, p 32.

Hommes R 2004 Indicadores de desarrollo social, alerta social. (Indicators of social development: a social warning) El Tiempo, Luio 16:1–19.

International Council of Nurses (ICN) 2000 Position statement: health services for migrants, refugees and displaced persons. ICN, Geneva.

Jameton A 1984 Nursing practice, the ethical issues. Prentice Hall, Englewood Cliffs, NJ.

de Laverde DI et al 2001 Redes Institucionales de apoyo a familias en situación de desplazamiento por violencia en la localidad de Fontibón, Colombia (Insitutional support networks for families displaced by violence in Fontibó, Colombia). Unpublished dissertation.

Morgan de Morillo G 2003 Comunidad Ecuménica Colombiana de Enfermeras Cristianas, cuidado a grupos especiales: desplazados y reinsertados (Ecumenical Union of Colombian Christian Nurses; Care of special people: those internally displaced and reinstated). Unpublished report.

Congreso de la República de Colombia, Ley 387 de 1997, por la cual se adoptan medidas para la prevención del desplazamiento forzado, la atención, protección, consolidación y estabilización socioeconómica de los desplazados internos por la violencia en la República de Colombia.
(Congress of the Republic of Colombia, Law 387, 1997 to adopt measures to prevent forced displacement, ways to attend, to protect, cosolidate and to stabilize the socioeconoic situation of people internally displaced by violence in the Republic of Colombia) Gaceta No. 292, pag.1-6, Julio de 1997 , Diario Oficial No. 43091, 24 de Julio do 1997, Bogotá, Imprenta Nacional
(Gazette No. 292 pages 1-6, Julio de 1997, Official Diary, No. 43091, July 24, 1997, Bogotá, National printing.)

Chapter **22**

Japan.
The teaching of nursing ethics
in Japan

Emiko Konishi and Anne J. Davis

Europeans believe that only what Europe invents is good for the entire universe, and everything else is detestable. So stop doing us the favor of telling us what we should do. Don't attempt to teach us how we should be, don't attempt to make us just like you, don't try to have us do well in twenty years what you have done so badly in two thousand.

(Simon Bolivar speaks in the novel, *The General in His Labyrinth*, by Gabriel Garcia Marquez, 1990)

INTRODUCTION

A major debate in healthcare ethics focuses on cultural diversity and its implications for ethical theory and action. One side of this debate takes the position that ethics is relative to a particular culture or society because of cultural diversity (relativism) while the other side maintains that an overarching, universal ethics can apply even with cultural diversity (universalism). Within this complex debate, some believe that ethical relativism may foster the idea that any action within a culture can be viewed as ethical simply because it occurs within a culture. All activity occurs within some culture, so does ethical relativism mean that no inside dissenter or a person outside a given culture can define a specific activity as unethical because it is in a culture? Those concerned about universal ethics ask whose ethics will become universal and suspect that western ethics will (Davis 1998). The Nazi government policy that killed more than six million people they defined as undesirables during the Second World War could not be viewed by non-Germans as unethical using ethical relativism (Macklin 1999).

All cultures have values and notions of right/wrong, good/bad and respect for persons but these differ across cultures. While agreement on this issue has not been reached in the west, for non-western countries grappling with the development of bioethics, such debates have theoretical and practical implications. Japan is a case in point. To what extent can Japan view western nursing ethics content as universal and therefore culturally appropriate for Japanese use?

Like other countries, Japan has complexities and contradictions created by many factors, including differences of opinion among individuals and groups, rural/urban adherence to traditional or modern values, and generational/gender perspectives that may differ on important matters. The juxtaposition of ancient and modern, a symbol of a strong traditional culture alongside the latest faces of modernity reflect the struggle to maintain the one while embracing the other. A gap between the ideal and the reality is not unique to Japan with its homogeneous culture and social and historical pressures for maintaining conformity (Davis 1999). For some years, Japan has engaged in public and professional debate focused on healthcare ethical issues. The concerns included such topics as brain death, informed consent, patient/family rights to information, and resource allocation (Davis et al 2002, Konishi & Davis 2001, 2003). One of Japan's realities on the international stage is its relationship with the west, whose global influence can overwhelm, especially in this globalization era. Influenced by the west in modern times, Japan has displayed great capacity to borrow from others and by modification to make that borrowed idea its own. At present, perhaps, Japanese nursing ethics reflects an early stage in this borrowing process. Years from now, this chapter might have a different focus.

A BRIEF HISTORY OF JAPAN

Japan's long history reaches back to the Paleolithic Period about 32 000 years ago. We begin this short history with the more recent twelfth century feudal period when samurai forced the emperor into obscurity and built a military dictatorship lasting seven centuries under a succession of generals (shoguns). Societal values during that time included the concealment of personality and rigorous loyalty to the group, which to some extent remain today. Before the 1500s many Chinese came to Japan and then in the early 1500s, a few westerners arrived, some bringing Christianity, which the ruling shogun viewed as a force to unite the feudal lords against him. In response, he issued the 1639 closed-country policy (sakoku) in which Japan allowed only a few Dutch merchants into limited ports and put to death any

Japanese attempting to leave. When the American naval officer, Commodore Perry, arrived in 1853, the shogunate was in an advanced state of decay (Smith 1998). During these years of isolation, Japan had almost no dialogue with the west and no Christian missionaries entered the country. However during these years, many changes occurred in the west. The seventeenth century – the Age of Reason – was a great formative era of modern philosophy marked by the decline of medieval conceptions of knowledge and by the rise of the physical sciences. The eighteenth century – the Age of Enlightenment – witnessed the emergence of science and philosophical influences on that development. These events laid the western foundation of liberal humanism and rationalism.

During the Meiji Restoration, which began in 1868, Japan opened up to the world after some 230 years of isolation. The country rapidly became economically modern but the Japanese people paid heavily for their leaders' decisions, which included no political freedom, much exploitation and the preservation of feudal customs that prevented the development of democracy and modern social arrangements. Japan, suffused with xenophobia and militarism, furthered its imperial ambitions and these factors, combined with victories in the Sino-Japanese war (1894–95), the Russo-Japanese war (1904–05) and internal unrest, led to Japan's involvement in the Second World War. The Meiji Restoration and the post-Second-World-War period, including the more than six years of American occupation, stand as two recent major historic events that have shaped present day Japan (Dower 1999, Keene 2002). These events of openness and defeat led to a reaffirmation of some traditional values and a serious questioning of others.

SOURCES OF JAPANESE ETHICS

Ethical traditions are born out of the ethos and mores that have been uniquely nurtured and accumulated in the long histories and cultures in the east and the west. Present-day ideas of right/wrong and good/bad receive some direction from the past, therefore ethics is neither ahistorical nor acontextual.

Western ethics, applied in western bioethics and nursing ethics, arises from the tenets in Judeo-Christian dogma and the western philosophical tradition first developed in ancient Greece. Parents teach children to love others, to do to others as they would have others do to them, to play fair and to share, not to harm pets and other people, to tell the truth, to be kind, thoughtful, and good and to be self-directed. These values represent some of the ideals that form western traditional virtue and principle-based ethics.

The following comments on the source of Japanese ethics cannot do justice to this complex subject, therefore they must be viewed as an introduction to the topic.

One fundamental stance of eastern ethics, Taoism or non-action (*mui*), does not recognize a dichotomy between good and evil. This distinction remains relative and not absolute. Non-action does not mean to take no action but rather to reach an enlightened state of personality (*jinkaku*). This fundamental idea differentiates eastern ethics from western ethical tradition. The West emphasizes will and actions directed to the external world. The Japanese word *jinkaku* (personality) signifies one whose psychological personality and moral character are fused together. The fourteenth-century Chinese *Book of changes* (*Ekikyo*), the philosophical origin for both Confucianism and Taoism that scholars consider a book on ethics, teaches how to live one's life in a given time. The answer, given only once, is not issued as an imperative. One receives the answer by intuition, not by intellectual judgement or by inference because the *Book of changes* does not give specific instructions to the inquirer (Yuasa 2001).

Shinto, the indigenous faith of the Japanese people from the mythological age, goes back several thousand years and has a historical role in the Japanese ethical tradition even today. Shinto, or kami way, remains more than a religious faith; it represents an amalgam of attitudes, ideas, and ways of seeing and doing. Kami, the objects of worship in Shinto, include not only objects but also phenomena such as nature. Today, the kami concept includes the ideas of justice, order and divine favour (blessing) and implies the basic principle that the kami functions harmoniously in cooperation with others (Ono 1962). Shinto, the Japanese people's sentiment of life, supports the deep structure of Japan's ethnic collective unconscious. The universal spirit did not create the world but it takes form as this world (Carter 2001). The spirit does not stand outside as a separate object but is in every object.

Confucianism, the characteristic Asian ethic, focused on political ethics and family ethics (filial piety), became modified in Japan to become neo-Confucianism (riki philosophy) that says one becomes a sage through learning. It emphasizes efforts to nurture an ethical, enlightened personality as an individual and incorporates meditation (*seiza*) methods from Buddhist and Taoist influences. This ethics places importance on the mind/heart relation with others. Some think that this neo-Confucian ethics finds similarities with Aristotelian virtue ethics.

Buddhism arrived from India via China in 552. Buddhist morality focuses on the fundamental process of self-cultivation aiming at the experience of nirvana (enlightenment). Meditation and retreat are preparation, not ends in themselves. The goal of nirvana cannot be attained independently by helping others through fully compassionate acts. Ethics (*sila*), an indispensable ingredient in the journey to enlightenment, cannot be reached without such action. Mahayana Buddhism insists on the cultivation and eventual perfection of moral and intellectual virtues (Carter 2001). Introduced to Japan in 1191, the Ch'an school of Chinese Buddhism, or Zen, had rules that became fundamental to samurai characteristics: discipline, austerity, aesthetics and adherence to an honour code with loyalty as paramount. In 1656, a Confucian scholar codified these ethical guidelines known as Bushido, the way of the warrior, for the first time (Sadler 1988). Once followed by warriors, ethics assumed a secular role as history moved the samurai into provincial administrator positions during the Edo or Tokugawa era, Japan's late feudal period (1603–1867).

The greatest interpreter and historian of Japanese ethics was Tetsuro Watsuji (1889–1960), who refers to the multi-layered Japanese culture in which newly introduced ideas do not obviate old ways but rather place themselves upon the old. Japanese ethics places marked emphasis on relationship so that ethics appears as a wholesale application of the Buddhist theory of codependent and Confucian cardinal relationships that constitute the grand relationships (*rin*) of human beings (Watsuji 1996). In his book, Kitaro Nishida (1870–1945), a philosopher and practitioner of Zen, defines the good as that which satisfies the internal demands of the self. The greatest of these internal demands is that of personality; therefore to actualize personality becomes the absolute good (Nishida 1990).

The Japanese sense of self defines individual autonomy as inimical to group cohesion and not by the western dualistic thinking that separates self from the other. The Japanese self (*jibun*) means self-part or self as part of a larger whole consisting of groups and relationships (Doi 1986, Nakane 1970, Rosenberger 1992). This self is always socially embedded. The ideal enlightened state of mind is pre-reflective and intuitively active as a compassionate state of awareness (Carter 2001). This means that external principles and rational decision making focused on the dual concepts of the common good and the autonomous self are not central in Japanese ethics as in western ethics.

What distinguishes the Far Eastern perspective on ethics, and echoes recent western feminist ethics, although for very different reasons, is the fundamental assumption that we are from the beginning in relation and only secondarily and dependently, individuals. These sources influencing Japanese ethics teach that humans are intrinsically interrelated and emphasize the centrality of compassion as the foundation of ethical theory and practice (Carter 2001).

In the west, the applied field of nursing ethics often uses secular philosophical ethics to discuss healthcare ethical problems. That historically this knowledge interacted with the Judeo-Christian tradition is not always acknowledged. In the west, philosophy and religion occupy two different arenas. Philosophy is an enterprise involving the intellect and reason while religion is a matter of faith. In India, China, and Japan philosophy and religion are originally undifferentiated and inseparable. Philosophical thought in these countries does not require demonstrative arguments and precise verbal expression. Communication of thought is often indirect, suggestive, and symbolic rather than descriptive and precise. The eastern way of thinking is qualitatively different from the western, which emphasizes verbal and conceptual expression (Abe 1990). Nurses in the west may not agree on every ethical issue in their textbooks or in clinical practice, but the virtues, ethical principles and content of relationship ethics they use have a general shared meaning for them and the underlying assumptions and values fit their world view. While one nurse may support abortion as ethical and another not, their disagreement stems from the same concepts of personhood, autonomy, rights and obligations. The export of western nursing ethics abroad for use in entirely different cultures such as Japan, raises questions for discussion within the larger context of universalism and relativist ethics mentioned earlier (Davis 2003).

SOCIAL NORMS IN JAPAN

Much has been written about Japanese society and its traditional social norms. A recent historical division places these norms in bold relief by describing them as pre-Second-World-War (*senzen*) and post-Second-World-War (*sengo*). Traditional norms, such as mutual dependence (*amae*) and reliance on another to make decisions (*omakase*) and filial piety (*oyakoko*) still function in Japan (Okuno et al 1999). However, multiple factors have weakened these traditional norms since the Second World War, especially the industrialization that brings younger people from small towns and villages to work in the cities, more women employed outside the home, and the increase of elderly people to 25% of the total population. After defeat in 1945, many Japanese people wanted to break with their militaristic past, with the cult of emperor worship and with the imprisoning past created by the social order (Smith 1998). Those Japanese people socialized before the Second World War do not merely represent an older generation that differs from younger ones, but perhaps the differences in Japan reflect deeper divisions in social norms than are often found in societies that have not embraced defeat (Dower 1999).

Case study

Mr S, a 68-year-old Japanese farmer, has lung cancer. Until recently he felt well but now he experiences shortness of breath and general weakness due to his cancer. He has lived all of his life in the same community with his family and is now a patient in the local hospital. After extensive tests, the physician says that Mr S is terminally ill and will not recover from this illness but rather will die from lung cancer. Mr S has two adult children who asked the physician not to tell their father about his diagnosis and prognosis. They want him to believe that he will improve so that he does not give up hope of a recovery. As usual, the physician did what the family asked and has withheld information from Mr S. This morning Mr S spoke with you, his nurse, and wondered if he is seriously ill and will not get well but he remains unsure about his situation. He turned to you directly and asked what you think about his condition. He specifically asked you to tell him what is wrong. What should you do ethically? How should you respond to Mr S?

Sixty-three third-year nursing students in a Japanese college responded to the case study, which represents a typical ethical problem found in Japan (Davis et al 1999). The findings showed: 27% said tell, 43% said do not tell, 14% said lie to him, 16% said they should tell but would not. When asked what they should do to help solve this ethical problem they responded as follows in order of frequency: (1) talk with the family to gather information and appeal to them to tell; (2) discuss with the family and physician; (3) discuss with other staff; (4) talk with the patient to get more information; and (5) talk with the physician and ask him to tell the patient. A major theme in these responses was that the role and responsibility of the family should override the patient's wishes. Such remarks as: 'we should not interfere in family affairs', 'the family knows him well and they are partners' reflect the Japanese socially embedded self of the patient and notions of harm and good (Davis et al 2000). This study did not ask what the nurse should do if the physician and family continue to withhold information from Mr S.

These findings suggest that nursing teachers in Japan need to think carefully and critically about the content of nursing ethics courses. Whether they can use the traditional western principle-based ethics that include patient autonomy, do no harm and do good and mean the same thing as in the west remains open to question given the sources of Japanese ethics. The larger question becomes whether in Japan the content of nursing ethics courses should seek to avoid confusion in value orientation for the students (Minami 1985). If ethics course content for undergraduates relies on nursing ethics with underlying values and definitions mostly or entirely from the West, will this create cultural, ethical, and clinical conflicts? How will graduates know the ethically right action to take in a given situation if these conflicts exist?

TEACHING NURSING ETHICS IN JAPAN: WHAT WE KNOW

At the Japan Association of Bioethics meeting in 2002, Junko Katsuragawa, a nurse, presented data from her Master's thesis, which focused on bioethics education in nursing (Katsuragawa 2002). At this time, Japan had 95 Baccalaureate nursing programmes and this researcher had asked each of them to send any materials, such as a course syllabus, that included nursing ethics, bioethics or patient rights. From the 95 programmes, she received 55 valid responses and, using the Bioethics Literature Classification Scheme, she identified key words in the materials she had received. She found the following: 52% (29 schools) had a bioethics or healthcare ethics course and, of these, 13 were compulsory, ten elective and six provided no data on this. The content in these courses covered such topics as: what bioethics is, the definition and meaning of life and death, informed consent, autonomy, self-determination, plus topical issues including reproductive medicine/technology and fetal diagnosis. The teaching method for these bioethics courses included lecture only (five courses), combination of lecture, discussion, group work and practical (12) and unknown (12).

In ten of these 55 schools, students could enrol in a nursing ethics course but only five (9%) programmes required an ethics course. These nursing ethics courses covered such content as: the relationship between bioethics and nursing ethics, historical perspective, concepts such as ethics, morality, values, law, codes of ethics, rights. Topics included gene diagnosis, fetal diagnosis, palliative care and ethical decision making. No course used lectures exclusively as their teaching; rather, teachers used a combination of lecture, presentations and group work. In addition, these data revealed that all 95 programmes taught about patient rights in numerous clinical courses, nursing administration courses, social science courses and nursing foundation courses.

This study represents an important beginning if we want to understand the nature of nursing ethics and the teaching of nursing ethics in Japan. Some important questions that go beyond the focus of this study are: Who teaches these courses? What knowledge base do they have and where did they learn it? How does this content fit with Japanese ethics, religion and the definition of the self? Does the ethics content taught fit with what the students observe and experience in the clinical setting? If not, how does the teacher explain these differences? Do the 40 programmes that did not respond teach nursing ethics or bioethics?

TENTATIVE SUGGESTIONS FOR THE TEACHING OF NURSING ETHICS IN JAPAN

In the final analysis, Japanese nursing must decide its own ethics content and methods of teaching nursing ethics. Here we raise some questions for possible reflection in that process. Some of the data reported in Katsuragawa's research seem to have been taken from the western philosophical tradition of ethics; however, without more information, this cannot be certain.

- How do such ethical principles as autonomy, self-determination and informed consent fit Japanese values and norms?
- What forms the basis of individual patient rights in Japan?
- Does this content reflect the borrowing-of-ideas-from-elsewhere phase and the beginning of 'making it Japanese'?
- Are students taught about their own long, remarkable culture and the value sources that might provide the theory for nursing ethics and bioethics?
- Do teachers in nursing ethics courses make it clear that these ethical principles are fundamental to Western bioethics and nursing ethics with its own rich value system?

Most of the reported specific topics taught appear more medical ethics than nursing ethics, except that nurses need to understand the ethical dimensions in all such issues. These medical issues include treatment decisions for terminally ill people and reproductive medicine that certainly influence nursing but these decisions are the obligation of physicians. This means that nursing ethics can become a critique of medicine and medical practices. Some questions that Japanese nursing must grapple with remain:

- What can and what should constitute the theoretical content for Japanese nursing ethics?
- Could some Japanese philosophers with a background in Japanese ethics and nurse educators teaching nursing ethics work together to develop a nursing ethics congenial to the Japanese ethos?
- If so, what might it look like?

Perhaps, Japanese nursing ethics would be an ethics of virtue and relationships rather than one of principles, which is so dominant in the west, and especially in the USA. Although such work would take Japanese values and norms as the starting point, could this work benefit from a review of virtue ethics and relationship ethics as depicted in this book and elsewhere? These comments focus on the need to develop Japanese ethics content in nursing with the realization that such an ethics would reflect Japanese values and norms while at the same time evolving as the society changes. Is it problematic for Japanese nursing simply to teach western nursing ethics without thinking through what this means and the nature of the ethical and cultural fit or lack of fit involved (Davis 2000)?

The second concern that Japanese nursing could examine relates to teaching methods used in nursing ethics courses. Historically, and continuing today in Japan, the teacher imparts knowledge and wisdom mainly through lectures. This method, an efficient way to teach large numbers of students basic knowledge, falls short if the teacher wants students to engage in critical thinking. In western nursing ethics courses, the objective is often the development of critical thinking and the ability to analyse ethical problems. This means that students need an understanding of ethical issues, such as lying to a patient and – more fundamentally – what constitutes a lie, along with how to think about these issues. Critical learning and analysis of ethical problems cannot be learned in a lecture because they require dialogue and debate. In Katsuragawa's (2002) research the ten schools reporting nursing ethics courses indicated that none used only the lecture teaching method. A teaching method that is explorative raises the question of what teachers hope to achieve. What are the course objectives and how can they be best attained?

These questions are not unique to Japan and need to be examined in all cultures, including those where nursing ethics courses have been available for some time. The world changes and these changes impact on individual cultures. As the world changes, values shift and modify to accommodate the new. We have only recently become uncertain of when someone is dead. This uncertainty stems from the use of technology that maintains the biological person indefinitely. To some extent, ideas and values change as they interact with each other during discourse on national and international stages. This means that ethics, bioethics and nursing ethics are not unchanging bodies of knowledge but continue to emerge and evolve. A recent doctoral dissertation by a Japanese nurse aimed to explicate the moral concerns of nurses caring for dying patients and to describe the ethical nursing practice that revealed nurses' moral concerns. She found seven moral concerns: (1) do not hurt the patient, (2) honesty, (3) isolation/loneliness, (4) regard for the patient's personhood, (5) respect for the patient's wishes, (6) comfort/relief from suffering, and (7) meaningful/pleasant time for the patient. These findings are similar to those in the USA and also make clear that cultural and social background meanings have an enormous impact on nursing practice and shape the practice (Izumi 2003). The present research conducted by Japanese nurses and that undertaken in the future will move Japanese nursing towards a fuller understanding of nursing ethics in Japan.

References

Abe M 1990 Introduction. In: Nishida K (ed) An inquiry into the good. Yale University Press, New Haven, CT, p vii–xxviii.

Carter RE 2001 Encounter with enlightenment: a study of Japanese ethics. State University of NY Press, Albany, NY.

Davis AJ 1998 Development of nursing ethics: are there universals? International Nursing Review (Japanese version) 21(5):69–72 [in Japanese].

Davis AJ 1999 Global influence of American nursing: some ethical issues. Nursing Ethics 6:118–125.

Davis AJ 2000 Ethics in international nursing: issues and questions. In: Chaska N (ed) The nursing profession: tomorrow and beyond. Sage, Thousand Oaks, CA, p 65–73.

Davis AJ 2003 International nursing ethics: context and concerns. In: Tschudin V (ed) Approaches to ethics: nursing beyond boundaries. Butterworth Heinmann, Edinburgh, p 95–104.

Davis AJ, Ota K, Suzuki M et al 1999 Nursing students' responses to a case study in ethics. Nursing and Health Science 1(1):3–6.

Davis AJ, Konishi E, Mitoh T 2000 Framework for information disclosure to the terminally ill in Japan. Journal of the Japanese Association for Bioethics 10(1):84–91 [in Japanese].

Davis AJ, Konishi E, Mitoh T 2002 The telling and knowing of dying: philosophical bases for hospice care in Japan. International Nursing Review 49:1–8.

Doi T 1986 The anatomy of self. Kodansha, Tokyo.

Dower JW 1999 Embracing defeat: Japan in the wake of world war II. Norton, New York.

Izumi S 2003 Nursing ethics in end-of-life care in Japan. Oregon Health Sciences University, Portland. PhD Dissertation Abstracts, University of Michigan, Anne Arbor, MI.

Katsuragawa J 2002 Bioethics education in undergraduate nursing curricula in Japan. Master's thesis, Waseda University, Tokyo [in Japanese].

Keene D 2002 Emperor of Japan: Meiji and his world 1852–1912. Columbia University Press, New York.

Konishi E, Davis AJ 2001 Right to die and duty to die: perceptions of nurses in the West and in Japan. International Nursing Review 48:17–28.

Konishi E, Davis AJ 2003 Physician non-disclosure and paternalism in terminal care: ethical issues for Japanese nurses. Eubios Journal of Asian and International Bioethics 13:213–215.

Macklin R 1999 Against relativism: cultural diversity and the search for ethical universals in medicine. Oxford University Press, New York.

Marquez GG 2003 The general in his labyrinth. Random House, New York, p 87.

Minami H 1985 East meets west; some ethical considerations. International Journal of Nursing Studies 22:311–318.

Nakane C 1970 The Japanese society. University of California Press, Berkeley.

Nishida K 1990 An inquiry into the good. Yale University Press, New Haven, CT.

Okuno S, Tagaya A, Tamura M, Davis AJ 1999 Japanese elderly in small towns reflect on end-of-life issues. Nursing Ethics 6:308–315.

Ono S 1962 Shinto: the kami way. Tuttle, Rutland, VT.

Rosenberger NR 1992 (ed) Japanese sense of self. Cambridge University Press, Cambridge.

Sadler AL 1988 The code of the Samurai (*Budo Shoshinshu*). Tuttle, Rutland VT.

Smith P 1998 Japan: a reinterpretation. Vintage Books, New York.

Watsuji T 1996 Japanese ethics (trans. Yamamoto S, Carter RE). State University of New York, Albany.

Yuasa Y 2001 Forword. In: Carter RE (ed) Encounter with enlightenment: a study of Japanese ethics. State University of New York, Albany.

Further reading

Aitken R 1984 The mind of clover: essays in Zen Buddhist ethics. North Point Press, San Francisco.

Ames RT, Dissanayake W, Kasulis T (eds) 1994 Self as person in Asian theory and practice. State University of NewYork Press, Albany.

Dharmasiri G 1989 Fundamentals of Buddhist ethics. Golden Leaves, Antioch, CA.

Fujiki N, Macer DRJ 1998 (eds) Bioethics in Asia. Eubios Ethics Institute, Tsukuba Science City, Japan.

Hamano K 1997 A report from Japan: human rights and Japanese bioethics. Bioethics 11:328–335.

Hardacre H 1994 The response of Buddhism and Shinto to the issue of brain death and organ transplants. Cambridge Quarterly of Healthcare Ethics 3:585–601.

Special Issue of Philosophy East and West 1990 Understanding Japanese Values 40(4).

Chapter **23**

Israel.
Teaching nursing ethics in Israel: ancient values meet modern healthcare problems

Nili Tabak

INTRODUCTION: ISRAEL AND THE JEWISH RELIGION

Israel was established in 1948 as a Jewish state. It is a mixture of ancient religious values and laws set in a modern, and to a large extent, secular society. Nursing ethics teachers in Israel must deal with the tensions created by this mixture of old and new as it penetrates every aspect of life.

The population of Israel is 80.1% Jewish, 14.6% Muslim, 2.1% Christian and 1.2 other (Central Bureau of Statistics 2004). Hebrew is the official language and the government is a parliamentary democracy with elected officials debating and creating the basic laws of the country.

Alongside these aspects of modern Israel stand the ancient Jewish traditions of belief and law. Judaism is a monotheistic religion with a belief in one God, who created and rules the world as all-powerful, all-knowing, in all places at all times. When God gave Moses the Ten Commandments on Mount Sinai, as depicted in the Bible, the Jews committed themselves to follow the code of law that regulates how to worship and how to treat others.

The Torah, the first five books of the Bible, contains 613 *Mitzvoth* (commandments) and serves as the primary document revealing God's instructions to the Jewish people teaching them how to act, think and feel about life and death. *Halacha* (Jewish law or the path that one walks) is made up of the *Mitzvoth* from the Torah and laws instituted by rabbis (*Takkanah*) and long-standing customs (*Minhag*). All of these have the status of Jewish law and all are equally binding. Essentially, Judaism is not just a set of beliefs about God, human beings and the universe but a comprehensive way of life. Judaism's ethics stems from these sources. Jews believe that people, while created in God's image, still have free will and responsibility for the choices they make. In the modern Jewish state these ancient beliefs and laws form the foundation for ethics and healthcare ethics.

Because each person is created in God's image, all are equal. Importantly, each person has free will and carries responsibility for the choices he or she makes. In Israel, people distinguish between general non-religious ethics and Jewish ethics, stressing the fundamental differences between Jewish law and secular ethical doctrines in all areas of life.

This chapter details selected aspects of Jewish law, the bases for Jewish ethics, and recent secular law that attempts to deal with present day ethical issues in health care. Some comments about teaching nursing ethics in Israel will also be made.

HEALTHCARE ETHICAL ISSUES IN ISRAEL

In some respects Jewish bioethics differs from general ethics in its attitude toward medical problems and research in the *Halacha* discourse and in the final conclusions. Ethical problems are decided according to *Halacha* principles, which are binding on patients and healthcare professionals, but not in cases where medical considerations are overwhelming. Jewish bioethics is based on obligations and prohibitions and the word 'rights' does not appear in Biblical or Talmudic literature, whereas general bioethics has a main focus on rights, autonomy and self-realization.

In Israel, the doctor–patient relationship binds the patient to seek treatment and cure and the doctor, as messenger of God, to treat and cure the patient. Patients are not autonomous with respect to decisions about their bodies. God granted individuals their bodies and lives, therefore human life is the supreme value. Where life is endangered, medical requirements overrule many prohibitions in the Torah (Steinberg 1998).

The Jewish tradition values the individual's free will to choose but that freedom is not absolute because a complex system of relations exists between the principle of Divinity and the principle of free choice. Once we accept that the individual must abide by the *Halacha*, then that restricts personal autonomy. This is a basic principle of the Jewish religion.

Case study   Mr AC, a 78-year-old Jewish man married for 50 years and father of four children, was born in Poland but immigrated to Israel. His wife is a homemaker and he worked for many years in a metal-coating plant. Several years ago he was diagnosed with bladder cancer and underwent surgery. He was then able to take care of himself. Lately, he had developed cognitive problems that included decline in memory, a thinking disorder, disorientation of time and place, speech problems, depression and apathy. At the same time he experienced a recurrence of cancer and his condition deteriorated. He received chemotherapy, which induced severe side effects, infections, and respiratory difficulties. In spite of his severe condition, and occasionally aware of his state, AC requested that his life not be prolonged by any artificial means because of his suffering.

He asked to be allowed to die with dignity.

How do the ancient Jewish laws and recent secular laws inform us as to the ethical action to take in this case? The next sections will demonstrate the complex issues in this case created by the fact that Israel has ancient laws that guide ethical actions as well as a secular society that questions aspects of this law.

HUMAN DIGNITY AND RIGHTS OVER ONE'S OWN PERSON

In Israel the basic law says the question of individual dignity and freedom raises issues of people's right over their body to a constitutional level. It further states that no harm must be done to the life, body or dignity of an individual as a human being and every individual is entitled to protection for his or her life, body and dignity (State of Israel 1994a).

The Patients' Rights Law and the Law for the Protection of Privacy also give individuals rights over their own bodies (Israel Medical Organization 1996, State of Israel 1994b). When a health professional acts against the will of the patient, this is defined legally as assault. The patient may refuse treatment, including life-saving treatment, on religious or ideological grounds. However, the doctor will not agree to this refusal if it conflicts with standards of medical practice (Carmi 1984). The *Halacha* takes the position that a health professional's duty is to take measures to prevent patients from making a decision that risks their lives (Ben Shlomo 1998), whereas in general, the freedom of an individual is limited when the person's action can harm another. Under *Halacha* law this restriction applies to not only causing harm to others but also causing harm to self. Any crucial medical decision cannot be made before consulting with greater experts. The consent of patients is not helpful according to *Halacha*, since they do not have possession over their bodies. The body is given to the person as a deposit from God and so the issue of consent is invalid. Saving human life is the supreme value because the value of life is indivisible and irreducible (Carmi & Sagiv 1986, Israeli Supreme Court 1982).

DYING PATIENTS

Today, *Halacha* has definitions for 'terminal patient' and criteria for dying by the standards of modern medicine (Shafran 2003).

In a draft law presented in the Israeli parliament (in 2001), a patient who is about to die is defined as one who suffers from an incurable medical problem and as one whose life expectancy, according to current medical knowledge, does not exceed six months (Steinberg 2001). From the *Halacha* perspective, this is a concept that describes a state of terminal illness and the subjective feelings of the person who is on the verge of death (Steinberg 1994). The Israeli parliament has not yet defined what a terminally ill patient is and what is meant by terminal illness. The first legal definition of terminal illness appeared in a legal case in 1999. Terminal illness was defined as a state in which medicine has no cure; the terminal patient was defined as one for whom medicine has no available treatment and whose medical condition will bring his or her life to an end within a few months as a result of the illness or its complications (Execution Proceedings 1990). In 2002, a draft law proposed to distinguish between irreversible terminal phases: (1) life expectancy not expected to exceed two weeks, and (2) life expectancy not expected to exceed six months (Steinberg 2002).

According to the *Halacha*:

- No act should be taken that accelerates the death of a patient about to die and whoever does so kills a healthy person.
- One should refrain from active treatment if the terminal patient is suffering great agony and asks to be left alone to die, but routine care such as food and liquids should be administrated.
- It is essential to administer antibiotics, oxygen and medications in every situation, even if the patient will die soon. It is prohibited to stop nourishment, including IVs, as long as the patient breathes. A person who does this will have starved another to death.
- A patient can be sent home to die but only with supportive treatment including food and liquids and pain medications.
- When a patient is defined as about to die, there is no obligation to begin a new series of treatments against his or her will or when this is only intensifying the patient's agony caused by the illness. However, treatments should be maintained if they are part of a series that was determined beforehand.
- If opinions differ among the treating medical personnel over the definition of 'terminal' then the opinion that the condition is not terminal should be adopted and the treatment adapted to the highest possible standard.

These guidelines stem from the orthodox religious view that God gave life and He alone has the authority to take a life. These remarks are tempered by the fact that the Jewish God is also merciful and just according to the Sanhedrin, the supreme legislative council and highest ecclesiastical and secular tribunal of the ancient Jews. While the emphasis here is placed on the supreme value of human life, there is some consideration of the quality of that life as well. The recent concept of quality of life, developed out of advancements in medical technology, had little place in ancient laws except in the discussion of patient suffering.

The rapid progress in medical sciences has contributed to the prolongation of life for many patients while reducing the quality of life for some who are dying. Recently, more people have become aware of this issue and have appealed to be freed of such a life and to be allowed to choose to die with dignity (Tabak 1996). Since the media and legal process have been involved in these questions, many Israelis have become more interested in their rights and more involved and assertive in the application of these rights, especially following the 1996 Patient's Rights Law. People show more willingness to refrain from what is considered medically futile treatment that prolongs the suffering and therefore extends a dying person's life. Social pressure is working to allow individuals to act autonomously in making unforced decisions not subject to *Halacha*. Numerous patients are refusing life-prolonging supportive treatments such as gastrostomy and regard it as their right to end their lives (Halperin 1997).

ATTITUDES TOWARDS TERMINAL ILLNESS

Traditionally, the ethical action was to extend human life by all and any possible means. That ethical position, established long before many means to prolong life existed, did not conflict with the quality of life principle to any great extent due to lack of medical treatment. Medical science and technology changed that and now the traditional ethics drawn from the *Halacha* is under discussion in a largely secular society. Today in Israel some people continue to follow the ancient Jewish law that regards human life as the supreme value, others have moved away from that to consider quality as well as quantity of life for dying patients, while still others support actually shortening the patients' life because of their suffering.

Active euthanasia is prohibited by law in Israel (Penal Law 1997). It is unethical and a criminal offence to accelerate death in an active manner. The controversy over passive euthanasia, the withdrawing of treatment and allowing a patient to die, revolves around the judicial precedent. Some people concerned for the ethics of treatment see no substantial difference between the two actions of not beginning any treatment at all (withholding) and stopping treatment after it was begun (withdrawing). According to the *Halacha*, passive euthanasia is 'the removal of the preventive' and that means the removal of that which prevents the departure of the soul and the death of the patient. Some health professionals think it ethical to stop treatment after it has begun but not to withhold it initially, while others view the interruption of treatment as an acute moral dilemma. According to one authority, passive euthanasia is legally and morally preferable to active euthanasia since the taking of another's life is considered a crime (Sellman 1995). For others, the duty to save lives and cure patients pertains as long as the dying person is considered alive and so long as he or she is considered alive, nothing should be done to hasten death (Steinberg 1994). Both voluntary passive euthanasia and non-voluntary passive euthanasia are considered ethically wrong by many people and should be defined as murder. The *Halacha* allows passive euthanasia under certain limited conditions. The opponents of voluntary euthanasia claim that a person's will to die is derived from social pressures and therefore should not be honoured. If the patient is in pain the wish is irrational and if there is no pain there is no justification to help the patient to die. The liberal view here is based on honouring the will of the patient but it is necessary to establish the reliability of that wish. Given these various ethical positions, it is safe to say that the attitude towards terminal illness varies from one medical centre to another, from one department to another and among physicians themselves.

The appeals to the courts express the will of some people to break away from life-supporting treatment at the end of life (Civil Appeal 1988). In recent years a more liberal wind has begun to blow through Israeli courts on the issue of terminal patients. Although these issues are of an ethical and moral nature, the courts nevertheless have assumed the role of balancing the conflicting interest between the individual and society (Israeli Supreme Court 1987, Kuhse & Singer 1993). This current situation raises the question: is the court the supreme authority to decide on these issues (Shelef 1994)? Physicians have avoided assuming responsibility for the issue because they were not in a position to accede to a patient's requests to refrain from prolonging life. Because of that, they referred cases to the courts, some of which have been reluctant to decide on the issue and often ruled in favour of the sanctity of life principle. Only as the years passed and the pressure of demand for a humane solution mounted has there been any indication of a tendency towards the realization of patients' rights to autonomy. Still, no consensus has been reached on this ethical question.

ISRAELI NURSES' ETHICAL STANCE ON EUTHANASIA: SURVEY FINDINGS

Several surveys have been conducted on the ethical stance held by Israeli nurses on euthanasia (Musgrave et al 2001). Generally speaking, there is widespread support for refraining from life-prolonging treatments in conditions of severe illness and complications. In addition, many nurses say that passive euthanasia can be ethically justified and should be made legal. In cases of passive euthanasia, these nurses advocate for full legal protection for the physician through legislation (Carmel & Zeidenberg 2000, Kuhse & Singer 1993). One Australian study found that senior nurses would be willing to participate in performing euthanasia provided the act is deemed legal (Kitchener 1998).

Undoubtedly, demographic factors that affect a nurse's stance about being involved in these situations can be found and nurses who came to Israel from different cultures are likely to have different views (Musgrave et al 2001).

A DRAFT LAW ON THE TERMINALLY ILL PATIENT AND THE LIVING WILL

Since 1992, the parliament has tried to draft a law dealing with end of life ethical and legal issues. Taking into account the *Halacha*, the secular law and ethics, several drafts relating to the right to die with dignity have been tabled but in 2001 were unified into a single draft law. Because this ethical issue has not been settled by legal means, the Minister of Health appointed a government committee to consolidate the law on the terminally ill patient. Under the draft law it will be permissible to refrain from nourishing terminally ill patients, but only if they gave their consent while mentally competent and now are enduring great suffering. In addition, the medical assessment must be that death will occur within two weeks. The termination of continuous medical treatment that could cause the terminally ill patient's death, whether he or she is coherent or not, is unlawful. However, refraining from administering a medical treatment for terminally ill patients is permitted. Such treatments include resuscitation, attachment to a respirator, chemotherapy, radiotherapy, dialysis, surgery. Any action that is medical treatment whose purpose is active killing is banned, even if done out of compassion or requested by the patient, a proxy, a family member, or any other person.

Along with these proposed legal changes, Israel developed the living will, a written instruction indicating what a person wants and does not want done to him or her at the end of life when no longer competent to make a decision. It is testimony to the individual's earlier wish, while still healthy, not to prolong life artificially (Hed 1989). This living will, first drafted in 1969, gives legal validity to a document that describes in detail the prohibition on life-prolonging treatments and the use of artificial means (Shelef 1994). Although the living will is not as yet recognized as a legal document in Israel, it carries much weight when a person is hospitalized or when a case is before the court.

At least one organization says that just as the State honours wills related to property and inheritance, they should equally honour wills that relate to the patient's person and allow that person to die with dignity by averting suffering.

TEACHING NURSING ETHICS IN ISRAELI UNIVERSITIES

The ethics course extends over the four years of the education programme, starting with an introduction to preclinical students. The focus is on universal values and principles basic to nursing care and includes discussions of rational behaviour, privacy, secrecy, the code of ethics (Israel Nurses' Association 2003), professional obligations, personal beliefs, mutual trust and moral philosophy. Students are exposed to a wide range of ethical problems so that they can define ethical problems and can deal with them in practice (Han & Ahn 2000, Wagner 1990).

The second year focuses on ethical issues in clinical encounters in which the teacher leads the discussion emphasizing values and preserving the principle of treatment. Topics include: unethical behaviour, unfair treatment, incomplete explanations, discrimination, lies, etc. In the third year, the ethics course is compulsory when students have had 18 months of clinical experience. Students discuss theoretical and practical issues. For example, a case of a terminally ill patient raises the following issues:

- What does 'respect for the person' mean and does this include the ability to choose and decide?
- Does the patient have the right to decide independently about his or her life according to medicine, the law, and the *Halacha*?
- What is the significance of terminating treatment from a patient's and caregiver's viewpoint?
- What is medical treatment without comfort for the terminally ill patient? Who decides about medical comfort? Should society invest in treatments to prolong lives of terminally ill patients?
- How do we deal with conflicting values, such as prolonging life, saving life versus preventing suffering, respect for the sanctity of human life?
- What are nurses' attitudes towards dying patients?
- What are nurses' attitudes about active and passive assistance to dying patients?
- What are the dangers to society in permitting individuals to choose death?
- What does Israeli and international research tell us about these issues?

Students use a case study to examine and analyse these issues. For example:

Case study

Mr S, an 80-year-old man, is in poor health and disoriented most of the time. Upon loss of function, he was transferred to a geriatric ward. His pacemaker battery was running down and, as a result, his cardiac output was deteriorating. It is clear that when the battery is finished, if it is not replaced, he will die. The doctor talked with the family saying that Mr S needed to be transferred for surgery to change the battery. The family strongly objected, saying that he was terminally ill and needed to stay in the geriatric ward. The doctor agreed not to transfer and focused on comfort care. The nurse objected to this decision and with the backing of the social worker, said that medically the patient should have surgery for the following reasons:

- Family objections were not medically based.
- The geriatric ward was not equipped to cope with this and was unwilling to accept responsibility for this patient since they could not treat him. The nurse thought the patient's life should be saved.

The course objectives are that students:

- Acquire tools to analyse, understand and cope with ethical problems.
- Examine factors affecting ethical issues based on specific ethical theories.
- Examine the significance of ethical problems at the clinical and national levels.
- Develop decision-making abilities and apply them in practice.

Teaching methods include lectures, group discussions, case studies and simulation.

In a class of 40 students, divided into eight discussion groups, these objectives can be met. Nurit Wagner's decision-making model is used in ethics courses (Wagner 1990). This model indicates that ethical decision making is linked to three sources: religious, rational and affective. Religion sets standards of behaviour and tells us what is right and wrong. The rational source means that we think rationally and logically and therefore ethics can be taught. Ethical judgements also stem from feelings and an intuitive moral sense which is the affective source. Some believe that nurses and doctors mostly solve moral dilemmas using their intuitive sense (Campbell 1975).

For evaluation purposes, students present an exercise in which they express their opinion about an ethical problem and analyse their decision in the light of what they have learned in the course. Students also evaluate the lectures and clinical discussions and have given high marks for them. Ethics has become an inseparable part of students' learning experiences. Students have mentioned that values need to be remembered even when the teacher is not present. In their words, dealing with ethics is one of the more significant events in their professional socialization.

The reality is that difficulties arise in Israeli nursing today because of changing attitudes in the nursing profession. Two apparent but conflicting attitudes are present. The traditional professional attitude from the past means that nurses accompany medical staff and perform medical directives in all aspects of their work, sometimes in contradiction with their values and personal philosophy. This progressive attitude relates to professional independence and taking responsibility for decisions related to ethical issues. Here, nurses request that they be involved in solving ethical problems. Some nurses are trapped between the traditional values of obedience and service and the recognition of professional independence.

Many teachers believe that education in professional ethics is essential despite the fact that many view nursing values not to be distinct from universal values. I believe that the emphasis and attention placed on ethical issues are increasing and that a message to this effect is being understood by students. I believe that this is not the time for Israeli nursing to cease dealing with complex and difficult ethical issues but to face them and attempt to find solutions. This is even more the case for mature professional practitioners who will take part in the research that is needed in nursing ethics in Israel.

References

Ben Shlomo A 1998 Hebrew law light table. Tel Aviv University, Tel Aviv.

Campbell A 1975 Moral dilemmas in medicine: a course book on ethics for doctors and nurses. Churchill Livingstone, Edinburgh.

Carmel S, Zeidenberg H 2000 Nurses' attitudes toward end-of-life of middle aged and old terminally ill patients. In: Tomer A (ed) Death attitudes and the older adult: theories, concepts, and applications. Brunner/Mazel, New York, p 193–210.

Carmi A 1984 The doctor, the patient, and the law. Tamar Press, Haifa.

Carmi A, Sagiv A 1986 Medical negligence in Judaism and in Israel. Tamar Press, Haifa.

Central Bureau of Statistics 2004, the State of Israel. Online. Available: http://www1.cbs.gov.il/reader/shnatonhnew.htm

Civil Appeal 1988 506/88 *Talila Shefer* v *Ziv Hospital*, Safad. 38(1):87.

Execution Proceedings 1990 1141/90 *Binyamin Eyal* v *Vilensky et al.* verdict (3) p 187–193.

Halperin M 1997 Withholding treatment from ALS patients and mercy killing – common characteristics and differences between Halacha ruling and a judge's decision. ASIA June:61–65.

Han SS, Ahn SH 2000 An analysis and evaluation of student nurses' participation in ethical decision-making. Nursing Ethics 7:113–123.

Hed D 1989 Ethics and medicine. In: The broadcast. Tel Aviv University, Ministry of Defense Publications, Israel.

Israel Medical Organization 1996 The Patient's Rights Law. Israel Medical Organization, Ramat Gan, Israel.

Israel Nurses' Association 2003 The code of ethics for nurses in Israel. Israel Nurses' Association, Education and Culture Ltd, Israel

Israeli Supreme Court 1982 30/82 *Maayan et al* v *the Director General*. Vol. 36 part 2.

Israeli Supreme Court 1987 820/87 *Nakash* v *Director General of Ministry of Health*. Vol 87 part 4.

Kitchener BA 1998 Nurse characteristics and attitudes to active voluntary euthanasia: a survey in the Australian capital territory. Journal of Advanced Nursing 28(1):46–70.

Kuhse H, Singer P 1993 Voluntary euthanasia and the nurse: an Australian survey. International Journal of Nursing Studies 30:311–322.

Musgrave CF, Margalith I, Goldsmith L 2001 Israeli oncology and non-oncology nurses' attitudes to physician-assisted dying: a comparative study. Oncology Nursing Forum 28(1):50–57.

Penal Law 1997 Amendment on the right to decide on prolonging life. Motion 4/309.

Sellman D 1995 Euphemisms for euthanasia. Nursing Ethics 2:315–319.

Shafran Y 2003 Definition of the terminal patient and medical treatment. Online. Available: http://www.edu.negev.gov.il/chemdat/adelayul/project/shafran.htm

Shelef L 1994 Between sanctity of life and human dignity: on physical agony, medical progress, human sensitivity, and criminal law. Laws 24(1):207–208.

State of Israel 1994a Basic law: the freedom and dignity of the individual. Gazettes 5754-1994.

State of Israel 1994b Privacy protection law. Gazettes 5741-1981.

Steinberg A 1994 Department of Medicine and Halacha. In: Encyclopedia of medical *Halacha*. Rabbinate and Jerusalem Religious Council, Jerusalem.

Steinberg A 1998 Value of life. In: Medicine and *Halacha* encyclopedia. Shlesinger Biblical and Medical Research Institute, Jerusalem.

Steinberg A 2001 Draft law on the terminally ill patient. The Knesset, Jerusalem.

Steinberg A 2002 Draft law on the terminally ill patient: a revised version. The Knesset, Jerusalem.

Tabak N 1996 Patients' right to an autonomous decision regarding their lives. Forum of Oncology Nursing September:7–11.

Wagner N 1990 Model of ethical decision-making in nursing. Dissertation, Tel Aviv University, Tel Aviv.

Further reading

Cohen H, Bruckstein AS 2003 Ethics of Maimonides. University of Wisconsin Press, Madison, WI.

Dorff EN, Newman LE 1995 Contemporary Jewish ethics and morality: a reader. Oxford University Press, London.

Dorff EN 2004 Matters of life and death: a Jewish approach to modern medical ethics. Jewish Publication Society of America, New York.

Chapter **24**

Turkey.
Teaching ethics in Turkish nursing education programmes

Leyla Dinç

Nursing is a women's profession in Turkey, and women's status is multi-dimensional, affected by the religion, culture, social, political and economical factors of any given country. As ethical orientation is strongly related to cultural background, it is worthwhile emphasizing several factors within this context and giving a brief historical background about the status of women and nursing education in Turkey.

RELIGION

The predominant religion in Turkey is Islam. Islam means submission and Muslims, the followers of Islam, practise the teachings of Mohammed, whom they regard to be the last great prophet, following the Jewish prophets and Jesus Christ. According to the Islamic belief, the will of God and the teachings of Mohammed are written in the Koran (Qur'an), the holy book (Siddiqui 1997). Islamic law provides guidance about what is right, or acceptable, and what is unacceptable for Muslims, and in this way it shapes the values, thoughts, choices, attitudes and actions of believers (Halstead 1997).

Although Islam lays stress on justice and equality, including between men and women, it emphasizes the importance of men. The Qur'an states: 'And they [women] have rights similar to those (of men) over them, and men are a degree above them' (Koran 2:228, Öztürk 1994 p 46). Islam emphasizes the concept of *ümmet*, a community of believers. The primary goal of education, family and social life is to be a good Muslim. The family is the foundation of Islamic society. The man is considered the head of the family and the primary role of women is to be good wives and good mothers. Women should cover their hair and body because these features attract men. By confining women to the private sphere, Islam divides the world into two, the public sphere, which belongs to men, and the private sphere, the domain of domesticity, which belongs to women (Müftüler-Bac 1999).

Muslim patients understand that illness, suffering and dying are part of life and a test from God (Rassool 2000). Caring is a natural outcome of loving God and the Prophet. Showing respect and compassion for elderly people and helping those who are powerless, orphaned, wounded or ill are merits and are encouraged in Islam (Dhami & Sheikh 2000, Halstead 1997). Islam does not prohibit Muslim nurses and other healthcare professionals from caring for both Muslim and non-Muslim patients. However, physical contact between a woman and man who are not close relatives is regarded as sin. Therefore, although midwifery was common because it involved women-to-women relationships and contact, caring was limited to the private sphere. In this respect, nursing as a profession does not have a profound history in Islamic countries. There are no Muslim models of nursing care in the literature and little has been written on developments of a theoretical framework of caring from an Islamic perspective (Rassool 2000).

CULTURE

The conventional, normative structure of Islam and the patriarchal Mediterranean culture, which rests on male superiority, shape the familial, social and political life of Turkey. That social life, especially in the eastern and south-eastern parts of Turkey, is mainly collectivist. Extended families, where the mother of the husband is influential in the family, are common. In such families, respect for elderly people according to their hierarchic positions and obedience to the man and his parents, is encouraged. Adherence to religious practices, norms and cultural values is promoted. Women are expected to be good wives and mothers, to care for their parents and never to break off their close relationships with their own families, even when they are married. As the image of God as father is sustained in the patriarchal social system, the father of the family, the husband, even the brother, are responsible for the protection of family honour (Gürsoy & Vural 2003, Yetim 2003).

THE ESTABLISHMENT OF THE TURKISH REPUBLIC

With the establishment of the Turkish Republic in 1923 under the leadership of Mustafa Kemal Atatürk, the country underwent radical administrative and cultural reforms in the direction of western modernization. According to Atatürk, modernity versus tradition, and science and rational thought versus indigenous knowledge were essential to reach the level of civilization attained by western countries. This meant that the traditional Ottoman–Islamic bonds had to be dissolved; the religious and ethnic identity of the citizens had to be subordinated to a new Turkish identity. Atatürk believed that the new Turkish identity should be secular, democratic, modernist and national. Education and secularism are considered as the most significant components of social, economic, scientific and technological development in the country.

With a number of radical reforms, which included abolishing Shar'iah (religious, Koranic law) and replacing it with a slightly modified Swiss Civil Code of Law (1926), adopting the Latin-based Turkish alphabet, instead of Arabic to increase the literacy rate (1928), and secularizing and monopolizing education, new institutions and ideals were all put into effect. The new civil code introduced gender equality in marriage, divorce and in matters of inheritance, and granted equal child custody to both parents. In 1930, Turkish women were granted the right to vote in local elections and in 1934, the right to vote for and to be elected to public office in national elections (Republic of Turkey 2003a). However, according to data of the Turkish State Institute of Statistics (Republic of Turkey 2003b), the proportion of female deputies in the Turkish parliament was only 4.4% in the year 2002.

Modern Turkey emerged out of a historical heritage embodying diverse cultural patterns and ethnic groups. While such social and cultural diversity is the source of societal enrichment, it is not free of tensions. The radical reforms in the Turkish Republic have influenced the cultural, social and political life of society; however, while giving rise to modernization, these reforms at the same time prompted the rise of religious and ethnic groups. Some Muslim and Kurdish groups engaged in a search for a self-identity and religious or ethnic sovereignty. Secularization might have stimulated religious movements to respond to the loss of their institutions, such as the caliphate, and nationalism might have stimulated the ethnic groups. The democratization process also led to an increase in political participation of religious conservative and ethnic populations and a rise in their demands, which included aspirations for a nostalgic past. It is noteworthy that economic decline, unemployment and inequalities in health, education and standards of living are some of the factors that provoke societal tensions and conflicts. However, it is also interesting that women are often at the centre of these religious and ethnic movements. There are now more veiled women in the ranks of Islamists than ever before and we have witnessed armed women in the ranks of Kurdish political groups and leftist fractions.

In fact, women's rights and making women public citizens are considered as the cornerstone of Turkish secularism and nation-state notions, wherein citizenship is based on the rights of individuals rather than on ethnic or religious identity. For this reason, women are the object and symbol of radical ideological movements against the current regime in Turkey. Another reason may be the opinion that women are the most powerless and are therefore groups that are easier to control. However, most of the women who join militant Islamist organizations do so voluntarily because of the alternative social and political power and autonomy they gain in these movements. This seems paradoxical, because Atatürk's reforms granted and promoted the rights of Turkish women. The underlying aim of his reforms was to make women visible in the public arena, active and competitive in education, employment and in all aspects of social and political life (Müftüler-Bac 1999, Republic of Turkey 2003a). Consequently, many women in Turkey were able to be educated and to have careers and jobs. Islam, on the other hand, as the sole authority in public affairs, cannot accept the supremacy of civil authority because it is considered divine and therefore unquestionable and unchallengeable; stemming from the belief that Islam is supreme and over all. This can lead to the restriction of individual liberty and rational thought. The forced covering of women in post-revolutionary Iran provides a striking example of the restriction of women's liberty. Despite this, it seems that women in the ranks of Islamist ideological movements in Turkey want to experience more political autonomy while living according to their religious beliefs and cultural values. This reveals that culture, religion and tradition are an important part of Turkish society despite the modernization efforts and legal regulations.

NURSING EDUCATION IN TURKEY

Nursing was invisible until the establishment of the Turkish Republic, because women were invisible due to their exclusion from the public sphere. Excluding women from the public sphere for hundreds of years meant excluding them from education and employment outside the home, and from formal power.

Following the establishment of the Turkish Republic, the first nursing schools were constructed by the Turkish Red Crescent Society (1925) and by the Ministry of Health (1946). The programmes run at these schools were at a high-school level and offered four years of education. Most of these schools were boarding, insulating students from societal relationships, and independent from the influence of universities. As such, nurses became captives of local hospitals where the primary authority was the male physician or the hospital administrator. Nursing care is perceived as supportive of physicians and nurses are expected to be the physicians' assistants or servants, their primary loyalty being to these physicians and institutions. The first school of nursing that offered a baccalaureate degree in a university was started in 1955. Meanwhile in 1985, associate degree programmes were opened at the universities, offering two years' education for students. In 1996 almost all of these programmes ceased to receive students and converted to licence under the establishment of nursing departments of Health High Schools. In general, there are now over 72 nursing programmes/departments of Health High Schools and ten schools of nursing at universities that offer bachelor-level degrees (Kocaman 2003). However, the quality and quantity of the nurse teachers, the equipment and physical facilities required for student education and the curriculum content vary widely. Consequently, until recent years it was difficult to say that there was a common understanding and cooperative effort among nurse educators, or at a national level, about what a professional nurse is and how she could or should be educated. Since 2002 there has been an effort to revise a nursing curriculum and to establish a nucleus curriculum according to European Union standards and norms.

ETHICS IN TURKISH NURSING PROGRAMMES

Until the late 1980s, morals and professional conduct were taught in several nursing courses in the context of nurses' obligations and responsibilities. The word 'ethics' and the scope of ethics were not popular, because obedience to physicians and loyalty to institutions without questioning was accepted as a role of the good nurse. In fact, obedience and loyalty were the two virtues expected from women in Turkish society. Women's rights, the efforts made to attain a higher educational level in nursing, the information explosion, and the demand for ethical decision making and behaviour in practice, as well as the consumer movement, raised nurses' sense of being responsible individuals in society and contributed to an expanded role and greater autonomy for nursing. Thus the moral context in nursing education developed in parallel with the development of nursing as a profession.

In the 1990s, more attention was given to ethics and most of the nursing education programmes began to introduce the subjects of ethics into their curricula as a unit of a required course entitled 'Nursing history and deontology', 'Nursing history and ethics' or 'Nursing history, deontology and law'. In addition, several nursing courses, in both undergraduate and graduate programmes, integrated ethics into their lessons. In general, however, insufficient time is allocated for ethical issues because ethics is taught alongside nursing history or nursing law.

Teaching ethics and applying ethical knowledge to the clinical experiences of nursing students requires the teachers to have ethical knowledge and skills. Ann Hamric (2001) stated that many clinical faculty members lack confidence in their knowledge of ethics or the process of ethical decision making and find it difficult to model this integration of theory and practice. This argument probably applies to ethics education in Turkish nursing programmes. In almost all of the nursing schools a faculty member whose experience is in a specialty area such as 'Fundamentals of nursing' is also responsible for teaching ethics. In nursing programmes and Health High Schools, faculty members with no nursing basis lecture in nursing ethics, although a few nurses working in these schools hold doctoral degrees from the Medical History and Ethics departments of Medical Faculties. By contrast, all the faculty members in nursing schools received their academic degree in areas of nursing specialties. Consequently, there is a lack of nurse educators with a formal education in ethics or philosophy at postgraduate level. Therefore, nurse educators who improve their ethical knowledge and skills through their personal efforts and initiatives, determine and shape the goals and content of ethics teaching. In most of the nursing programmes the ethical content includes ethical concepts and principles, human and patient rights, ethical problems in health care and in nursing practice, and codes of ethics for nurses (mostly the ICN code), but students are taught by teachers with limited skills in value analyses and ethical decision-making processes.

In addition, because of the fact that traditional nurses are still preferred in many of our healthcare institutions, and many new graduates adopt the traditional role, there is a lack of role models in practice. Nermin Ersoy and Fügen Göz (2001) found that bedside nurses have ethical sensitivity but that their knowledge of ethical decision-making models and processes is insufficient.

Although ethics is now commonplace on nursing curricula in Turkey, the question of why ethics should be taught is uncertain. Peter Allmark (1995) suggested that these uncertainties in nursing are due to not knowing if we are teaching ethics to professionalize or because we are a profession. This point of view reflects the status of Turkish nursing education programmes. Most of the nurse educators will claim that their objectives of ethics instruction are to increase nursing students' knowledge of ethical concepts and principles, to enable them to identify ethical problems in health care, and to improve their skills in ethical decision making. Indeed, all of these objectives are important and are indicated in many nursing ethics courses, but what should be the primary aim and moral context of nursing ethics? Can this be generalized and standardized for every country?

THE AIM OF TEACHING ETHICS IN NURSING

Professions like medicine and nursing, which centre on human beings, provide services mostly for ill, wounded and injured people – 'the vulnerable' – with the aim of preserving life, alleviating suffering and promoting health. It is therefore a requirement that healthcare professionals are sensitive to humanistic values and ethical principles. In addition, ethics is already inherent in nursing because of the concept of caring. Chris Gastmans et al (1998) point out that caring activities presuppose a reciprocal interaction between human persons who enter into relationships with each other, based on their uniqueness. Thus, nursing care is an ethically loaded endeavour, a moral practice primarily geared to making explicit, and accomplishing whatever is good for the patient.

However, in Turkish society cultural, religious, economic and political factors determine our values, attitudes and behaviours. These factors also affect the goals and content of ethics education. Verena Tschudin (2003 p 183) writes 'The content of ethics education cannot be restricted to a few principles and theories. Ethics concerns how society functions, the concepts of power and its use, the impact of terrorism and war on health care, discrimination of all kinds, the use of resources, globalisation, the use and abuse of toxic substances and the impact on society, and many more aspects.' Geoffrey Hunt (1997) states that professional ethics will mean little if nurses are not acquainted with the political and legal dimensions of the struggle for greater democracy and accountability in our public institutions. These views reveal the importance of developing a consciousness in students of social, cultural and political issues because all of these factors affect their decision-making capacity and actions. Such a consciousness is especially important for Turkish nursing students for several reasons.

First, Turkey is the only secular and democratic country in the Muslim world. This special feature makes it a land of religious, cultural and political conflicts. Women are often at the centre of these conflicts; they are used to symbolize both the aspirations of the secularist and modernist elite and Islamists, or they are volunteer pioneers of ideological movements.

Second, religious, cultural and traditional practices are very important in the life of Turkish society. In fact, religion and culture have a moral dimension because as human beings we are not only brain and reason; we have emotions and beliefs that impregnate our rational thoughts, choices and actions. Virtues such as compassion, charity, patience, respect and caring for powerless and vulnerable people are inherent in Islam and Turkish culture. However, culture, religion and tradition are often gender-biased and Turkish women are still oppressed by the patriarchal system. The dominant role of men remains present at individual, family, community and national levels. In a study by Behice Erci (2002), women were found to make decisions more slowly than men. Yetim (2003) found that male university students become more autonomous and more individualistic than female students. Decisions, such as using contraception, having a child or an abortion, are still made by the husband rather than the woman, in particular within extended families; and domestic violence, virginity tests, sexual harassment in the streets and honour crimes based on the patriarchal cultural values are still the focus of women's debates in Turkey.

The following case provides an example of a cultural and traditional practice that contradicts both human rights and Turkish laws.

| *Case study: a virginity examination of a bride* | SA was 19 years old. She was married to MD by arrangement with her parents. During the first attempt at sexual contact with her husband on the wedding night, there was no bleeding. Because the bloodstained sheet on the wedding night is perceived as proof of the virginity of the bride, she was accused by her husband and his parents of not being a virgin, and immoral. She insisted on her virginity and stated that she never had sexual contact before marriage. However, they did not trust her and demanded a virginity examination. In the morning, the couple was at the hospital for a hymen examination. Nurse B met the couple, with SA crying. The nurse explained that sometimes there is no bleeding due to the structure of the hymen and that SA had the right to refuse the examination if she wanted. SA said that she had no other choice. If she objected, she would be regarded as admitting a premarital sexual relationship, in which case she would have to return to her father's home and live with the stigma. She |

signed the consent form. Nurse B helped her to undress in privacy and gave her a gown for the examination. A gynaecologist performed the hymen examination.

This case is adapted from a news item that appeared in the newspaper *Hürriyet* (Anonymous 2002).

CASE STUDY AS A METHOD OF TEACHING NURSING ETHICS

Being a responsible professional requires ethical decision making in practice. Case study analysis is an effective method for improving the ethical decision-making skills of students. It facilitates easy comprehension of the theories and principles of ethics; it helps students to analyse the moral nature of problems and to evaluate the ethical choices involved in the case.

Case studies should be analysed in the light of the information about ethical theories and principles, human and patient rights, laws and codes of ethics for nurses, and by taking into consideration the cultural, social and political factors offered by the teacher through a series of lectures and discussion sessions.

The case story above reveals an ethical dilemma that can be used as a case study example in teaching nursing ethics. The first step in a case study should be to enable students to distinguish the moral problem from the non-moral problems, and to raise their awareness of the cultural and traditional values involved in the case.

A family's honour rests on a woman's chastity and fidelity in the patriarchal Turkish culture. Therefore, one of the choices of the bride in this case was to accept the hymen examination, which includes a violation of her bodily integrity and privacy. The other choice was to reject such an examination and to bear the consequences, such as divorce, stigmatization, shame and social isolation.

The second step should be to enable students to identify the relevant ethical principles, laws and codes in this case. This case reveals the violation of ethical principles, because the autonomy of the bride was violated and she was psychologically harmed. Hymen examination without the consent of the individual contravenes Article 10 of the Turkish Constitution, which states equality for every citizen, and Articles 17 and 20, which state that the bodily integrity of a person cannot be violated. It also contradicts the human rights, patient rights and international agreements of the Republic of Turkey (Anonymous 1997).

As the last step of a case study, students should be encouraged to evaluate the cultural, religious, social and political factors related to the case story and their roles as citizens and as nurses. Their moral reasoning and choices in resolving the moral problem should be assessed in terms of ethical principles and codes, human rights, laws and nursing responsibilities, as well as the cultural, social and political factors.

CONCLUSION

Nursing remains a women's profession in Turkey. As such, its position in society and the moral content in nursing education programmes are influenced by women's status. In spite of the high educational level, nursing still strives for professionalization. Professionalism requires accountability and autonomy in education, management and service, and this in turn necessitates individual autonomy.

Ethics requires a sense of community and a respect for the religious, cultural and social aspects of that community, but not without respect for individual autonomy. In this respect, along with the objectives stated in many nursing ethics courses, the emphasis of nursing education programmes and nursing ethics should be on democracy, secular and rational education, equality of genders, and the acceptance and tolerance of cultural and ideological diversity. Cultural, religious and traditional values should be respected but they should also be reconsidered and reinterpreted in the light of contemporary social and political realities and human rights, as some values and practices that are rooted deeply in religious and patriarchal values contradict human rights, in particular women's rights.

References

Allmark P 1995 Uncertainties in the teaching of ethics to students of nursing. Journal of Advanced Nursing 22:374–378.

Anonymous 1997 Türkiye Cumhuriyeti Anayasasi (Constitution of the Turkish Republic). Sel Ofset Matbaacilik (Sel Publisher), Ankara.

Anonymous 2002 Bekaretime esim bile inanmadi (My husband didn't believe my virginity). Hürriyet (Hürriyet newspaper) 29 October 2002.

Dhami S, Sheikh A 2000 The Muslim family. Western Journal of Medicine 173:352–356.

Erci B 2003 Women's efficiency in decision making and their perception of their status in the family. Public Health Nursing 20(1):65–70.

Ersoy N, Göz F 2001 The ethical sensitivity of nurses in Turkey. Nursing Ethics 8:299–312.

Gastmans C, Dierckx de Casterlé B, Schotsmans P 1998 Nursing considered as moral practice: a philosophical–ethical interpretation of nursing. Kennedy Institute of Ethics Journal 8:43–69.

Gürsoy E, Vural G 2003 Nurses' and midwives views on approaches to hymen examination. Nursing Ethics 10(5):485–496.

Halstead JM 1997 Muslims and sex education. Journal of Moral Education 26:317–329.

Hamric AB 2001 Ethics development for clinical faculty. Nursing Outlook 49:115–117.

Hunt G 1997 Moral crisis, professionals and ethical education. Nursing Ethics 4:29–38.

Kocaman G 2003 Türkiye'de Hemsirelik Egitim Sorunlari. In: Ülker S, Kocaman G, Özkan Ö (eds) Dünya Hemsireler Günü Ö Baski. (Nursing Education Problems in Turkey) Hemsirelikte Arastirma ve Gelistirme Dernegi (Association for Research and Devolopment in Nursing). Odak Ofset, Ankara, p 71–91.

Müftüler-Bac M 1999 Turkish women's predicament. Women's Studies International Forum 22:303–315.

Öztürk YN 1994 Kur'an-i Kerim Meali (Commentary on the Qu'ran). Türkçe Çeviri (Turkish translation) Hürriyet Ofset, Istanbul.

Rassool GH 2000 The crescent and Islam: healing, nursing and the spiritual dimension: some considerations towards an understanding of the Islamic perspectives on caring. Journal of Advanced Nursing 32:1476–1484.

Republic of Turkey, Ministry of Foreign Affairs 2003a From 1923 to the present. Online. Available: http://www.mfa.gov.tr/grupc/ca/cai/2.htm [accessed January 2003].

Republic of Turkey, Prime Ministry State Institute of Statistics 2003b Women's indicators and statistics. Online. Available: http://www.die.gov.tr/toyak1/cover1/index.html [accessed January 2003].

Siddiqui A 1997 Ethics in Islam: key concepts and contemporary challenges. Journal of Moral Education 26(4):423–431.

Tschudin V 2003 Ethics in nursing; the caring relationship, 3rd edn. Butterworth Heinemann, Edinburgh.

Yetim U 2003 The impacts of individualism/collectivism, self-esteem, and feeling of mastery on life satisfaction among the Turkish university students and academicians. Social Indicators Research 61:297–317.

Chapter 25

Norway.
Some ethical challenges faced by health providers who work with first-generation immigrant men from Pakistan diagnosed with type 2 diabetes

Eli Haugen Bunch

The ethical and clinical issues encountered by Norwegian nurses when working with men from Pakistan diagnosed with type 2 diabetes are culturally demanding. Ethical principles of distributive justice are discussed in the light of patients' legal right to health care within a culture grounded on solidarity, equality and equity and an expectation that patients will follow recommended medical regimes. An estimated 17% of all Pakistani men living in Norway are diagnosed with type 2 diabetes. Explanatory factors for this high incidence rate are genetic, cultural and intermarital.

BACKGROUND

The perception of Norway as a country with a homogeneous population is long gone. Today Norway is multi-cultural and people from more than 100 ethnic backgrounds live here. By the year 2003, 110 000 Norwegian citizens were defined as immigrants from non-western countries, which is 7.3% of the entire population of 4.6 million (Kommune 2003 p 55). Also in 2003, 74.2% (6676) of all Pakistanis in Norway lived in Oslo (Kommune 2003 p 58). Madeleine Leininger (1995) reminds us that 'our rapidly growing multicultural world makes it imperative that nurses understand different cultures to work and function effectively with people having different values, beliefs, and ideas about nursing, health, caring, wellness, illness, death and disabilities' (p 6).

Communication and ways of thinking are unique to each culture. When Norwegian nurses meet patients with a non-western background, such differences can cause confusion and misunderstandings. Even conflict solving might be different for the two populations (Hanssen 1996). People diagnosed with type 2 diabetes are in need of education about the illness, to include necessary dietary changes to prevent secondary complications, and recommended alterations in lifestyle. To teach people with a different cultural background can be challenging because of language problems, different religious beliefs and attitudes towards chronic illness. A feeling of failure, not doing a good job and sheer frustration at being unable to pass on relatively simple information about a medical regime is common for nurses working at outpatient diabetes clinics in Oslo with first-generation immigrants.

This chapter will focus on ethical dilemmas Norwegian nurses must recognize when working with first-generation immigrant men from Pakistan diagnosed with type 2 diabetes. The foundations of the Norwegian healthcare system and patients' rights, and the causes and effects of type 2 diabetes are briefly explained. Specific aspects of Pakistani culture are compared to Norwegian culture. A constructed case is presented to examine the ethical and clinical issues. Some solutions are suggested in the conclusion.

THE NORWEGIAN HEALTHCARE SYSTEM

Norway's healthcare system is based on rights and laws. The foundation for the national healthcare system is equality, solidarity and legal rights to treatment regardless of race, age and place of domicile (Helsedirektoratet 1987). The system is financed by indirect taxes and small patient fees for certain treatments (e.g. cosmetic surgery for non-therapeutic purposes). Two White Papers (1986, 1994) defined how patients are to be prioritized. A patient's Bill of Rights, passed in 1999, gives each patient a legal right to treatment and choice of where to be treated within the country. The system is benefit based; the model promotes welfare (Beauchamp & Childress 1994).

All citizens have a designated primary physician and access to specialist healthcare centres, such as mother–child care, centres for elderly people and low-threshold teen centres. For more specialized care, the primary physician must refer to a specialist and/or a diabetes outpatient clinic. In Oslo there are two diabetes clinics where Pakistani men diagnosed with diabetes are referred for follow-up treatment. The primary providers at the clinics are nurses with some type of specialization, i.e. public health nursing.

The ethical principle of justice is woven into the Norwegian healthcare system. Justice is here defined according to Tom Beauchamp and James Childress (1994 p 38) as 'a group of norms for distributing benefits, risks, and costs fairly'. From the mid-1930s there has been a heavy emphasis on preventive health and care within a social democratic model. Strong societal expectations and sanctions continuously promote healthy lifestyles in the media. For instance, all alcoholic beverages are sold in state-licensed stores and are heavily taxed. Norway was one of the first countries to ban alcohol and tobacco advertising in the 1980s. In 2004 all public places were designated as smoke free. However, a study on high technology and ethics from 1999 found that 'once a patient was inside a hospital door, money was never an issue of whether to treat or not. Further, no age limits were found for complex cardiac surgery even when the expected outcomes were doubtful' (Bunch 2000). I think one can say that the Norwegian healthcare system advocates autonomy, a norm for respecting the decision-making capacities of its citizens, and also has subtle expectations and restrictions in its structure and policies.

Persons diagnosed with type 2 diabetes are offered medical treatment and follow-up care at outpatient clinics. Medicines and any medical equipment are given at reduced prices. The Norwegian Diabetes Association, an organization that receives funding from national and local budgets, offers free courses and supports groups throughout the country.

TYPE 2 DIABETES

Diabetes mellitus is a metabolic disorder of multiple aetiologies characterized by chronic hyperglycaemia (WHO 1999); type 2 diabetes is one of the components in this metabolic syndrome. Type 2 diabetes is usually diagnosed in people over 40; they often do not feel sick but may have hypertension, feel thirsty and be overweight. Treatment of type 2 diabetes is a balance of eating the right foods, exercise and taking medications. The disease is chronic and, if ignored, is likely to cause long-term arterial complications to kidneys, eyes and nerves. Kristian Johansson and Tor Skinner (2003) say that the goal of type 2 diabetes treatment is fitting the care into the patients' life and not the other way round. A person with such a diagnosis must make daily dietary choices and get enough exercise to control the body's glucose levels. A recommended regime is three meals a day with snacks in between; such a regime often differs from the person's usual eating habits.

How many people with a Pakistani background living in Norway are diagnosed with type 2 diabetes is difficult to establish. Johan Jervell (2000) estimated that 17% of men with a Pakistani background are diabetic. Explanatory factors for this high incidence are genetic, cultural, environmental, nutritional and caused by intermarriage.

FAMILY STRUCTURES

Many generations living together is not the norm in Norway. Today's families live with few relatives nearby, both spouses have jobs outside the home, preschool children attend daycare and schoolchildren attend multiple organized after-school activities like bandy and soccer playing, dancing, horse riding or playing in a band or orchestra.

The typical Pakistani families in Oslo live together with many generations; women rarely have outside jobs and non-Pakistani contacts. The men are the breadwinners while the women take care of the home, children and daily meals. To promote integration, Pakistani children are offered reduced rates for child care. Special language classes are given to all children with a non-Norwegian mother tongue.

Norwegians are born into a State Lutheran church whereas most Pakistanis are Muslims and have their own mosques. Pakistani food also differs from the typical meat, potato and gravy that Norwegians eat. People from Pakistan use different spices, much white meat and rice. A major difference is also the evening meal in the Pakistani family, which is rare among modern Norwegians.

CULTURES

Culture, values, ways of communication and traditions vary and at the same time protect us. Cultural differences define how we communicate and look at issues such as authority, individuality, group membership and identity. Different cultures decide what people notice, what they overlook and are a determinant for how we think of health and illness (Hanssen 1987, 1996).

Norwegians are future oriented, whereas research shows that people from Pakistan are here-and-now oriented. They see their future as being entirely in the hands of Allah and all chronic illnesses like diabetes are treated with a focus on cure. Research also shows that present-oriented people tend not to take medications when feeling well, and persons with type 2 diabetes do not necessarily feel sick (Jølf 2004). Within the cultural system of Unani medicine from which most Norwegian-Pakistani people come, the treatment of type 2 diabetes has the goal of cure. The western health system's classification as chronic/not chronic is not compatible with the Unani tradition, which has a holistic perspective. Pakistani people do not separate physical and psychological aspects of a disease and they engage in cure-oriented treatment systems (Hanssen 1987). As they are mostly Muslim by religion, their beliefs are that the future is completely in the hands of Allah. The plans Allah has for each person cannot be influenced, thus one must live as best as possible today (Carlsen 2001). According to Islam (Hanssen 1996), illness is something God has given as punishment for sins. At the same time, God and his grace will help the sick and through medial treatment restore to well-being.

THE NORWEGIAN CULTURE AND HEALTHCARE SYSTEM

A belief system that does not think one can live a healthy life with a chronic illness, where the concept 'chronic' is equated with death, and where the future is in Allah's hands frustrates duty-oriented Norwegian nurses. Norwegian patients are expected to be obedient and show solidarity, and in turn they expect to be treated as autonomous persons with equality and equity. Autonomy is defined by Knut Erik Tranøy (1997) as a person's right to self-determination and shared decision making. For the most part, patients follow a suggested medical regime. A person following the recommended guidelines for type 2 diabetes can expect medical expenses to be subsidised and live a good-quality life.

ETHICAL AND CLINICAL DILEMMAS

Case 1 *A typical referral to the* *diabetes clinic*	Mr Z came to Norway from Pakistan in the 1970s. Before leaving his country he married his second cousin. Today they have five children, all living at home. Mrs Z's elderly but well parents are also living with the family. Mr Z is a first-generation Pakistani in Norway. His wife is illiterate and never learned to read or write either Norwegian or her own language. She is dependent on her husband for all interactions with public services, such as the children's schools, visits to the family practitioner, public health nurse and so on. Mr Z has a good and steady income as a bus driver in the city of Oslo. The Z family owns a large apartment in downtown Oslo. Mr Z was diagnosed as having type 2 diabetes more than three years ago and now attends the outpatient diabetes clinic every three months to test his glucose levels, learn more about the illness, talk about dietary requirements and learn how to balance diet and exercise. Nurse Ellen has worked with Mr Z for the last year and feels frustrated. His blood pressure continues to be high, he has not lost any weight despite being 15 kilos overweight, and his glucose levels show he continues to eat fatty foods, carbohydrates and lead a sedentary lifestyle. During the Muslim month of Ramadan he continues to fast, eating one big meal a day. Nurse Ellen has encouraged Mr Z to bring his wife to the clinic so they can discuss dietary changes together but so far without response. Nurse Ellen's frustration is also caused by the long-term side effects she knows the patient will most likely acquire. In her previous work place, a cardiac unit, she met many Pakistani men undergoing complex cardiac surgery caused by untreated type 2 diabetes.

There are many ways of examining this scenario. The obvious clinical issues are how Mr Z can learn more about type 2 diabetes and adhere to a recommended medical regime. The ethical dilemmas I want to focus on are the nurses' duties and obligations, distributive justice and a person's legal right to healthcare services.

Dilemmas are defined by Martin Benjamin and Joy Curtis (1994) as 'a situation requiring a choice between what seem to be two equally desirable or undesirable alternatives' (p. 4). An ethical dilemma according to the same authors means choosing an ethical principle where either seems a violation, yet a choice must be made' (Benjamin & Curtis 1994 p 5). The clinical issues to which Nurse Ellen must find resolutions are how she can explain type 2 diabetes so that Mr Z understands this as a chronic disease and that by following the diabetes guidelines his quality of life will not be at risk. In adhering to nutritional and medical regimes along with preventive measures, for instance walking to work, he can reduce or postpone secondary complications.

THE NURSES' CODE OF ETHICS

Nurses have an obligation to patients, the physicians and the institution in which they work (Davis et al 1997 p 63). The nurse's primary responsibility is to patients; as the ICN *Code of ethics for nurses* (ICN 2000 p 2) says, 'the nurse's primary professional responsibility is to people requiring nursing care'. Nurse Ellen therefore has a duty to provide Mr Z with knowledge about his disease so he can make essential life adjustments. Nurse Ellen knows how to do this for persons with a similar cultural background as her own. But how she can convey the same information to a person who believes any illness can be cured, and that if his type 2 diabetes is chronic he will not live, becomes a clinical and ethical dilemma. She must find solutions to both obligations.

One can argue that as all decisions are made in a social context, Nurse Ellen's employer has an obligation to make sure she has the knowledge necessary to carry out her professional duties and obligations. An answer to her frustration could be to request education on Pakistani belief systems for all staff members at the clinic.

Another proposal could be to ask second-generation Pakistanis with a background of health provision in Norway to come and talk about how the two cultures can be synchronized. The goal must be for the staff members to understand better how Mr Z can make lifestyle changes that are bound to improve his quality of life. The ICN *Code* says that 'the nurse carries a personal responsibility and accountability for nursing practice and for maintaining competence by continual learning' (p 3). Another point to explore is how nurses' professional obligation can be fulfilled and how the organization's duty for hiring qualified employees can be ensured.

A third factor that must be addressed is the personal responsibility Mr Z has 'for his own health and for moderation of health risks that can be changed through choices of healthy behavior to claim a right to health care' (Davis et al 1997 p 83).

DISTRIBUTIVE JUSTICE AND A PATIENT'S RIGHTS

Beauchamp and Childress (1994) define distributive justice as a group of norms for distributing 'benefits, risks, and costs fairly'. The question is how one can balance benefits, risks and costs. The authors offer several systematic theories on how social benefits and burdens can be distributed. One example is the utilitarian approach that 'sees justice as involving trade-offs . . . for instance in establishing benefits in prepaid health maintenance programs'. The authors do add a cautionary note that 'problems emerge if utilitarian principles of justice are accepted as sufficient in themselves' (Beauchamp & Childress 1994 p 335).

Health care became a legal right in Norway in 1999, and one should perhaps ask if justice also expects that a person has a moral obligation to pursue a healthy lifestyle. Health authorities addressed some of the distributive issues in two White Papers in 1986 (Norges Offentlige Utredninger (NOU) 1987) and in 1997 (NOU 1997), justifying ways of prioritizing healthcare services. The two White Papers led to fruitful national, Nordic and international discussions on issues of just distribution of health care. Questions that remain unanswered are:

- Who defines health rights?
- Who defines a patient's needs?
- Who balances values of where to draw the line?
- What constitutes adequate levels of healthcare benefits?

Specific questions are beginning to be asked, such as whether people who ignore health guidelines and medical regimes after (for example) organ transplants have a right to a new organ if failure is caused by this neglect. Patients suffering from type 2 diabetes have a high probability of needing expensive cardiac, vascular or eye surgery if the illness is ignored. Thus far there is a reluctance to question whether or not this is a just way of distributing limited health resources. All citizens have a right to health, but can the country afford the same standard of care to all when limited resources must be distributed sparsely, although justly? Norway's health services are generous and few have yet been brave enough to raise this as a national debate and query the cost of unhealthy lifestyles. Perhaps Nurse Ellen's employer has an obligation to engage people who have the clinical and ethical knowledge of working with Muslims.

The lack of knowledge of how to harmonize aspects of all cultures is a growing problem, and providing in-service courses for all health providers who encounter patients with non-Norwegian backgrounds is not an unreasonable expectation. If society has an ethical obligation to ensure equitable access to health services (Davis et al 1997), then an employer might have an obligation to provide nurses with the necessary knowledge so that they can fulfil their social mandate. This is certainly an issue that needs to be addressed.

Nurse Ellen conjectures that Mr Z will claim his right to costly treatment when his secondary complications occur because of his inability to adhere to the recommended guidelines for type 2 diabetes. The Norwegian healthcare system has a clear ethical principle of distributive justice because all citizens have legal rights regardless of lifestyle. As the healthcare system is costly and serves young and old alike, resources are limited. Mr Z will most likely obtain the cardiac surgery he might require but the follow-up rehabilitation capacity might be limited because there are limited resources for rehabilitation. The Patients' Bill of Rights (White Paper 1998–1999a), and the professional law for health providers (White Paper 1998–1999b) are unclear in their interpretations of which has precedence, the patients' right to refuse treatment or the nurses' duty to provide health services to all.

According to Nurse Ellen's professional code of ethics, she has a duty to explore how patients with other cultural backgrounds can receive medical information they have a legal right to obtain. A complicating factor for Nurse Ellen is that although Mr Z has lived in Norway for nearly 30 years, his comprehension of the Norwegian language and culture is limited and he speaks Urdu most of the time. Mr Z keeps saying that he is 'unable to change his diet' as his mother-in-law does the cooking. For him to request a special diet will reflect poorly on her as a good housewife.

Mr Z works shifts and the irregular hours make it even more difficult to follow the recommended three meals a day.

SUGGESTED SOLUTIONS

Nurse Ellen could explore several avenues to reduce her frustration and feelings of inadequacy. One is to make contact with second-generation Pakistani nurses educated in Norway. Talking to them might help Nurse Ellen to learn how to understand Mr Z's background and lifestyle better. She could also make a home visit and talk to the whole family about Mr Z's diabetes and how they can all contribute so that he can improve his life by following the recommended guidelines.

The ethical and clinical issues in this case are not new to Norway and many western countries are having similar experiences. In the past, issues around pre- and postnatal care led to projects financed by the Department of Health to distribute pamphlets with culture-appropriate pictures to pregnant women and their families. Midwives working with pregnant immigrant women are given special education so that they are better prepared to meet the patients' needs. Type 2 diabetes, although not a new disease among first-generation Pakistani men, has only recently been defined as ethically and clinically demanding. There are ongoing projects interviewing second-generation health providers educated in Norway to explore how the two cultures can be harmonized. Harmonization here means how the best from the two cultures can be woven into educational modules for Norwegian nurses and physicians who work with people from other cultures living with type 2 diabetes. Making available pamphlets with culturally sensitive pictures and videos in Urdu, Arabic, etc. and distributing them to meeting places frequented by immigrants might be helpful. Making home visits to the families of first-generation Pakistani family members with type 2 diabetes might be courteous, and would enable the nurse to learn more about their dietary customs.

There are no good solutions to how Nurse Ellen can fulfil her ethical and clinical duties to Mr Z in terms of him changing his lifestyle and following the recommended guidelines for type 2 diabetes. Much more information about people whose families originated in Pakistan must be collected so that health providers can offer services that harmonize key elements from both cultures. Nearly all western countries struggle to integrate immigrants and refugees with very different cultural backgrounds, health beliefs and spiritual needs. Talking to second-generation persons and making use of the knowledge of anthropologists is one way of understanding and integrating vastly different belief systems.

References

Beauchamp TL, Childress JF 1994 Principles of medical ethics. Oxford University Press, New York.

Benjamin M, Curtis J 1994 Health care ethics. Temple University Press, Philadelphia.

Bunch E 2000 Delayed clarification. Information, clarification and ethical decisions in critical care in Norway. Journal of Advanced Nursing 32:1485–1491.

Carlsen B 2001 Sykepleie til flyktninger og invandrere (Nursing refugees and immigrants) In: Gjengedall E, Jacobsen R (eds) (Sykepleie) Nursing. Cappelen Akademiske Forlag, Oslo, p 1250–1265.

Davis A, Aroskar M, Liaschenko J, Drought T 1997 Ethical dilemmas in nursing practice, 4th edn. Appleton & Lange, Stanford, CT.

Hanssen I 1987 Islamic patients in Norwegian hospitals. University of Oslo, Master of Nursing Science.

Hanssen I 1996 Health providers in a multicultural society. Oslo University Press, Oslo.

Helsedirektoratet (Health Directorate) 1987 Helse for alle i Norge (Health for all in Norway). Kommuneforlaget, Oslo.

International Council of Nurses (ICN) 2000 Code of ethics for nurses. ICN, Geneva.

Jervell J 2000 Diabetes blant innvandrere (Diabetes among immigrants). Oslo University Press, Oslo.

Johansson K, Skinner T 2003 Empowerment and the diabetes patient. Clinical nursing, Copenhagen.

Jølf S 2004 Is it a question of will? Experiences Greenlanders with diabetes 2 have. University of Oslo, Master of Nursing Science.

Kommune Oslo (Oslo City) 2003 Statistisk Årbok for Oslo kommune, 2003. (Statistical Yearbook for Oslo 2003). County of Oslo.

Leininger M 1995 Transcultural nursing. McGraw Hill, New York.

Norges Offentlige Utredninger (NOU) 1987 23. Retningslinjer for prioriteringer i helsetjenesten i Norge (White Paper). (Guidelines for prioritizing health care services in Norway). Department of Health, Oslo.

Norges Offentlige Utredninger (NOU) 1997 18. Prioriteringer på ny. (White Paper). (Prioritizing health again). Department of Health, Oslo.

Tranøy K 1997 Medisinsk Etikk (Medical ethics), 2nd edn. Sigma, Bergen.

White Paper 1998–1999a Pasient rettighets loven, (Patients' legal rights) 1998–99.

White Paper 1998–1999b Helsepersonell loven. (Law for health providers) 1998–99.

WHO 1999 Definition, diagnosis and classification of diabetes mellitus and its complications. WHO, Geneva.

Further reading

Hylland Eriksen T, Sørheim A 2000 Kultur forskjeller i praksis (Cultural differences in the clinic). ad Notam, Gjøvik.

Chapter **26**

Malawi.
Ethical challenges of HIV and AIDS
in Malawi, southern Africa

Adamson Muula

INTRODUCTION

Southern Africa is the region most affected by the HIV and AIDS pandemic. In most of the countries in the region, at least 10% of the adult population is already infected by HIV. AIDS is now among the common causes of morbidity and mortality among children under the age of five years and adults between the ages of 19 and 49 years. Most of the HIV transmission in the region is by heterosexual and vertical (mother-to-child) means. The significance of unsafe blood transfusions and injections (therapeutic or recreational) and homosexuality is presumed to be small, although a growing concern.

In most countries in the region, nurses are the front-line health workers whom patients consult for either acute or chronic illnesses, but also for health promotion and disease prevention. The multiple roles of nurses in clinical care have also resulted in nurses being the preferred health workers to be involved in recruiting research participants. This chapter will discuss the various ethical challenges that nurses face in the performance of their duties in teaching patients, in clinical care, in research and in community care.

THE COUNTRY OF MALAWI

Malawi is a country in the south-eastern part of Africa with an estimated population of eleven million inhabitants. It is bordered by Tanzania to the north and north-east, Zambia to the west and Mozambique wraps around it from the east, south and south-west. Most of the health problems result from poverty and deprivation. Communicable diseases such as diarrhoea and malaria are exacerbated by undernutrition and are major causes of both adult and paediatric morbidity and mortality. Of particular note is the fact that southern Africa is the region of the world with the largest prevalence of HIV and AIDS and Malawi is no exception.

HIV in Malawi was first described in 1983 and it is estimated that at least 10% of the adult population was infected by the end of 2003. As a result of the HIV situation in the country, there has been an upsurge in the prevalence of tuberculosis, with about 29 000 recorded patients at the end of 2003, and increased occurrence of other opportunistic infections such as *Pneumocystis carinii* pneumonia (Kamiya et al 1997). AIDS-related malignancies such as Kaposi's sarcoma are among the most common cancers in Malawi (Banda et al 2001). There are an estimated 800 000 orphans in the country, half of whom are 'AIDS orphans', i.e. children whose parents have died from AIDS.

The general health status of Malawi's population is poor, and this is particularly shown in the extremely high maternal mortality ratio of 1120 deaths per 100 000 live births (Muula & Phiri 2003), an infant mortality rate of 104 deaths per thousand live births and a life expectancy at birth of about 37 years.

However, the situation regarding HIV/AIDS is not all dismal. In the past few years, Malawi has identified a lack of political will, limited resources being provided to the health sector and other social sectors, and lack of treatment for HIV and opportunistic infections as some of the gaps that needed to be attended to. The country has therefore mobilized resources internally but has also benefited from HIPC (Highly Indebted Poor Country) initiatives and the Global Fund against AIDS, Tuberculosis and Malaria (GFATM) to enable it to improve the health status of its citizens (Harries et al 2004).

HIV COUNSELLING AND TESTING

Voluntary counselling and testing for HIV is recognized as an important entry point for sexual behavioural change but also for care and support of people who test positive for HIV. Testing for HIV in Malawi is fraught with ethical and programmatic or logistical challenges. Despite the recognition that HIV testing is important for stemming the HIV pandemic, testing is not widely enough available to enable many people who require it to benefit. Until recently, HIV testing was available only in regional or provincial centres run by non-governmental organizations (NGOs). Testing in public health facilities was only possible for diagnostic reasons in already symptomatic individuals and for the testing of blood donors. As part of the antiretroviral 'scaling-up' initiative, HIV counselling and testing facilities have been established at each of the country's district and mission hospitals.

Practising nurses are often responsible for ensuring that counselling and testing is done. This may be intrapartum to facilitate antiretroviral administration to reduce mother-to-child transmission of HIV, during outpatient visits and for inpatient treatment.

For HIV testing to be justified, it should be carried out only if it is in the best interest of the patient, i.e. the potential benefit must outweigh the risks. How, then, do we know that testing would be in the best interest of the patient when many patients also prefer not to know the results after the test? Who should decide if and when testing is in the best interest of the patient? For patients to make informed decisions regarding testing, they must have information that is relevant and appropriate to them; information must therefore be individualized. The biological model of HIV, where the HIV infection is explained as *kachilombo* (a little beast) might not be easy for the majority of illiterate Malawians to understand. Even those who are literate might not do any better. Ensuring that our patients are fully informed is therefore fraught with significant challenges as the question arises, how far have nurses to go to ensure that patients and clients are well informed?

HUMAN RESOURCES

Nurses are currently the largest cadre of health workers being lost from Malawi as they migrate to other countries and from the public sector to the private sector and to NGOs (Muula et al 2003). The suggested reasons for the migration include: lack of promotional opportunities and general poor working conditions, poor remuneration in Malawi and attractive remuneration packages in the recipient countries and organizations. While indeed working conditions for nurses in most of the developing countries must be improved, the present brain drain raises questions of the 'commodification' of the nursing profession. Is the principle that nursing is a vocation to serve, rather than being for personal gain, still relevant today? Or should nursing be lumped together with any of the professions whose aim is simply to have bread on one's table at the end of the month? Some nurses from Malawi who have migrated to the UK have found themselves in job positions there which they would not normally have liked and might not have taken had they known in advance.

ACCESS TO ANTIRETROVIRAL THERAPY

Only about 6000 people in Malawi were receiving highly active antiretroviral therapy (HAART) by mid-2004, out of an estimated 150 000 people who might have been clinically eligible (Muula 2004). Two main reasons for this small number of people being on antiretrovirals (ARVs) are that in the public health sector treatment was available in only four centres, two urban and two rural, and the rural areas that were covered by antiretroviral therapy (ART) were the neighbouring districts of Thyolo and Chiradzulu in the southern region of the country. A few mission hospitals were also providing care but the number of people enrolled in these programmes was less than 200. The other reason why ART was not widely accessible to many people was the fact that, except in Thyolo and Chiradzulu, ART was mostly available only for a fee. Although the fees patients were required to pay were heavily subsidized, the majority of the population in need could still not access treatment. ART was the privilege of the minority rich people.

The Ministry of Health in Malawi planned to scale up the access to ART, having obtained funding from the Global Fund. This 'scaling-up' of ART access has already meant that, by October 2004, there were about 9000 patients on free ART in Malawi, i.e. in three months the number had grown by about 50%. The question then arose, who was going to be able to access this therapy? The simple answer to this had been that ART would be available on a 'first-come first-served basis'. There were obviously concerns over equity and who would eventually end up benefiting from this programme.

So far, the system had been that free ARVs had begun to be given to those clients who had been on the paying system. Inevitably, these were the 'haves' who could afford ARVs when everyone else could not. New patients or clients, and those who were clinically eligible but could not afford to pay when the ARVs were being provided at a fee, had access, but only when the 'haves' had been served. Even when all the centres were operational at the same time, ARVs were not accessible to everyone who needed them, based simply on proximity to the centre and accessibility of the centre itself.

The policy of first-come first-served was arrived at after failing to find a suitable alternative. Preference for special groups such as health workers, military personnel and teachers was discouraged because it had been argued that such a practice discriminated against those not belonging to the suggested population groups. The first-come first-served basis was preferred because, in a sense, the environment and other factors would militate against who would get ART and who would not. No one would, in the end, be blamed for deciding on who should receive therapy and who should not.

However, the scaling-up of the numbers of patients receiving ART did not go according to plan; the government could not procure all the ARVs in the quantities that had been planned. As a public health measure to prevent drug non-adherence and development of community-wide HIV resistance towards ARVs, it was decided that all those patients who were on ARVs would continue being on therapy but that adding new patients to the programme would be done gradually.

CULTURAL CONSIDERATIONS

Among the many reasons that have been suggested as contributing to the lamentable HIV/AIDS situation in Africa are the 'harmful' cultural or traditional practices of many of the Bantu tribes in the region. These cultural practices include initiation ceremonies, sexual practices, treatments for infertility, widow inheritance and funeral rites.

INITIATION CEREMONIES

Traditionally, adolescents are expected to go through an initiation process, which is a ritual passage from childhood to adulthood. The boys and girls camp either in a house or in the bush where specially identified and trained people, *ngalibas* and *nakangas*, impart knowledge about adulthood to the initiates. This training into adulthood comprises sessions on how to behave in society as an adult, but inevitably also includes sex education (how to have sex and how to satisfy the opposite gender sexually). On release from the initiation camps, the initiates are advised to have sexual intercourse, or else they will die or bring calamities on their families. Such practices, called *kuchotsa fumbi* (removing the dust) or *kudzola mafuta* (smearing the oil), are considered non-negotiable. Many young people believe that not having sex will result in the suggested adverse effect, and are therefore encouraged to have sex.

The initiation ceremonies for males also involve circumcision. In the event that cutting blades are shared among the initiates, they can be vehicles for the transmission of blood-borne infections.

While these harmful initiation practices exist, some NGOs run programmes to influence change. For instance, instead of the local elders circumcising the boys, health workers at the government or mission hospitals will do this, using sterile and disposable surgical blades.

SEXUAL PRACTICES

The literature on 'dry sex' suggests that, in many southern African cultures, this behaviour is widely practised. Dry sex implies that the woman's vagina is artificially dried with wads of cloth or cotton, or powdered herbs in order to make sexual intercourse more pleasurable. Smit et al (2002), have reported that women in South Africa who use Depo-provera (a combined injectable contraceptive) complain of excessive vaginal wetness. Zachariah et al (2003) also reported that female commercial sex workers complained that the extra lubrication associated with female condoms results in loss of sensation. In the traditional Malawian psyche, more friction means more pleasurable penetrative sex.

The main concerns over dry sex in the HIV era are:

- Dry sex creates the environment where abrasions of the genital organs are much more likely. Open sores thus created can therefore operate as portals of entry for HIV.
- Abrasions in the genitals can also be associated with inflammation, resulting in increased concentration of white cells and hence a higher likelihood for HIV transmission.
- Dry sex is also associated with non-use of condoms and yet consistent and correct condom use is associated with reduction in the transmission of HIV.

Many women are encouraged to use herbs or other methods to dry the vagina in order to 'please' their spouses. It is not unusual for a man to complain about the increased vaginal wetness of a sexual partner.

INFERTILITY TREATMENTS

As in many other southern African countries, in Malawi, childlessness – from whatever cause – is presumed to be a 'curse'. When a couple has been married for at least year and there is 'no gift of a child', the extended family becomes concerned. In some tribes, a male relative who is himself married is asked to have sex with the woman without the knowledge of her spouse. If the couple's childlessness was due to male infertility, it would be possible for the woman to conceive. The husband, without realizing it, might therefore think that he has sired a child.

WIDOW INHERITANCE

Widow inheritance (*chokolo)* is the practice where a widow is given in marriage to a relative of her deceased husband. This was a common practice among many tribes in southern Africa. The intention was that there continued to be someone in the husband's family who would take care of the economic needs of the widow after the death of her husband. This practice has potential to spread HIV if either of the parties to be married is HIV infected.

Related to the practice of *chokolo* is the practice of *kuchotsa imfa* (chasing death away). In this practice, when a man dies, the village is supposed to destroy the family's house as a way of chasing away the bad spirits. There are anecdotal reports that such practices, which leave the widow and children destitute, could be driving some widows into sexual relationships that would not have happened if they were not so impoverished.

FUNERAL PRACTICES

AIDS has resulted in an increased occurrence of deaths. When death has occurred, it is customary for the elders of the clan to organize the bathing of the body. Even in the era of AIDS, this practice of 'bathing the body' (*kusambitsa thupi*) is yet to be fully modified. Unless the body is embalmed by commercial undertakers, the practice is that the dead body is bathed by either relatives or the elders of the community, without any gloves. Such practices may spread HIV (if those who wash the body have sores on their hands) and other infections spread through body fluids.

ETHICS OF HIV RESEARCH

HIV and AIDS are probably the most researched areas in Malawi. Much of this research is conducted by international research organizations with partners in Malawi. In an environment in which healthcare workers' conditions of services within the public health sector (the major employer of health workers in Malawi) are far from ideal, an increasing number of health workers are moving from the public health service to research organizations. There is some evidence that the deterioration of the quality of care within the public health sector is partially created by the loss of health workers from the public health sector to research and other HIV/AIDS care organizations. Professional nurses are a much-sought-for cadre of health worker in Malawi among research organizations. Because of their training and skills in patient care and support, the nurses find themselves recruiting study subjects. The nurses' appreciation of health research ethics is therefore being used.

AIDS is challenging the way that Malawian society has functioned in the past. New methods and thinking, which society perceives as alien, have been introduced. An example of this was a study where the viral load of seminal fluid was quantified among clients attending a sexually transmitted diseases clinic (Dyer et al 1998). Clients had to submit semen through masturbation. The prevalence of masturbation among Malawian males is not known and it is therefore difficult to suggest how common the practice is. Even if the practice were to be common, asking a research participant to do it for collection of a research specimen is a challenge on its own. Such situations put nurses in the position of dealing with the training, fears and concerns of research subjects.

TEACHING ETHICS TO NURSES

Ethics is taught through didactic lectures where usually the principles of ethics are introduced. Case studies are also used to highlight a particular principle. A case study can now be presented:

Case study   Janet (not her real name) has been married for four years. She has just been diagnosed as HIV-infected at the fertility clinic, where she had gone without the knowledge of her husband, to find out 'what was wrong with her'. She fears she may be beaten up or divorced if she informs her husband about her HIV status. She is not sure whether her husband has ever tested for HIV, as they do not spend much time talking to each other. She still wants to have a child.

This case study highlights the principles of justice, autonomy, beneficence and non-maleficence. To make a reasonable ethical assessment of Janet's situation, we need to isolate certain aspects of her case. Janet is childless and this state is abhorred in the local Malawian cultures. Having a child who dies is perceived to be better than childlessness from primary infertility. Janet knows her HIV situation but her husband does not. She still wants to have a child. She faces two evils, i.e. childlessness and disclosure of her HIV status, which could both expose her to violence and/or divorce.

The primary responsibility of any health worker is to serve the best interest of their patient. Janet decides not to tell her spouse about her HIV status. In order to 'keep her marriage' and therefore personal happiness and a meaning in life, she is persuaded to have a child. In so doing, however, she may forfeit her opportunity to inform the spouse about HIV in the family, the possibility of the husband also considering testing and possibly also using condoms when having penetrative sex. If she does not disclose to her spouse about her HIV status, she may be putting her spouse in harm's way. Janet's spouse might not be infected with HIV, and not telling him could be harmful. The onus should be on the partner who knows her or his HIV status to tell the other and encourage him or her also to undergo testing. If this is not done, there is a real possibility that the non-infected partner will be infected in the long run (Porter et al 2004).

There is the dilemma of double effect, i.e. doing a thing that has potential for harm just as it has potential for good. Janet might also forgo an opportunity to request a non-vaginal delivery should she become pregnant. There is evidence to suggest that babies of HIV-infected mothers born by caesarean section have a reduced chance of getting infected. More importantly, by her non-disclosure of her HIV status to her spouse, Janet prevents him from making informed decisions as to whether the couple should continue pursuing the idea of being biological parents. The husband cannot therefore exercise informed decision making. On the other hand, Janet's action could prevent the violence and divorce that might occur if she were to disclose, thus potentially saving her own life from possible abuse and in some cases grave physical violence. Janet is an autonomous being and entitled to make decisions regarding her own life.

WEB-BASED TEACHING

With the improved access to internet-based information services, teaching is increasingly being offered through web-based approaches. Case-studies and reading materials can be provided electronically. Interactive teaching and learning programs on cases can be an important part of teaching nursing ethics for those that have access to such facilities.

REFLECTION

Reflection, which encourages critical thinking, is another way ethics could be taught (Price 2004). In this approach, situations that are posed as ethically difficult or challenging, are narrated by the nurse trainees in a class for discussion. How the situation was handled is also presented. The group or an individual then reviews the case, identifying what was done well, what was done not so well and how best the situation could have been handled. A nurse trainee could present the following case:

Case study   'I was in the operating theatre one day when we had a child being operated on for cataract. As the inner lens capsule was opened, it was not just an opacified lens. Pus was coming out. We all knew that the parents of the child had given us consent to operate on the child based on their understanding that the child would gain her sight after the 'cataract' treatment. But now it was a different thing. Just draining the eye and giving antibiotics could predispose the child to cavernous sinus infection and thrombosis, with very little chance of survival. One of the options, and this was done, was removal of the eye ball. I was sent to inform the mother, who was just outside the operating room, where many of the parents or guardians of our patients wait when the patient is being operated on. She accepted the procedure. However, things changed when the girl's father came. The mother denied having giving us permission to go ahead with removal of the eye ball. The family went on to report to the hospital complaints committee after a few days.'

From a case like this, a group of nurse trainees, or even just one nurse, can be asked to review the case by first isolating what could be described as the facts of the matter, then what went well, and then what could have been handled better. We can start by looking at the following:

- Did the healthcare team and the child's parents act in the best interest of the child?
- It would appear that, for the healthcare team, the necessity to save life was supreme.
- For the parents, it would appear that the necessity to have both eyes, even if the child died, was supreme. However, the discrepancies in choice could result from different levels of understanding between the two groups. To the healthcare team, the child had a slim chance of survival by just draining the eye and take antibiotics. The parents might not perceive the issue in that way.

We have also used on-line discussion groups for the teaching of ethics to medical students. There is no reason why this approach cannot be used for nurses. Leppa and Terry (2004) report a similar on-line discussion group among post-registration nurses in the UK and the USA. However, there are problems with the availability and accessibility of internet services in Malawi, and this will be more critical in developing countries. However, where possible, this mode of instruction should be considered.

CONCLUSION

Nurses tend to find themselves in ethically challenging environments, be they in clinical research, care or counselling. As in many societies, Malawian cultural beliefs and literacy levels will have a bearing on how the principles of justice, beneficence and autonomy are going to be manifested. Teaching ethics makes use of didactic methods, interactive problem-based approaches and web-based methods.

References

Banda LT, Parkin DM, Dzamalala CP, Liomba NG 2001 Cancer incidence in Blantyre, Malawi. Tropical Medicine and International Health 6:296–304.

Dyer JR, Kazembe P, Vernazza PL et al 1998 High levels of human immunodeficiency virus type 1 in blood and semen of seropositive men in sub-Saharan Africa. Journal of Infectious Diseases 177:1742–1746.

Harries AD, Gomani P, Teck R, et al 2004 Monitoring the response to antiretroviral therapy in resource-poor settings: the Malawi model. Transactions of the Royal Society of Tropical Medicine & Hygiene 98:695–701.

Kamiya Y, Mtitimila E, Graham SM et al 1997 *Pneumocystis carinii* pneumonia in Malawian children. Annals of Tropical Paediatrics 17:121–126.

Leppa CJ, Terry LM 2004 Reflective practice in nursing ethics education: international collaboration. Journal of Advanced Nursing 48:195–202.

Muula AS 2004 Ethical and programmatic challenges in anti-retroviral scaling-up in Malawi: challenges in meeting the World Health Organization's 'Treating 3 million by 2005' initiative goals. Croatian Medical Journal 45:415–422.

Muula AS, Phiri A 2003 Did maternal mortality increase in Malawi between 1992–1998? Review of Malawi demographic and health surveys and other data sources. Tropical Doctor 33:182–185.

Muula AS, Mfutso-Bengo JM, Makoza J, Chatipwa E 2003 The ethics of developed nations recruiting nurses from developing countries: the case of Malawi. Nursing Ethics 10:433–438.

Porter L, Hao L, Bishai D et al and the Rakai Project Team 2004 HIV status and union dissolution in sub-Saharan Africa: the case of Rakai, Uganda. Demography 41:465–482.

Price A 2004 Encouarging reflection and critical thinking in practice. Nursing Standard 18(47):46–52.

Smit J, Mac Fadyen L, Zuma K, Preston-Whyte E 2002 Vaginal wetness: an underestimated problem experienced by progestogen injectable contraceptive users in South Africa. Social Science & Medicine 55:1511–1522.

Zachariah R, Harries AD, Buhendwa L et al 2003 Acceptability and technical problems of the female condom amongst commercial sex workers in a rural district of Malawi. Tropical Doctor 33:220–224.

Chapter **27**

Hungary.
Nursing and nursing ethics after the Communist era

Elizabeth Rozsos

INTRODUCTION

In 1989 Hungary emerged from the control of the Soviet Union; the political changes that took place when this occurred influenced health politics. The Health Law of 1972 was abolished and a new modern law was issued (Act 1997), which is specifically concerned with patients' rights. There were also big changes in nursing education.

Malpractices became public that, until then, had been carefully concealed by the courts, and abuses of patients' rights were discussed in the newspapers, on radio and on TV. These information sources showed that:

- Nurses who had spoken up for the interests of patients had either been silenced or lost their jobs
- Paternalism and physician-centred practices were common within health care
- Miserable salaries were the norm for all healthcare workers
- There was a total lack of respect for workers and patients
- Exhaustion and burn-out were common among the nursing staff
- There was a total lack of any nursing ethics education

These issues became sources of moral problems. Since 1990, huge efforts have been made in teaching ethics to nurses to bring about changes in practice. The reasons why the cases described could exist at all lie in the past, in the previous regime.

HUNGARY IN BRIEF

Situated in the Carpathian basin of Central Europe, the Republic of Hungary has an area of 93 033 square kilometres, i.e. 1% of the area of Europe. The official language is Hungarian (Magyar), which belongs to the Finno-Ugrian family of languages. In 2002, the population of Hungary was just over ten million. For the purposes of public administration, the country is divided into 19 counties and the capital city, Budapest, consists of 23 districts.

In AD 1000, King Stephen was crowned, and thus the year 2000 marked the millennium of the existence of Hungary as a State. After the Second World War, Hungary became one of the Communist countries. After the disintegration of the Soviet Union, Hungary changed her political establishment peacefully.

With the promulgation of the Constitution on 21 October 1989, and the ensuing formation of the government, the Republic of Hungary became a parliamentary republic in the European sense. In 1990 there were the first free elections to a six-party single-chamber Parliament; 386 members of Parliament elected were for four-year terms.

Hungary is a member of the World Health Organization, Council of Europe, Organization for Economic Co-operation and Development (OECD) and, since 1 May 2004, the European Union. The Hungarian Nursing Association (HNA) has been a member in the International Council of Nurses since 1981 and, as such, is actively engaged in various collaborative activities internationally. The Hungarian Nursing Association published its own Code of Ethics for Nurses in 2000.

AFTER THE CHANGE IN 1989: FROM COMMUNISM TO DEMOCRACY

In 1989, the Communist Party system was replaced by a multi-party system and a democratically constituted State in Hungary. The healthcare system had never been under political direction but the political influence prevailed on those working in it: head physicians, chiefs of department or principals of hospitals were appointed only if they were politically reliable; one of the members of the ethics committee of a hospital was always the District Party secretary.

Nurses depended entirely on the doctors and were placed in a very rigid hierarchical system, in which they were forced into a 'servant role' and expected to carry out the doctors' instructions without question. Those who criticized the system were either severely punished or lost their job. Nurses who were trained under this system simply agreed to whatever the senior physician said. In some places, this meant that nurses were giving intravenous injections without being competent to do so (Rozsos 2003); in other places, the informed consent form that needed to be signed before an operation was presented to the patient by the nurse, not by the doctor, because that was the instruction. This still happens sometimes today (personal communication).

NURSING EDUCATION IN HUNGARY

BEFORE 1975

Direct entry into nursing education was after age 17. There were two models: a full-time course of 24 months or on-the job training for three years, which led to a certificate in general/adult health nursing, child health nursing or psychiatric nursing.

FROM 1975 UNTIL 1993

Age at entry was 14 years, with 8 years of primary school completed. There were two options: a three-year programme of basic nursing education and a four-year programme to train as a nurse and to obtain the secondary-school leaving certificate (baccalaureate). This led to the general nursing and healthcare technician certificate. Specialization was mandatory for those in nursing, with a ten-month on-the-job course (e.g. medical–surgical nursing, infant and child health nursing, psychiatric nursing, district/community nursing, midwifery).

FROM 1993

There is now an alignment to the Directives and Recommendations on nursing education from the European Union. Age at entry has to be at least 18 years, with a secondary-school leaving certificate (baccalaureate, GCE, similar to colleges and universities). There is a three-year full-time basic nursing education of 4600 hours, leading to a Diploma in nursing. Specialization is possible with post-basic courses in nursing, which means essentially on-the-job courses to train in various nursing specialties (e.g. critical care nursing, oncology nursing, operating theatre nursing) (Ministry of Health 2002).

In addition to the three-year programme, nine colleges of nursing offer a four-year bachelor programme in nursing that provides graduates with a BSc degree in nursing, gained during academic education (colleges are institutions of higher education). Graduates of these programmes can continue their studies at various university programmes to become, for example, nurse teachers and managers. Those training in the three-year programme can enrol in one of the colleges of nursing and obtain an academic education. A Masters in Nursing programme was launched in 2000 in Pécs and in 2002 in Budapest.

EXAMPLES OF NURSING PRACTICE AND PROBLEMS

The two examples below have been much in the news in Hungary. Because of the low status of nurses and their equally low salaries, nurses were driven to desperate measures to make ends meet, as the second example shows. The caged beds described in the first example were first used in Hungary in 1940. The human rights issues were not considered for many years, but a new law in 2004 prohibited their use.

THE CAGED BED

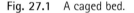

The health care of psychiatric patients in Hungary bears in every respect the 'crimes of the former system'. To lock in, punish, terrify and hide forever some patients was in the interest of society and the family, and was the most comfortable practice for public health. The most terrible product of that system was the so-called 'caged bed': metal cages attached to beds in psychiatric units, which were used by nurses to punish patients (Fig. 27.1).

A caged bed: *'measured 2.08 m × 0.93 m, (approximately 7 feet × 3 feet) and was covered with a strong net, fixed on a tubular metal structure 1.26 m (approximately 4 feet) in height, an articulated opening with a padlock having been made on the left side. The individual enclosed in such a bed cannot stand up and has to eat, sleep and defecate in the caged bed'* (Lewis 2002)

Fig. 27.1 A caged bed.

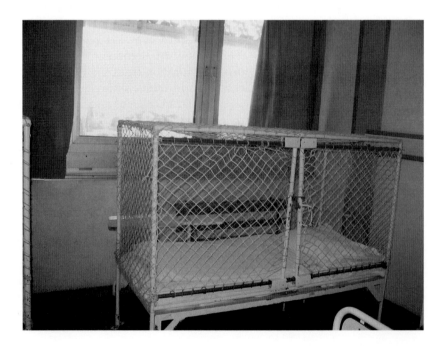

National and international organizations and the Office of the Parliamentary Commissioner for Human Rights (the Ombudsman) regularly examine and criticize the situation of persons living in psychiatric institutions and hospitals. After their inspection in 1989, the European Committee for the Prevention of Torture (CPT) asked the Hungarian government to outlaw immediately the use of caged beds. However, despite the revelations and reports of the tragic situation, not much changed. The crowded institutions, lack of morale and shortage of nursing and medical staff, as well as the grave inheritance concerning the treatment of psychiatric patients, continued largely unchanged. Some patients were there on the wishes of their family; there was no release until they died (Bakonyi 1983); this was a form of life imprisonment.

The situation – at the level of the law and, in reality, regarding the circumstances of referral and treatment – changed in line with international regulations. Since 1997, the CLIV Health Law (the chapter on Patients' Rights) and many more laws and orders have protected patients, especially those who are deemed defenceless. However, the inheritance from the past, the experiences of the people concerned, the behaviour of staff and the lack of clear orders from the governing bodies have prevented openness about these problems, and the law is not yet well recognized.

In Hungary, if a doctor incorrectly adjusts a dose of a medication, the nurse does not recognize this as a sign to advocate on behalf of the patient; or if a patient who should not be admitted to a psychiatric hospital, but there is no other appropriate accommodation available, has his or her right to privacy breached and becomes agitated, the person who is in power takes steps to deal with the situation, as is shown in the following.

In 1996, a statement from the Ombudsman concerning the effectiveness of human and civil rights of patients in institutions and psychiatric wards found that the fundamental human dignities included in the Constitution were breached in the care of patients in one (named) institution. At the time of the investigation neither a specialist nor any other doctor was available to care for the 301 patients in the institution. A part-time specialist nurse visited the patients once in a while; there were two head mental health nurses, 42 qualified nurses, seven assistant nurses and 21 auxiliary staff (manual workers) (Ombudsman 1996). At that time, the patients' stories and the diary notes of the investigators (Ombudsman 1996) revealed that nurses carried out different punishments in cases of 'disorder', i.e. they removed the patients' clothes and shoes, did not allow them to bathe, or they put the patients in caged beds without the knowledge of the doctor. The following statements are a selection from these notes; only the first letters of the names have been changed:

AA is drunk, the purse and cupboard key is taken away, he is dressed in pyjamas, his wound is treated, has been in pyjamas for one month (i.e. the patient has to stay in pyjamas).

BB is very noisy, wants to go to X. When I did not let him go, he became even louder, he was sitting for two hours in a caged bed.

CC was up the whole night. He cried, moaned and said he was unwell and we should help him. Twice he was led to the bathroom from the caged bed.

DD provoked his eye to get stuck (oculogyric disease: causing or concerned with movements of the eye). When he was promised the caged bed, he recovered. He is excitable.

EE woke up at 1 in the morning, then he cried and woke also his fellow patients, got one tablet of Nitrazepam and I put him in a caged bed. Then he fell asleep with difficulty.

FF took his dinner from the fridge without permission: 1 litre of milk and salami. Was put into the caged bed.

JJ and KK were drunk in the morning, they were in the caged bed before lunch.

LL had a visitor, a little disturbed, put into caged bed. (Ombudsman 1996 p 22, 27, 31)

The Office of the Ombudsman closed this institution immediately (Ombudsman 1996). Despite this, the caged bed was used elsewhere as a punishment in psychiatric wards even in 2003. In such institutions, who determines what human dignity is?

These stories clearly show that nurses were left to their own devices. They had to take responsibility for the problems caused by lack of staff, unqualified staff, lack of medical supervision and lack of moral knowledge, and they took desperate measures. Their actions injured the physical and mental health of the patients and their rights to human dignity. Such nursing practice includes injury and torture. It infringes totally the rights to self-determination and to information. It is clear from the statements that the patients were not informed about any prognosis or treatment and did not have any choice or right of consent or refusal.

In the course of their work, nurses should act according to their code of ethics. It is therefore necessary that psychiatric institutions are controlled by civil bodies. The teaching and training of nurses should be such that they work to protect the interests of society; the work of the Ombudsman needs to be made more efficient.

AN UNUSUAL INHERITANCE CONTRACT

In the 1990s, not a year went by when we did not hear on the radio or TV or read in the newspapers about the miserable situation of nurses in Hungary. Health workers even entertained the idea of strike action. The salary of bedside nurses, working in three shifts, was HUF 39 000 per month (US$ 190). Research on the living standard of nurses carried out by the sociologist Bettina Pikó in the county of Csongrád concluded that nurses under 25 years of age living with their parents were best off.

Single, widowed or divorced nurses were in the worst financial situation, with one-third of them having no home of their own. The poorest were those living in lodgings or in nurses' homes (Pikó 1999). The question is whether these circumstances influence the moral behaviour of nurses.

The next story is about a special inheritance contract between a heavily sedated patient cared for in an intensive care unit and who later died, and the matron of the department. The patient had a family but had no contact with them (Köbli 2002). This is not only a nursing situation, but involves the law. The matron of the intensive care unit said she wanted to demonstrate that nurses can inherit money from patients and that they are therefore able to rise above penury.

Case study	A patient lying in an intensive care unit received less than the minimal dose of morphine because of possible respiratory irritability. At 19.00 hours the head doctor, who treated the patient, called the matron of the unit according to the wishes of the patient. The matron was told that the patient felt he was dying and wanted to leave all his property to her. The head doctor helped with drafting and typing the will. He stated that the patient was completely conscious and that this was also the opinion of the two enrolled nurses who signed the will as witnesses. The family learned about this event a month later; meanwhile the matron let the deceased person be buried. The family asked the court to verify the validity of this will on the basis of whether the patient was of sound mind at the time (Köbli 2002).

The ethical aspects of the case involve some of the following. The work of a nurse is outlined in the introduction of the Hungarian Code of Ethics, which is similar to the ICN Code of ethics for nurses (ICN 2000). We read in the Hungarian Nursing Association's Code of Ethics (2000) that: 'The fundamental responsibility of the nurse is to restore health and to alleviate suffering. The starting point of nursing is a holistic approach.' Nurses enter into a contract with their employer and therefore must act according to the rules of the health institution and be competent in their work. Nurses maintain the professional, ethical and legal standards of the profession; but nurses enter into a contract with patients, too. Patients accept the course of treatment and nursing care and the often painful interventions, and have full confidence in the people who look after them.

This contract is the clearest declaration of trust among the people involved. The contract to be adhered to by the staff of the intensive care unit is to accompany dying and defenceless patients who are preparing for their last journey. This agreement cannot be changed to a 'double relationship' whereby, besides caring and nursing, a different type of contract is also established in the same situation with the same person.

CAN AN INTENSIVE CARE MATRON INHERIT FROM A DYING PATIENT NURSED IN THE UNIT?

This double connection can be a particular worry for elderly people, who may be under the influence of medication at the time of decision making. The capacity for self-determination is then questionable. The staff of the intensive care unit did not inform the patient what type of will is possible in his case and did not contact anybody whose advice could have been justified. It is not known whether they made any effort to contact the relatives. Under the present circumstances, the patients' rights representative, as the legal representative of the hospital, the leader of the ethics committee or the association representing the interests of patients could have given the right answer. In this story we see the active and informed matron who is in a powerful position, as well as the hapless patient, who is at the other's mercy, without knowledge of the facts.

This is reflected in the Code of Ethics (HNA 2000) in the statement: 'The nurse does not abuse the dependent situation of the person in her or his care and does not expect material recompense for her or his work' (Clause III.4). Also, 'The nurse acts according to the norms of practice and professional expectations such as strengthen and protect the honour and good reputation of the profession' (Clause III.10).

In the text of the Oath of Graduation in the supplement to the Code we read: 'I refuse all demands that would abuse my professional activity and count them as illegal or immoral activities' (HNA 2000).

To the very self-assured matron, 'whose conscience is clear and who will end the affair' and who said that 'it is possible that a nurse can inherit' I would give the following advice in the words of József Imre (1925), who wrote in his first Hungarian medical ethics text for doctors:

> 'The ethical and legal rules apply on two fronts: one is the inner conscience of a person, which is always moving and engraving on one's mind the consequences of one's activity. The other is the ethical judgement given by public opinion when there is an immoral influence.'

The nurse should have refused this sort of inheritance because of her ethical duty in this situation.

PATIENTS' RIGHTS IN HUNGARY

In 1997, the Hungarian Parliament adopted a new Health Care Act (Act 1997). This new health law defines nursing for the first time ever and specifies that only qualified practitioners can engage in the practice of nursing. The Act also outlines a registration system for nurses and other healthcare workers.

This Act had become necessary in view of the changes that had occurred at the level of the European legal system: the act was written with an eye to adjusting to European norms. The Act proclaims patients' right to self-determination and all other rights in connection with this notion. Patients' rights were incorporated into the Act as a separate chapter, thus creating the official position of Patients' Rights Representative. There are 54 such representatives in the country, attached to hospitals and under the control of the Surgeon General's Office.

It is obvious that the traces of the old regime had not disappeared with the political changes. The struggle in 1990 to introduce ethics into the nursing curricula was neither easy nor safe. The publication of laws, the introduction of educational programmes and the publication of textbooks were just a framework for the change in the way of thinking.

NURSING ETHICS EDUCATION IN HUNGARY

Until 1990, nurses had no opportunity whatsoever to learn nursing ethics or to lecture on the subject. Doctors did not understand why *medical* ethics was appropriate for *nurses*. Nurses educated under the former system were puzzled and horrified at the changes they experienced because of the new laws and training prescriptions, and were accustomed to somebody else making decisions for them. Nurses with some degree of moral responsiveness soon realized that 'something was wrong' with them if they behaved differently, and they felt the result in their salary or in work arrangements. Despite this, all those courses that advertised ethics for practising nurses received many applications. The first course in ethics for basic nurse training began in 1990, and that for qualified nurses in 1994. The first years were very difficult because those teachers who until then had taught Marxist ethics and philosophy were watching incredulously. However, other colleagues recognized the importance of nursing ethics.

According to Marxist teaching, the social milieu determines the social consciousness and, with it, morality. In the book that was compulsory reading for every nurse in 1979 we read: 'The basic law of a socialist society is to maximize satisfaction by constantly encouraging the material and cultural demands of the population . . . This effort is expressed in the principle of socialist public health, worked out by the Soviet Union' (Marosi 1979 p 35). For nurses, this included the order: 'The best professional work fails unless it is inspired by dialectical materialism and activity based on strong basic principles. This teaches the nurse to see the social implications beyond the hospital bed' (Marosi 1979 p 25). The text linked almost every sentence to instruction and is typical of textbooks of the period. In what follows the author thinks that the nurse 'helps in the understanding of daily political events and bringing about the right attitudes' (Marosi 1979 p 26). The nurses who learned from this textbook until 1987 say that they did not understand a single sentence of it, and forgot it as soon as possible.

PRACTICAL TEACHING METHODS

As a teacher of ethics, I consider it most important that we assist and encourage nurses to recognize the moral conflicts that arise in nursing or clinical practice. To do this, I use lectures, role play and case analysis. My students and I prefer the role play and case analysis. They can read the scientific literature when convenient and they then participate actively in solving a problem. My goal in teaching and learning of ethics is to:

- Raise the students' sensitivity to ethical problems
- Help students recognize how decisions are made
- Enable students to be aware of their responsibility
- Help students learn to reflect, discuss and question values and practices

ROLE PLAY

The aim of role play is that students should recognize the ethical problem in a situation and the decisions nurses can take to prevent future similar events. I work up the unethical behaviour of nurses in a case and ask my students to choose a role. Two examples are: nurses who force a patient into a caged bed; a nurse who does not agree with others on a decision. One nurse takes the role of the head nurse, one of the patient, one of the patients' rights representative.

I ask the students to try to identify themselves with the role they are playing and to defend their point of view in a discussion. They are then asked to prepare a presentation to the class. Students thus learn about psychiatric care and restraint orders.

The patients' rights representative and the nurse who recognizes the appropriate ethical conduct then outline the ethical principles and ideas used to defend their arguments. In the class I start the discussion by first asking the nurses to say why they chose the method they did for punishment. Then everybody declares their point of view. The students can join the various players to strengthen the discussion.

I stop the discussion when it is necessary to clear up an important ethical concept.

CASE ANALYSIS

After the role play discussion, I distribute to everyone a paper with the following headings:

- Autonomy
- Information
- Self-determination
- Incompetent patients and self-determination
- Civil commitment procedure
- Quality of care
- Quality of life
- Conditions of physical restraint
- The right of psychiatric patients to consent and information
- Codes of ethics
- Responsibility for professional standards
- Non-maleficence in health care
- Justice
- Beneficence

- Patients' rights
- Torture

I ask the students to tell me what the connection is between their story and these ideas, principles and issues. I ask them to answer the following questions:

- On the basis of which symptoms can nurses recognize that a lack of caring leads to unethical procedures?
- What alternatives do they propose to prevent unethical procedures?
- What are the sources from which they can seek help (patients' rights representative, ethics committee, others)?
- What does responsibility mean to them?

I reinforce their positive answers and encourage them to speak up and protect patients against unethical procedures.

I then ask students to select a case from their own experience and analyse it by the same principles, while maintaining patient privacy.

These methods enable me to evaluate the following:

- The sensitivity of students for ethical problems.
- Whether the students can recognize certain values.
- If they are able to recognize when they transgress nursing ethics.
- Whether they can apply the concepts of bioethics and nursing ethics.
- Are they able to apply deontological and utilitarian models in the course of analysis?
- Based on their knowledge of nursing ethics, whether they are able to arrive at a correct decision in the given situation.
- In the course of analysis, whether they have used literature that assisted in the solution of the problem.

The students have the opportunity of consultation and I evaluate every student's work orally and in writing. At the end of the programme, a test serves to evaluate general ethical knowledge. Many students are thus enabled to give lectures in Scientific Student Circles, write relevant theses, carry out research and see their results employed in practical applications.

I select situations or short video presentations for young students who have little experience in health care.

I have found that nurses who have never studied nursing ethics and are at the bottom of the hierarchy are unable to handle ethical problems. The system quite simply suppresses them. In hospitals where the nurses have gained higher education and studied nursing ethics, the attitude is much more effective in tackling unethical situations.

CONCLUSION

In the cases detailed we have to recognize not only the responsibility of the nurses but the system in which they were brought up. Nurses often have to do like the others to remain equal; therefore their stories are very sad.

The comfort is that today nothing can prevent the spread of knowledge of nursing ethics. It is now expected that nurses will speak up in the interests of patients if they see that others do it, and will be able to judge when something is unethical and harmful for the people whose care is entrusted to them:

> *Unless nursing, through the reform of the institution in which the majority of its members practise, acquires a balance of controlling power in that institution or creates new structures for the organization of practice, it cannot effectively implement standards of care for its own practice. If it cannot realize reform it will compromise the integrity of the nurse–patient relationship, which is the moral foundation of nursing, and it will have lost its status as a profession.* (Yarling & McElmurry 1986)

Central and eastern Europe is learning the democratic, free and independent way of thinking, and the place of moral values in public life and in the professions. Nursing as a profession is sharing this journey.

References

Act 1997 CLIV on health care. Magyar Közlöny 119:9503–9558.

Bakonyi P 1983 Téboly, terápia, stigma (Madness, therapy, stigma). Szépirodalmi Könyvkiadó, Budapest, p 374–375.

Hungarian Nursing Association (HNA) 2000 Magyar Ápolási Egyesület (MAE). Etikai kódex (Code of ethics). HNA, Budapest.

Imre J 1925 Orvosi etika. (Medical ethics). Studium Kiadó, Budapest, p 12.

International Council of Nurses (ICN) 2000 Code of ethics for nurses. ICN, Geneva.

Köbli A 2002 Can an intensive ward matron inherit from a patient? Népszabadság (newspaper) 23 November:22.

Lewis O 2002 Performance in the International Workshop on Health Care and Human Rights. 26–27 April 2002. In: CPT report on visit to Hungary 1999. Ref. CPT/Inf (2001). Hungarian Civil Liberties Union, Budapest, p 22.

Marosi J 1979 The place of nurses in public health (Chapter 1) and The organization of the Hungarian Public Health (Chapter 2). In: Schwarczmann P (ed) Ápolástan (Nursing). Medicina, Budapest.

Ministry of Health 2002 Official publication of the Department of Nursing and Professional Education, Republic of Hungary (compiled by Katalin Vittay Fedinecz). Ministry of Health, Budapest, p 31.

Ombudsman 1996 Report of the Parliamentary Commissioner for Human Rights on the human and civil rights of patients in psychiatric in-patient institutions and psychiatric care homes (Number OBH 2255/1996). Office of the Parliamentary Commissioner for Human Rights, Budapest.

Pikó B 1999 Survey about the social status of nurses in Csongrád county and the judgement of professional prestige of their career. Egészségügyi Gazdasági Szemle 34:79–100.

Rozsos E 2003 Hungary's 'black angel' and her 'dragons'. Nursing Ethics 10:428–432.

Yarling RR, McElmurry BJ 1986 The moral foundation of nursing. Advances in Nursing Science January:63–73.

Chapter **28**

Spain.
Professionalism and issues within nursing and between nursing and other health professions

Maria Gasull

INTRODUCTION

This chapter tackles the concept of professionalism. By using a specific situation, the questions and problems that can arise with regard to a difference of opinion within a health care team – particularly between a nurse and a doctor – are analysed. Beginning with the moral responsibility of each, an analysis of the case will be carried out, bearing in mind the principles of bioethics, the virtues and ethic of caring. The importance of human relationships, teamwork and the need for dialogue and consensus in conflict situations are here stressed.

For centuries the healthcare world was governed by the classic concept of medical power. Doctors, judges and priests exerted authority and, in turn, society demanded that their behaviour and decisions be excellent. In the last few decades, health institutions have democratized and, due to the complexity of the health problems and scientific advances, the incorporation of new professions has been necessary. These professions, like the rest of society, have been obliged to redefine the concepts of profession and professionalism.

Nurses have stopped being mere executors of medical orders and, thanks to better academic training, can now assume a degree of responsibility that was unthinkable a few decades ago. Nurses have stopped simply performing a job and have transformed themselves into professionals and they are assuming the responsibilities that come with this change. Now nursing can be considered a profession that, besides reuniting the characteristics that define the concept of the profession, requires autonomy in its performance. This autonomy must be limited to avoid the defence of nurses' rights harming the rights of the patients. Nurses would like to determine the correct way to carry out their profession without forgetting the rights of the people being cared for to make decisions. Maintaining an equilibrium between public demand and professional expert criteria is not easy and requires that professionals bear both in mind. On the one hand, the demands must be valued, whereas on the other hand so also must the professionals' specific knowledge. Thanks to their knowledge and expertise in making decisions, nurses have demonstrated their competence and won themselves the respect of people. No-one any longer doubts that nursing is an autonomous profession. However, most countries have not yet legislated for this change to an autonomous profession.

Being an autonomous profession does not imply that nurses can care without taking into consideration all the professionals who contribute to the welfare process. This teamwork is not always easy, given that the different professionals who take part in the process might not share the same opinions and values. Determining who practises authority and how the various professionals' different areas of competencies are established can often be arduous, as we can see from the description of the following case story.

Case study	Ana was a 30-year-old mother. She was a highly cultured married woman and had just given birth to her first child. She had been suffering from epileptic seizures for 7 years, for which she was obliged to have treatment with two low doses of Tegretol (carbamazepine), even during her pregnancy. The dose was not considered to produce an accumulative effect. During gestation Ana underwent all the medical check-ups and did not show signs of any adverse health problems. As well as finding information on the internet, she consulted paediatricians about the possibility of breastfeeding while being treated with Tegretol. At the time, nobody considered it to be counterindicated.
	She gave birth at the weekend to a boy weighing 3100 g, in the 39th week of pregnancy. There were no problems and he had an Apgar score of 9-10-10. After the birth, the gynaecologist and the paediatrician on the weekend shift thought they should inhibit breastfeeding and that the child should be bottle fed because the mother was taking Tegretol. The mother did not accept the medical order and expressed her disagreement by refusing to take the medication. Her husband shared his wife's beliefs and supported her decisions. The nurse responsible for her care was also a midwife and shared the woman's opinion. She disagreed with the doctor and argued that there are scientific publications to support her opinion. The nurse was presented with an ethical dilemma: she believed that medication could not be given forcibly to an autonomous person able to make decisions, and she also questioned the decision to bottlefeed the newborn, who was a minor

and therefore not free to make decisions. She knew that if bottlefeeding began it could result in the child being unable to continue breastfeeding. Besides, the mother insisted that no feeding bottle should be given to him. The other nurses in the unit, who were not midwives, thought the nurse should obey medical orders. The nurse herself was afraid that if she did not follow the medical instructions she would be sanctioned.

The different aspects and problems in this situation will be analysed separately, bearing in mind the various protagonists and the different approaches to ethics, such as the principle-based approach of bioethics, the ethic of care, deontological norms and the prevailing legislation upon which the protagonists base their decisions.

AUTONOMY OF THE MOTHER AND SON

The mother is a 30-year-old married woman who has a good life and no financial or social worries. She is well educated and has a degree in biology. She displays full mental faculties and is considered to be totally capable of making decisions. She wants the best for her son and feels responsible for everything that happens to him. She does not think she has to obey the medical orders because, according to her information, her breast milk is not a danger to her son. Because the baby is under age he is not autonomous and the paternal authority belongs to the parents, but according to existing legislation they cannot put the life of the child in danger. An ethical conflict therefore exists between the wishes of the mother, who wants to offer her child what she considers to be the best food – breast milk – and the doctor's view, which considers that breastfeeding can cause the child serious harm.

THE CONCEPT OF RESPONSIBILITY

In this situation one can appreciate the differences of opinion between the doctor and the nurse. These differences cut into the moral responsibility of both professionals. Before determining the competencies of both, it is useful to analyse the concept of responsibility and, above all, professional responsibility. Being responsible is intrinsic to human nature; as people we are constantly justifying what we do. We justify to ourselves (ethical responsibility) just as much as to others who ask us to justify our actions (legal responsibility). As professionals the same thing also happens: we can only have legal responsibility when we also accept ethical responsibility; something that Diego Gracia (1998) calls 'quality', 'excellence' and the *ethic of maximums*, which considers the respect for and happiness of each person. This is balanced by the *ethic of minimums*, which is demanded of everyone and expressed in the form of public law. Being professionally responsible means making moral decisions that not only respect current legislation, or the *ethic of minimums*, but also promote the happiness and well-being of the people who are being cared for or looked after.

The case story thus presents a problem of responsibility. The nurse-midwife and the doctor both feel responsible on a moral level: each not only wants to comply with the law (*ethic of minimums*), they also want the care to be excellent and to promote the maximum well-being (*ethic of maximums*).

THE DOCTOR'S REASONING

The doctor, who is influenced by a long medical paternalistic tradition, does not consider the mother's autonomy or that her rights may have priority; he is worried only about not harming the child. The doctor acts according to his conscience and with a paternalistic attitude. By prescribing artificial milk he is looking after the well-being of the child because he thinks that artificial milk is the best thing for him, in case breastfeeding damages his health. On making this decision he does not take into consideration the conflict of conscience within the mother who, as a consequence of study and prior consultations, has a different opinion. In this situation a problem of power arises; the doctor thinks that he is responsible for the health of the mother and the child and imposes his criteria without taking other opinions into consideration. By acting in this way he does not acknowledge the autonomy of the mother, who is fully able to make ethical decisions. In this situation the relationship between the mother and the doctor becomes conflictive because both are acting as autonomous, free and responsible beings. Each intervenes according to his or her opinion and moral beliefs that are protected by the right to freedom of thought. The doctor resolves the existing conflict by imposing his beliefs but without consulting other professional doctors, because it is the weekend.

One could conclude that the doctor bases his decisions on the theory of bioethical principles, but he only upholds the principles of non-maleficence and beneficence, without respecting that of autonomy. He thinks of the nurse-midwife as full of good will and intentions and as someone who can be relied on to obey authority and practise the virtues of submission, trust and solicitude. According to his criteria the nurse-midwife is not capable of making decisions on her own. The doctor denies her the capacity to be autonomous as he considers himself the only one with the capacity to think; it is up to the nurse to obey!

THE REASONING OF THE NURSE-MIDWIFE

The stance of the nurse-midwife is totally different. She knows the Spanish Nurses Association's code of ethics well and she knows that this defends her duty to protect the patient and respect her freedom when she is in her care. The nurse knows that she must recognize the patient's capacity to deal with her own needs and health problems in a very personal way. For this reason she will help the sick to maintain, develop or acquire personal autonomy, self-respect and self-determination. However, codes do not cover all the ethical problems that could arise in the daily work of the nurse. The problems related to the moral professional commitment can be resolved by following certain principles or observing given values. Lidia Feitó (2000) says 'a code of ethics states only the minimum obligations and situates itself within the field of duty, thus establishing the demands the professional group considers fundamental to its practice'. The code of ethics therefore corresponds to the *ethic of minimums,* pointing only to the necessary minimums. Not all actions that professionals must carry out in accordance with the *ethic of maximums* are regulated by codes. The *ethics of maximums* is more in agreement with the sense of responsibility for upholding the happiness and well-being of the people being cared for. One must not forget that the codes were born of the professions themselves – including nurses – as a means to control themselves, as the members of the profession consider themselves to be the experts who best know their jobs. The codes determine the professional norms and duties related to the people for whom the professionals care and they do not consider all the problems derived from teamwork or major ethical dilemmas.

At the same time, the nurse-midwife does not ignore professional competencies or the current legislation in Spain, which indicates that nurses and midwives alike must obey medical orders. As midwives possess more obstetric knowledge than nurses in terms of the normal gestation process, birth and puerperium, they are authorized to make decisions in a normal, non-pathological process. In this case, given that the woman suffers epileptic seizures and is taking Tegretol, the midwife is not considered to have the competencies to go against the decision of the doctor.

The nurse-midwife, from her moral standing, is presented with dilemmas that affect her conscience, freedom and responsibility. One can say that all the actions carried out by nurses have a meaning that endows them with importance. According to Feitó (2000) 'this meaning is determined by one's own conscience which positions the action in a framework of options alongside the one chosen in freedom and for which responsibility is taken for the future consequences'. In professional work, to take these points into consideration is to assume that one is dealing with a moral practice and therefore this demands a vital compromise. This is the root of the term 'responsibility'.

The nurse-midwife agrees with the woman's opinion and considers the solution given by the doctor to be inappropriate because it does not offer any other option or resolve the problem. The woman therefore carries on thinking that her decision is the right one. The doctor is sure of his decision and records it on the medicine chart, where he indicates the inhibition of breastfeeding but does not consider the related existing problems. In her ethical analysis, the nurse-midwife considers the principles of bioethics and perhaps from this perspective she agrees with the doctor. At the same time, she keeps in mind what it is that determines the code of ethics and the current legislation, but remains consciously unsatisfied with the decision that has been taken. This is because the analysis carried out up until now has not been considered from the perspective of caring ethics.

According to Chris Gastmans (2002), this *caring ethic* runs counter to the principle-based approach of clinical ethics because it is concerned with a way of life that stresses the ethical side of health care. The concept of a person, according to a caring ethic, is characterized by the great importance given to the *relationships* between human beings and the integration of human actions and human beings. From the perspective of the caring ethics, the relationships between human beings are considered in terms of bond and responsibility.

Gilligan's works have influenced caring ethics and have served as a starting point for the discussion on the ethical dimension of the *relationships of human beings*, where emotions and reasoning are intertwined (Milmoe McCarrick & Darragh 1996). When persons act, they do this in a complete way, as a whole, using reason and affective skills and therefore human conduct cannot be divided into rational and irrational parts. Emotions and intuition must be integrated and emotional sensitivity cultivated in order to observe shrewdly the moral aspects of a situation when faced with the demands of another person. This emotional sensitivity, together with intellectual discernment, will show a caring attitude, altruism and compassion (Gastmans 2002).

The nurse-midwife feels responsible and does not accept the duty of submission and obedience that has been assigned throughout history to the feminine role and to nurses, the majority of whom are women. Perhaps in the answers given by the doctor and the nurse the two different voices described by Gilligan (1993) are appreciated. On the part of the doctor, the voice of formal logic prefers the values of masculine language and those values that shape autonomous individuals capable of making decisions about what is right and wrong from a state of impartiality. On the part of the nurse-midwife, the voice of the psychological logic of relationships upholds the values of feminine language, that is, those values that protect human relationships and look after the weak as well as caring for specific people in specific contexts of action. These two voices were traditionally identified with the masculine and feminine roles respectively. The reason they have not been fully accepted is because in a caring relationship the elements of justice and autonomy (traditionally masculine) and those of compassion and responsibility (traditionally feminine) are indispensable in order to reach moral maturity (Cortina 1996). Following the elements of justice, autonomy, compassion and responsibility, the nurse-midwife always accepts the doctor's authority when coherent and well-founded reasoning is sustained in the classic sense of the authority assigned to men. The nurse-midwife believes that, according to caring ethics, she must bear in mind all the points in question and respond to them morally in her relationship with the patient. She feels that the mother could have conflicts of conscience in the future if she obeys the medical orders because the mother's milk is, in her opinion, essential and she does not want to deny her son this most precious gift. The nurse-midwife, with her caring attitude, feels obliged to protect the mother. Despite being an autonomous and independent woman, the mother is vulnerable and weak because she has just given birth and therefore she must be helped. This feeling of solidarity and respect towards the mother on behalf of the nurse-midwife is the basis of her moral behaviour because she is required to respond to the situation in a free way, justifying her acts.

TEAMWORK

The social, economic and technical changes that have taken place in the last few decades have cut into the heart of the healthcare world. The complexity of technology and the extent of scientific advances have meant that it is no longer possible for a professional individual to possess the knowledge and skills necessary to cure and pay attention to a person with a health problem. Professionals from different areas of knowledge are required to work in a team with the same objective: to promote the healing or well-being of the person for whom they are caring. Working in a team presents many difficulties because it means contact with other human beings and arranging and reaching agreements on the different opinions and values that come into play. In the case study, the doctor and the nurses have a different point of view to that of the nurse-midwife regarding whether or not the mother should breastfeed her son. Faced with this divergence of beliefs, the nurses do not discuss it among themselves or with the doctor and they do not come to any agreement. The doctor does not recognize the moral integrity of the nurse-midwife and imposes his beliefs with his reason that he knows more about the effects of Tegretol. He does not value the fact that the nurse-midwife also has some knowledge, experience and – thanks to her close relationships with the mother – more knowledge of her values and beliefs. It was an ethical duty to find a solution together with the mother.

RESOLUTION OF THE CASE

Faced with this dilemma, the nurse-midwife found herself in a crisis of whether to follow her conscience, defend the woman and respect her beliefs, or obey the medical orders. She did not receive any help from her fellow nurses, who thought she should obey. Faced with the mother's request for guidance on what she should do, the nurse-midwife advised her not to be given Bromocriptina (to inhibit lactation), but manually to extract the milk and authorize the baby to be fed with a feeding bottle until Monday, when her case might be reconsidered.

The conflict was resolved 36 hours later when the doctor responsible for the neonatology unit revoked the weekend duty doctor's orders because he believed that the latest studies on the effects of carbamazepine on the health of the child did not justify the counterindication of breastfeeding. He authorized the child to be fed with the mother's milk. The nurse-midwife did not receive a warning.

This situation obliged the doctors and nurses to analyse the meaning of professionalism and the grey areas where responsibility can fall upon different professionals. Some guidelines were drawn up to serve as orientation in relation to similar situations and the importance of working as a team was stressed.

CONCLUSION

It is easy for ethical dilemmas to arise in our hospitals and healthcare centres. Cultural diversity and changes in values in western society, together with changes in different professionals' roles, are the fruits of professional evolution. It falls particularly to the nursing profession to ensure that the principlism defended by bioethics cannot be considered the only possible argument on which to base ethical decisions when faced with situations that predict a conflict or an ethical dilemma. It is essential that when decisions are made they be made with consideration of all the principles that support caring ethics and human relations. Situations such as the one described can be of great help to analyse and think twice about the relationships between professionals and patients.

Nurses influenced by feminism and the writings of Gilligan, Noddings and other authors have made a profound study of care and, in particular, the caring relationship (Milmoe McCarrik & Darragh 1996). Nurses no longer accept the role of passivity and submission that they assumed for centuries in their relationship with doctors, and they consider themselves autonomous to make decisions relating to their field of knowledge and competencies. This new caring relationship bears in mind the rational aspects, affective skills and particularly the emotional sensitivity that facilitate the capacity to listen to, maintain a conversation with and promote the well-being of the person being cared for. The sense of responsibility should stimulate healthcare professionals into acting not only according to the *ethic of minimums* but also in line with the *ethic of maximums*, favouring in this way the well-being of the population.

References

Cortina A 1996 El ethos: el carácter moral de las personas y las profesiones (The ethos: the moral character of people and professions). In: Arroyo MP, Cortina A et al (eds) Ética y legislación en enfermería. (Ethics and Law in nursing). McGraw Interamericana, Madrid, p 29–30.

Feitó L 2000 Ética profesional de la enfermería (Professional ethics of Nursing). PPC, Madrid, p 186.

Gastmans C 2002 Towards integrated clinical ethics approach: caring, clinical and organisational. In: Lie R K, Schotsmans P (eds) Healthy thoughts. European perspectives on health care ethics. Peeters, Leuven, p 84.

Gracia D 1998 Profesión médica, investigación y justicia sanitaria. Ética y vida. Estudios de bioética 4. El Buho, Santa Fé de Bogota, p 39, 43.

Milmoe McCarrick P, Darragh M 1996 Feminist perspectives on bioethics. Kennedy Institute of Ethics Journal 6(1):85–103.

Further reading

Beauchamp T, Childress J 1994 Principles of biomedical ethics, 4th edn. Oxford University Press, New York.

Codi d' Ètica (Code of ethics)1986 Collegi Oficial Infermeria de Barcelona, Barcelona.

Código Deontológico de la Enfermería Española (Deontological code of Spanish nurses) 1989 Consejo General de Colegios de Diplomados en Enfermería, Madrid.

Cortina A 1997 Ética aplicada y democracia radical (Applied ethics and radical democracy), 2nd edn. Tecnos, Madrid.

Edwards S 2001 Philosophy of nursing: an introduction. Palgrave, Hampshire.

Gilligan C 1993 In a difference voice, 2nd edn. Harvard University Press, Cambridge, MA.

Noddings N 1984 Caring: a feminine approach to ethics and moral education. University of California Press, Berkeley.

Tadd W 2004 Ethical and professional issues in nursing: perspectives from Europe. Palgrave, Basingstoke

Tschudin V 1992 Ethics in nursing: the caring relationship, 2nd edn. Butterworth-Heineman, Edinburgh

Vielva J 2002 Ética profesional de la enfermería (Professional ethics in Nursing). Descleé de Brouwer, Bilbao.

PART 4

The future of nursing ethics

Chapter 29

An international perspective

Miriam Hirschfeld

INTRODUCTION

In this chapter I shall focus on two major issues that take ethical theory and teaching into a wider global perspective. The first relates to globalization and the implications for a professional ethic that transcends the traditional view of patriotism and love of one's closest reference groups as community and country. The second issue focuses on dependency and the growing need and responsibility for long-term care (LTC).

Both of these issues are linked to human and social capital that include the well-being of individuals, viability of families, strength of communities, employment, education, health and welfare and the crucial importance of care and interdependency. With the new reality of globalization and the old reality of patriotism, the question arises, as to whom we consider in need and deserving of our care and concern. In LTC, dependency and interdependency stand at the heart of any ethical consideration of what is just and fair. I believe that these two issues have become inescapable and vital concerns to all of us due to global demographics and epidemiological and social developments. I will first address the issue of globalization that has become such an important concern in recent years.

GLOBALIZATION: THE CONTEXT

Globalization resulted from a worldwide integration of economic and financial sectors. This development was made possible by technological progress (e.g. computers), geopolitical changes (disintegration of the Soviet Union) and the dominant ideology of regulation by the market. It has resulted in a phenomenon illustrated by an anecdote a well-known journalist relates. A Bangkok taxi driver told him 'When you sneeze in New York, I catch a cold' (Friedman 2000).

While valid arguments praise this development and other valid arguments consider it the root of much evil, no doubt exists that globalization is here and a phenomenon people worldwide must learn to live with. The facts are that, on the one hand, globalization unifies the world and fosters economic development, but that on the other hand, large parts of the world's population remain excluded and their living conditions have become even more miserable.

However we choose to think about globalization, there is no doubt that we live in one interconnected world. In addition to capital, bacteria and viruses, terrorism and fear do not respect national borders. These are not phenomena that can be ignored or discounted by finding them distasteful.

A growing literature and increased discussions by people the world over ask whether globalization is overall a positive or a negative development. These discussions range from academic exercises to articles in the press, to violent street protests that address questions of how globalization impacts on poverty, living standards, cultural uniqueness, the roles of women, as well as national and ethnic identities, to name just a few of these issues.

I cannot discuss globalization in any depth here but I do recommend readers to look at the vast literature examining this development. The answers to these questions are manifold and often inconclusive, dependent on the specific context.

GLOBALIZATION AND ITS IMPACT ON NURSES' WORK

The reality of globalization has considerable impact on nurses' daily work. International travel and trade bring us within weeks of the viruses and bacteria from far away, with SARS being a recent vivid example. International terror exports fear and injuries with new infringements on civil liberties. All these realities affect our health, our need for health services and the way nurses work.

People develop expectations of health services from various sources, including television programmes such as 'Emergency room'. Financial experts on health care from international agencies and private consulting firms provide answers, both knowledge-based and fads, that profoundly impact on the financing of healthcare services and their availability to poor people. The widespread introduction of user charges over the last two decades is just one well-known but misled example of an expert solution spread globally. The cost of this is paid for, in part, by poor women and children with diminished access to health care or old people with chronic diseases now unable to afford prescription drugs.

Globalization, with expert solutions that may or may not fit the situation or, if they do, have a high cost for some if not all people in developing countries, has become the context in which we live and provide nursing care. Another facet of this phenomenon is the often uncritical transfer of knowledge. This seems especially problematic as the knowledge flow is almost exclusively one way from the Anglophone countries to the rest of the world. There is no doubt that we must learn from one another and that theories and research can have relevance for others than those who initially developed the knowledge. However, nursing theories and conceptual frameworks, as well as research results are often translated from English into other languages and transferred from one cultural context to another without the crucial critical discourse needed to ask how these theories and results fit in a different cultural context and how they might need to be adapted or changed. Self-care theory is but one example. In Dorothea Orem's (1971) nursing theory of self-care developed in the USA, the concept 'self' relates to the individual. However, in Japan and in Arab culture 'self' relates to the family, and in Jewish tradition 'self' relates to the community. There is no doubt that Orem's and other nursing theories cannot be applied in other cultures without carefully considering how they need to be adapted (P. Underwood personal communication). This responsibility rests with those who are borrowing nursing theory or other knowledge from another culture.

One specific area all nurses need to deal with in the context of globalization is migration. This includes migration of our patients and their families, of our colleagues and – often – our selves. Most migration takes place within countries and internal migration of skilled workers from rural to urban areas is an issue of concern in many developing countries where the migration of health professionals has reached crisis proportions. Worldwide, the loss of health personnel from needy to wealthier countries is a serious problem, as poor countries are losing their best health professionals. The General Agreement on Trade and Services (GATS) regulates, among other things, the movement of personnel, the movement of consumers and the provision of private healthcare facilities in developing countries. Corporations can open hospitals for profit that will provide services to those who can afford them. These private services will often also attract the best prepared professionals, as pay and working conditions will be superior to others in the country (Adams & Kinnon 1997).

Illustrations of health personnel migration can be seen in many countries. The outflow from Jamaica means that 50% of registered nurses' posts and 30% of midwifery posts remained unfilled in 1995; in Ghana, some two-thirds of the Ghana Medical School graduates had left the country by the late 1990s (Adams & Kinnon 1997). The Gulf States attract nurses and doctors from Egypt, India and the Philippines, while Austria and Germany recruit nurses from eastern Europe, as well as from many other countries with a significant salary differential. The migration of highly skilled workers represents a large component of total migration and although medical practitioners and nurses make up only a small proportion of professional migrants, the loss of human resources in the health sector of developing countries usually results in the loss of capacity for the health system to deliver health care equitably (Stilwell et al 2003).

One of the major ethical concerns in nursing today is the recruitment from poor to rich countries. In several countries there are aggressive and targeted international recruitment initiatives (Kingma 2001). In the UK, for example, the government has stated that international recruitment is part of the solution in meeting its staffing needs (Buchan 2002). The total work permits approved for foreign nurses in Great Britain in 2001 was over 23 000, of which 10 050 were for nurse graduates from the Philippines and 2612 from India, two countries that produce nurses for export. South Africa (2514 permits), Zimbabwe (1801), Nigeria (1110), Ghana (493) and Trinidad and Tobago (357), however, do not overproduce nurses (Stilwell et al 2003). While 'push factors' such as very low salaries and poor working conditions are important causes for international migration, the ethics of aggressive international recruitment needs to be re-examined and policies developed.

Remittances are the portion of international migrant workers' earnings sent back from the country of employment to the country of origin. For the last decade, these earnings returned home have exceeded the total of global development aid. This source of income benefits the individual families of migrants and their countries' economies. However, poor countries shoulder the cost of publicly financed health professional education and suffer the loss of taxation, loss of work contribution of the migrant person, and loss of health care to the population as a result. Rich countries that recruit human resources from poor countries thus owe a considerable unacknowledged debt to these developing countries. Although remittances provide some compensation for poor countries that 'export' health professionals, these countries will usually experience a net loss of human capital in the health system, with serious implications for quality, coverage and access to services. The World Health Organization (WHO) is now studying fair ways to compensate poor donor countries (Stilwell et al 2003).

In summary, globalization is not something we have the luxury to ignore. Globalization impacts on living standards and on the ability of people to afford health care, as well as on the provision of health care in different countries and on the availability of health personnel. Globalization also impacts on people's expectations of healthcare services and the different health professions' perceived duties in providing health care.

THE WAY WE VIEW OUR WORLD: COSMOPOLITAN EDUCATION

When considering nursing ethics and nursing education within the broad context of globalization, I believe there is a need to rethink the way we view the world and the way we view our work. Globalization creates tremendous diversity and change in 'the known' and 'the familiar' in addition to the above ethical issues. Many of our basic assumptions of what patients, doctors or nurses should know, say, or feel are no longer compatible with new realities. Reactions of people are different and are often hard to understand. While contact with strangers may enrich us, it often creates insecurity and fear. One essential way to address this fear is awareness and cosmopolitan education. For us to realize that we live in one world is the first step. The call for a cosmopolitan education goes beyond the respect for every individual's human rights. It asks us to consider all human beings as our true reference group. This implies that we need to listen to and learn from each other, to learn about them and learn about ourselves. The philosophical arguments about the limits of patriotism seem most relevant to the way we see the world. Martha Nussbaum (1996) suggests that we should be taught first to be citizens of a world of human beings, and only then to be citizens of a specific country. With respect to the most basic moral values, such as justice, we should regard all human beings as our fellow citizens and neighbours.

In educational terms, this implies that students in country x, for example, may continue to regard themselves as defined partly by their families, religious, ethnic and racial communities, or their country. They must also, and most importantly, learn to recognize and understand human beings in all their different, often strange (to others) and unfamiliar guises. They must learn enough about the different cultures and nationalities also to recognize the similarity of all humanity in the wishes for health, happiness and well-being. Making one's fundamental allegiance to the world community of human beings, of justice and reason, does not mean that we need to give up our special affections and identifications, whether social, ethnic, gender-based or religious. Our identity is constituted partly by these factors, but we should also work to make all human beings part of our community of dialogue and concern (Nussbaum 1996). This does mean that as nurses we need to be connected and accountable to our own communities, including the minorities and 'special groups' such as homeless people or illegal immigrants. In addition, our concern must include the well-being of people in far away lands.

Nussbaum (1996) calls this the 'concern of cosmopolitan education'. It seems to me that there are small beginnings to this educational approach whenever equity and cultural sensitivity are learning objectives in nursing education. A broader discussion on cosmopolitan education is beyond the scope of this chapter, but it is no doubt an area that will require more serious thought in the future.

GLOBALIZATION AND CONCERN FOR THE WORLD COMMUNITY

Consider how commitment to the world community of human beings links to globalization and its five sources of capital:

- Financial capital
- Man-made capital
- Basic resources capital
- Human capital
- Social capital

It seems to me that the one major problem of globalization is that of these five sources of capital, only financial capital (e.g. the dollar, yen or euro), man-made capital (e.g. factories, products such as cars or pharmaceuticals) and basic resources capital (e.g. oil, uranium, water) constitute today's globalization focus. Human and social capital (the well-being of individuals, viability of families, and strength of communities, employment and education) have been not only ignored but sacrificed to the globalization of these first three capital sources (Stiglitz 2003). The welfare of people who have migrated seems to be beyond public and policy concern. In the majority of countries, large parts of populations have become excluded from decent living standards. Unemployment is widespread and resources for education, health and welfare are dwindling. Poverty is growing and gaps in income within and among countries are widening.

The Human Development Report (UNDP 2003) documents the interconnectedness of countries and the present lack of concern for human and social capital, i.e. the well-being of all people. The agricultural export markets of poor countries have been severely curtailed and many families go hungry because of the exploitation of producers by large, often multi-national companies and the subsidy policy of rich countries. The annual dairy subsidy of the European Union (EU) is US $913 per cow, while the annual aid to sub-Saharan Africa from the EU is US $8 per African person. The annual dairy subsidy in Japan is US $2700 per cow, with annual aid to sub-Saharan Africa from Japan of US $1.47 per African person. The US domestic subsidy is US $10.7 million per day for cotton as compared to US $3.1 million per day in US aid to sub-Saharan Africa. In addition, agricultural subsidies in rich countries benefit about 5% of farmers: the large producers. The Human Development Report 2003 concludes that this 'leaves a few rich-country farmers as the sole true beneficiaries of subsidies, with a multitude of losers across the globe' (UNDP 2003). The trend of out-sourcing jobs from developed to developing countries is a case of job migration that has increased unemployment in some developed countries. This trend in the USA, where there is no national health system, adds numbers to the already large list of those uninsured for health care. This too has serious implications for healthcare services and nurses. The ebb and flow of globalization is dynamic.

While I do not argue that any one economic or political measure leads to growing poverty, widening gaps and social unrest, there is no doubt that injustice and exclusion experienced and perceived by so many human beings around the world feed crime, unrest, widespread insecurity and terror. All of us have experienced these effects on our daily lives. Perhaps this need not be so. A world in which everyone has decent living conditions that include food, housing, education and health care, is a world safer for everyone. As nurses, we belong to the one profession that claims to have 'care' at the core of our endeavours. If this is true, we need to educate towards care and concern for all human beings, regardless of their ethnicity, religion, gender, age or social and economic status, not merely on an individual clinical level but on a political level as well. This demands the active participation of each and every nurse in the political process influencing a society's actions regarding the country's equity, coverage and quality of health and social services and the country's actions towards poorer countries and their citizens. Openness to such involvement and acquiring the skills for effective participation in the policy development and implementation process is, in my opinion, the measure for successful cosmopolitan education in nursing.

CARE: THE ESSENCE OF NURSING

Although globalization is the context in which we live and cosmopolitan education is one means to deal with this reality, care remains the essence of our professional work as nurses. According to Eva Kittay and Ellen Feder (2003) care is a multi-faceted term. It is labour, an attitude and a virtue (see also Chapter 10). As labour, it is the work of maintaining ourselves and others when a person is in a condition of dependency and need. It is most noticed by its absence. As an attitude, caring denotes a positive, affective bond with and investment in another's well-being. The labour can be done without the appropriate attitude, but labour, unaccompanied by the open responsiveness to another, cannot be good care.

It seems to me that care and a concern for others are prerequisites to justice. Without care for those who are poor, dependent, different or weak, a society cannot be just. Whereas justice is the broader concept, care is an essential component of justice in the family, the community, a country and among nation states. Care is what gives hope to globalization with a human face. It is the essential component to human and social capital. In national and international deliberations and policy forums, care and justice need as much concern, consideration and respect as the pure economic commodities of financial and other capital. If globalization is to benefit all, or at least not to exclude large sectors of the population, there is a need for attention and concern for human and social capital as of equal importance to the purely economic commodities. This is not merely a question of attitude and *Weltanschauung* (world view), but an issue of knowledge and action. National and multi-national policies need to set clear goals and develop strategies on how to reduce gaps and provide every human being with the capabilities to tend to their basic needs (Stiglitz 2003). One area where inequities are most glaring and widespread is in the area of disability, chronic disease and LTC.

LONG-TERM CARE: A PRIORITY IN NURSING EDUCATION

My choice of LTC as a priority for nursing education does not deny the need for more efforts to be invested in health promotion and the prevention of disease. These should undoubtedly constitute social, economic and public health priorities everywhere. In addition, there is a need to improve the availability, accessibility and affordability of acute health care in most countries. However, given the demographic, epidemiological, social and economic developments worldwide, and the unique responsibility of nursing for care, I consider LTC the first priority for nursing education.

Given the issues of globalization outlined, care and justice are the concerns and responsibilities of everyone. However, as nurses, we have special expertise and responsibility for care, where there is functional dependency. We share this responsibility for care with families, communities, and other health and social professions with complementary expertise. The ethical concerns in LTC are what justice requires and demands of us to teach and learn. These are the crucial issues I want to address, but first to the scope of LTC.

THE SCOPE OF LONG-TERM CARE

Long-term care refers to the provision of services for persons of all ages who have long-term functional dependency. Dependency creates the need for a range of services that are designed to compensate for their limited capacity to carry out activities of daily living. Dependency also results in difficulties in accessing health care and in complying with healthcare regimes. It impacts on the ability of individuals to maintain a healthy lifestyle and to prevent deterioration in health and functional status. Dependency creates additional emotional needs and strains that must be addressed because relationships among patients, family and other 'informal' caregivers and professional care workers are often complex and fraught with ambivalence. Social needs also arise from limitations in maintaining regular social contacts. For example, people who are bedridden and/or confused, as well as their caregivers, often face great difficulties in maintaining social and supportive relationships.

Further health problems arise from either single or multiple chronic diseases that may be the source of the disability. These health problems in themselves require complex health services and special regimes of chronic care management. Moreover, when combined with functional limitations, the challenge becomes even greater. To give just two examples: mobility limitations may require considerable measures to enable a person to move freely inside and outside the home and may need services brought to the home. Cognitive impairments can prevent individuals from maintaining compliance with complex medical regimes or accurately judging dangers to themselves and others (Brodsky et al 2003).

Dependency creates a complex range of needs for services, which in turn creates a need to coordinate access to and management of these multiple services. This care management function creates still another need in itself. Central to the care of those dependent is the role of the family in providing that care, and the resultant needs of the family. The need to address dependency impinges not only on various aspects of family function but also on relationships within the family. It creates a necessity to manage relationships between the disabled person and the family, as well as those between and among family members according to their respective roles in providing care. The need to address such dependency also has emotional consequences for family members and for their relationships with one another (Brodsky et al 2003).

Stated broadly, a LTC system comprises a comprehensive range of services, some based in the home and others based in the community, in healthcare institutions and elsewhere. In an optimal and rational model, all of the services and structures that form a system will be designed to allow individuals to lead lives of dignity and, where possible, independence, without placing intolerable burdens on their families. Timely planning offers the best opportunity for policy makers to define the fundamental values on which their LTC systems should be built and then to move forward with the actual design (Brodsky et al 2003).

THE GROWING NEED FOR LONG-TERM CARE: FORECASTS

The growing need for LTC policies is generally associated with industrialized countries. Less widely acknowledged is the fact that LTC needs are increasing in the developing world at a rate that far exceeds that experienced by industrialized countries. For example, WHO estimates that China and India will experience a 70–120% increase in the prevalence of dependency by the year 2050, and that the dependency ratio will nearly double in China, because far fewer young people will be available to care for disabled and frail elderly persons due to the one child policy (WHO 2002a).

In Latin America, the Caribbean, the Middle East, sub-Saharan Africa and the Pacific Islands, WHO estimates that the number of dependent people will double or triple. In Somalia, Uganda, Liberia, the Palestinian territories and Yemen the increases will be 400% and more. Moreover, the developing world is experiencing increases in LTC needs at levels of income that are far lower than those that existed in the industrialized world when these needs emerged (WHO 2002a).

These large increases in level of dependency will occur in countries that are just beginning their demographic and epidemiological transitions. This denotes countries or societies passing from a state of high fertility and high mortality to one of low fertility and low mortality. This transition is characterized by increasing life expectancy and population ageing, and it involves progressing from a time when infectious diseases predominate, with high maternal and child mortality, to a state where premature mortality is low and chronic diseases predominate. Such diseases include ischaemic heart disease, cancer, stroke, arthritis, chronic obstructive lung disease, dementia and depression. The prevalence of these diseases typically increases with age and those who suffer from them often have multiple, co-morbid pathologies.

LONG-TERM CARE POLICY ISSUES

On the international, national, regional, district and community levels, nurses must understand the key policy issues of LTC and be involved in searching for sound solutions, such as linking preventive, acute, chronic and long-term care. Some of the questions related to this issue are:

- Should LTC be considered an integral part of a country's healthcare system and, if so, how does LTC link to a country's social system?
- How does one make sure that a person who needs LTC will also receive appropriate care for acute illness when they are cared for either in their home or in an institution?
- How do we make sure that patients receiving and families providing home care get the necessary health education and disease preventive measures, such as guidance on how to lift or turn a paralysed person, or obtain flu vaccinations?

Another important policy issue is the level of professionalization of the health workforce. While we might be in favour of an all-university edu-cated nursing staff on a hospital ward or in a health centre, few of us find it realistic to argue for a highly educated nurse providing the bulk of home care, which includes bathing patients, feeding them and perform-ing household chores or doing necessary shopping. Sensitivity and expertise are needed to do these tasks well but the cost of such a service, if provided by highly educated professionals, would be prohibitive. The question therefore arises: who are these front-line workers and what responsibility do nurses have to support, educate and supervise them? Should these front-line workers have career paths, and if so, what are they?

Yet another broad LTC policy issue must question how the burden of care is shared among the individual, the family, the community and the state. Should taxes be used to support family caregivers and in what way can or should a community be involved in caring for their weakest and disabled members and how should this be done?

The provision of quality LTC involves complex professional skills in the areas of:

- Understanding policies
- Planning, providing and monitoring appropriate community, family and individual services
- Hands-on skills, including interpersonal and cultural sensitivity

On both a clinical and a public health level, significant knowledge is necessary to guide, educate and inform disabled persons, their family, other health professionals and the community at large. All this implies the need for an ethical imperative for competence, which dictates a broad range of requirements for nursing curricula and life-long learning for nurses.

ETHICS AND LONG-TERM CARE

The looming crisis in LTC makes it essential that governments every-where place a higher priority on finding strategies for providing care. If societies abdicate their responsibilities, the burden of care will remain entirely and unfairly on the shoulders of a few people, and for some no care will be available at all. While the issue of fairness in allocating the burden of care will become more acute when the ratio of caregivers to those in need worsens, we must also assess the justice of present practices.

Whether judged by the ethical standards within traditional societies, or by universal norms of equality and human rights, present systems of allocating the burdens and benefits of caring for chronically ill and disabled people are unfair. While traditional moralities are a basis for the obligations that most people accept to provide care for dependent family members and others in need, the contribution of deeply embedded cultural, ethical and religious values that perpetuate this unfairness also need to be re-examined. Women, and in particular poor women, often pay a huge price in the form of their own health and well-being for being assigned, and assuming, the major burden of care for their own and others' families.

Society needs an infrastructure – schools, roads, clean water and the other common requirements for healthy and dignified living – and the benefits from these public goods are shared by all who need them. We all come into the world in a completely dependent condition. Later in life, some individuals will need additional care whereas others will not. Yet everyone gains when care that is consistent with respect for the individual is available to all. A society that treats its most vulnerable members with compassion is a more just and caring society for all.

In considering the future role of nurses and future LTC, a society must first begin a dialogue on how to address the human needs of all of its members with dignity and respect. Our teaching must initiate this dialogue and educate nurses to be not only competent and skilful practitioners, but knowledgeable partners in these ethical discussions.

After answering the questions of what LTC needs exist and what resources are available to provide them, the discussion should focus on these ethical questions:

- What does justice require?
- Who should provide for these LTC needs?
- How should the responsibility and burden of care be shared among individuals, families, communities and the state?
- How should responsibilities be shared between men and women?
- How should responsibilities be shared among generations?
- How should responsibilities be shared between the public and private sectors?
- How should responsibilities be shared among rich and poor countries?

The answers to these questions will then point the way to systems that are fair, responsible, accessible, efficient and accountable.

Fully addressing these questions can move the respect for human dignity to the centre of the LTC policy paradigm. This implies a need to recognize that all people – including those with disabilities – have the right to function as fully as their condition permits. Respect for human dignity at the centre of the social paradigm means protecting weak and vulnerable persons from domination, exploitation, and neglect (WHO 2002b).

To date, most discussions of ethics in LTC focus on clinical decision making in individual cases, professional responsibilities and obligations, or dispute resolution. While questions of justice, broadly defined as the equitable distribution of costs and benefits, have been discussed regarding overall priorities in resource allocation, these questions are relatively new to LTC, and especially the role of incorporating ethics into education conveys a respect not only for the importance of weighing options and choosing among them, but also for the process of doing so.

One way to begin this process is to gain in-depth knowledge and a better understanding of what the LTC situation is in our own community and country. LTC needs to be put into the social situation of countries and areas and there considered in terms of demand and supply.

What are the long-term care demand factors?

The amount and kind of LTC needed in the future will depend on the technologies that enable people with disabilities to remain independent, and on the environments that foster independence, such as wheelchair access. Other variables are the future prevalence of injuries, such as preventing road injuries, occupational injuries and violent behaviours that lead to injuries. Variables that can potentially prevent severe chronic illness are also important in considering future demand, such as changes in lifestyle to reduce smoking, and increase good nutrition, safe sex, physical activity, etc.

What are the potential supply factors for long-term care?

The resources needed to provide care include the availability of families and informal caregivers. In countries where HIV/AIDS has decimated young populations, or in countries where there is a one child family policy, as in China, this future supply of caregivers will be very limited. Other supply factors are family income. With growing poverty, the ability of families to provide care is restricted. The growth in female participation in the labour market (in many developing countries there is a steep increase in women now working outside the home) limits the potential supply of caregiving labour. Additional supply factors are dependent on future health and LTC funding policies. Will countries support and pay for LTC?

The World Health Organization, in collaboration with the Institute for Alternative Futures, Washington, DC, has developed a long-term care futures tool kit, that enables a guided discussion on the future of a country's LTC based on national disability estimates and forecasts for nearly all countries (WHO 2002c).

A FINAL WORD

Finally, to link the main issues of globalization with the resulting need for cosmopolitan education and LTC as a major focus for nursing ethics and education worldwide, let me state my basic credo. Society functions best as a harmonious whole when care that is consistent with respect for the individual is available to all, enabling those who have resources to enjoy their full benefits, while providing security to people who are less fortunate. Cost is one consideration, as we need to be able to indicate how services could be financed and who should cover the cost. Such discussions always include trade-offs that are value based. However, other ethical considerations of solidarity, genuine concern and respect for all are of no less importance. As nurses, we have a major responsibility actively to participate in creating conditions where everyone has the capability and social acceptance to be a full citizen with equal rights.

References

Adams O, Kinnon C 1997 Measuring trade liberalization against public health objectives: the case of health services. Health Economics, Technical briefing note, WHO/TFHE/TBN/97.2 World Health Organization, Geneva.

Brodsky J, Habib J, Hirschfeld M (eds) 2003 Key policy issues in long-term care. World Health Organization, Geneva. Online. Available: http://www.who.int/ncd/long_term_care/index.htm and http://www.who.int/chronic_conditions/en/

Buchan J 2002 International recruitment of nurses: United Kingdom case study. Royal College of Nursing, London.

Friedman TL 2000 The lexus and the olive tree. Anchor Books, New York.

Kingma M 2001 Nurse migration: global treasure hunt or disaster in the making? Nurse Inquiry 8(4):205–212.

Kittay FE, Feder EK (eds) 2003 The subject of care – feminist perspectives on dependency. Rowman & Littlefield, New York.

Nussbaum MC with respondents 1996 For love of country – debating the limits of patriotism. Beacon Press, Boston.

Orem D 1971 Nursing: concepts of practice. McGraw-Hill, New York.

Stiglitz JE 2003 Globalization and its discontent. Norton, New York.

Stilwell B, Diallo K, Zurn P et al 2003 Developing evidence-based ethical policies on the migration of health workers: conceptual and practical challenges. Human Resources for Health. Online. Available:http://www.human-resources-health.com/

UNDP 2003 Human Development Report. Oxford University Press, Oxford, p 156.

World Health Organization (WHO) 2002a Current and future long-term care needs. WHO/NMH/CCL/02.2. WHO, Geneva. Online. Available: http://www.who.int/ncd/long_term_care/index.htm

World Health Organization (WHO) 2002b Ethical choices in long-term care: What does justice require? WHO, Geneva. Online. Available: http://www.who.int/ncd/long_term_care/index.htm

World Health Organization (WHO) and the Institute for Alternative Futures 2002c A long-term care futures tool-kit. WHO, Geneva. Online. Available: http://www.who.int/chronic_conditions/en/ and http://www.altfutures.com/ltctoolkit

Further reading

Brodsky J, Habib J, Hirschfeld M (eds) 2003 Long-term care in developing countries. Ten case studies. Geneva: WHO. Available: http://www.who.int/ncd/long_term_care/index. htm

Family caregiving: current challenges for a time-honored practice. Generations. 2003–2004; 27(4), Winter (whole issue)

Stiglitz JE 2003 The roaring nineties: a new history of the world's most prosperous decade. WW Norton, New York

Human Development Report 2005. International cooperation at a crossroads: aid, trade and security in an unequal world. New York, UNDP (available for free download on http://www.undp.org)

Chapter 30

The future: teaching nursing ethics

Anne J. Davis, Verena Tschudin and Louise de Raeve

CHAPTER CONTENTS

INTRODUCTION

This book pursued two aims. The first of these was to provide four different conceptual ways of thinking about ethics, and to critique these in such a way that would be useful in teaching health care ethics to nurses, whether students or clinicians. The second aim was to present numerous ethical issues and case studies from selected countries, to show some possible similarities and differences in ethical problems cross-culturally. These chapters, written by colleagues in industrialized and non-industrialized countries, range over ethical problems that you might experience in your own country or they may assist you to understand more fully the ethical quandaries facing nurses in other places around the globe. By including various ethical issues from diverse places, we have also raised the thorny question as to whether the world, and therefore nursing, has universals in ethics or whether our values and ethics are more narrowly defined by being embedded in specific cultures.

The English author, Rudyard Kipling, once said that east is east and west is west and never the twain shall meet (Kipling 1889/1982). In one way he was wrong, because east and west have met for many years and in our era of global communication and rapid travel they meet constantly in myriad ways. However, Kipling might have been right in another way. If he was referring to the foundations of societies, their values and ethics, then he might have a point. As indicated in some of the chapters, the foundations of eastern ethics are predominately Confucianism, Buddhism or Islam, whereas those societal foundations in the west are Judeo-Christian and ideals from the western philosophical tradition and the eighteenth century Enlightenment (Arrington 1998).

Although the conceptual frames for teaching nursing ethics presented, critiqued and commented on in this book do not necessarily cover the entire range of ethics in the western philosophical tradition, they do give readers the major structures or theories used or being further developed for application. Nursing ethics, like bioethics and medical ethics, is applied ethics. To apply ethics in nursing, we believe that individuals need a knowledge base. This book demonstrates many types of knowledge in ethics and points out some of the strengths and weaknesses of the theories presented. This chapter is both a summary of some ideas previously mentioned and an extension of some of them.

Some of this ethics knowledge has been derived from the western philosophical tradition and has been taught for many years and long before nursing became a profession. Other ethics content presented here did not evolve in the same manner but rather represents a fairly recent reaction to the more traditional ways of framing and conceptualizing ethics and subsequently, nursing ethics.

In teaching ethics, several points need to be highlighted. First, ethics does have knowledge bases, therefore our ideas of good and bad or right and wrong are not just vague notions with no history or general agreement but are ideas that can be articulated, taught and learned as a body of knowledge. Some people say: 'ethics is so difficult and vague and it does not make any difference anyway'. Clearly, we do not agree with this statement and believe it to be uninformed and either cynical or naive. The same point can be made about other fields of knowledge from an uninformed point of view. If you do not know anatomy and physiology, it is difficult to understand the body and how it functions. There are some differences in these two examples, however. Anatomy and physiology, in most cases and to a large extent, are the same for humans everywhere; and although there are many folk beliefs about the body, those who hold these beliefs would agree at least on what has been proven by science or observed by long experience to date. This knowledge base changes as we know more but there is a core of agreed-upon knowledge that we use in making decisions. The recent genetic mapping is an example of developing knowledge that has the potential to change much in our understanding of the biological and medical sciences. It also brings with it some profoundly difficult ethical questions.

Although we have ethics knowledge, it is often perceived as not as clear cut as many people think the biological sciences are. In our opinion this attitude is biased, perhaps because ethics is moral philosophy and philosophy has a reputation in the public mind of being difficult, academic and fuzzy. Yet, ethics is present in every aspect of daily life. One cannot read the newspapers without seeing ethics either clearly or between the lines. A third reason for misguided belief is that science has dominated how we have thought about knowledge for the last several centuries. For many people, logical positivism is the essence of science and the only valid knowledge. This philosophy says that science is objective and systematic, and experimentation is needed to test hypotheses. Such disciplines as literature, history and philosophy provide us with a more humane view of the world, ourselves and others, but remain suspect as 'real' knowledge (Gaddis 2002). Research can be undertaken on ethical issues but such research is no longer ethics per se. This does not mean that all our ethics knowledge is cast in concrete, never to change. The body of knowledge we call ethics must accommodate and find ways to understand the rightness or wrongness of acts in our brave new and ever changing world.

We have presented four conceptual ways of thinking about ethics that could indicate the possibility for disagreement as to how we should frame what we think of as ethics, ethical issues and ethical solutions. Nevertheless, we take the position that some agreement about ethics does exist. First, people who have spent time thinking about this agree that ethics does have a base in knowledge. Ethics is a body of knowledge that provides us with guidelines for decisions and also a creed as a guide in life. We would encourage teachers of nursing ethics to use more than one theory to frame, guide discussion, reason through a problem and reach an ethical conclusion.

Some colleagues who teach and write about bioethics and nursing ethics also believe that most people develop their codes of ethical behaviour without knowing much about this body of knowledge. The values that form the foundation for our ethics are learned in daily life and more indirectly through word and deed at home, in school, and from people in our families and from others, who leave their mark on us. For example, many cultures have some version of the golden rule that says: do unto others as you would have them do unto you. How that translates into behaviours might differ across cultures but the basic values and ethics remain. Values and ethics are somewhat like the wind in that we see their effects and results but we do not see them directly because they are abstractions and not concrete objects like a table or chair. If we have such knowledge, we may not know the original source of these ideas. Parents and teachers do not resort to Kant or Mill or Confucius, the well-known philosophers from the past who greatly influenced ethics, because they usually lack this knowledge. Parents, teachers and others use what they have been taught to socialize the next generation.

- What values and ethics were you taught as a child?
- Did some or all of those ideas and values change as you grew to adulthood?
- What do you think are the major sources of your ethics as a person, as a nurse, and as a teacher?

It is our contention that people in society with special roles entailing responsibilities towards others need to have a firm grasp of their own values and ethics, and also those espoused by their profession. A code of ethics stands as one mark of a profession and serves as an openly stated social contract between the profession and the public.

AIMS OF TEACHING NURSING ETHICS

We teach ethics in several ways: in formal courses, during clinical supervision and in our own interactions with students, colleagues and patients. A formal course in nursing ethics resembles any other course in that it relies on a knowledge base for its content. This content may be used directly or indirectly, depending on what the teacher wants to achieve. In many cases, the aim of teaching ethics to nurses is to provide them with the knowledge and language to enable them to think through an ethical problem and reach some ethically right action. Some people believe that nurses have ethical concerns that differ from those of other health professionals and therefore should not rely entirely on principle-based ethics as their only knowledge source. We take the position that nurses need several ways of conceptualizing ethics, including principle-based ethics, because of the broad array of ethical issues that emerge in their professional role. However, to deal with ethical issues that arise predominately in nursing, principle-based ethics might not be sufficient to participate in discussions of ethical problems that concern all health-care professionals. In teaching content as complex as ethics, teachers need to think through their own values and ethical positions as much as possible. Disagreements in various branches of science and the humanities occur, and such disagreements also arise in ethics, bioethics and nursing ethics. In some instances, these disagreements occur because people base their positions on different premises. For example, in the abortion debate some people believe that personhood begins at conception and therefore abortion is ethically wrong. Others believe that, until viability or when the fetus can survive on its own, the fetus is not a person and therefore abortion is ethically permissible until the end of the second trimester of pregnancy. Another example can reveal differences in beliefs within and across health professional groups. Some health professionals define artificial feeding and hydration to terminally ill patients as treatment and believe they can ethically justify the withdrawal of the tubes from patients to allow death to occur naturally. Others define such nourishment as food, and the withdrawing of it as killing the patient, which cannot be ethically justified.

In 2004, one of us attended a conference on teaching nursing ethics convened at Yonsei University, Korea. A speaker used a case study of a father, his son and daughter having gone mountain climbing. The three roped together on one rope experienced great difficulties and were about to fall. The father was on the bottom of the rope, the son in the middle and the daughter on the top as they went up the mountain. The father asked the son to cut the rope. This meant that the father would fall and be killed but possibly the son and daughter would be saved.

After some anguished moments, the son cut the rope and the father fell to his death. The other two survived. We were asked what we would do in this situation. A Chinese colleague said, 'He is my father. I have a duty not to kill him. I would never cut the rope.' A western colleague said, 'If you did not cut the rope, all three would die and that is an unnecessary waste of human life. The father has made an autonomous decision, so I would cut the rope. This is not a new idea. We call it triage.' The speaker said that the Chinese colleague made her decision based on Confucian values of family and the ethics of duty while the westerner made another decision based on the greatest good. Neither decision was wrong, only different and reflective of the two cultures. This is a good example of what is called 'life-boat ethics' in which some will die to save others.

- What do teachers do with their own values and ethical positions on abortion, terminally ill people and other ethical issues that students need to reflect on?
- Can teachers put their values aside?
- Should they try to put them aside when they teach?
- How does the teacher interact with a student who holds an ethical position that differs from that of the teacher?

TEACHING NURSING ETHICS: WHO, WHAT, WHEN, HOW?

Nursing ethics, like all ethics courses that deal with problems and not only theory, is best taught when the teacher builds in time for dialogue. For this reason, a seminar format in which students engage with each other and the teacher to address the issues can be most useful. This is especially good for undergraduates who are in their last year of the programme, and for graduate students.

One question that arises is when to teach ethics to undergraduate students. Some of the chapters in this book address this question. If the course is taught too early, students have little or no clinical experience and do not necessarily understand the issues involved. Yet if nursing ethics is taught late in their educational programme, then they have not benefited from this content while students. There are several possible solutions to this. Some schools have two formal courses: the first is given early and introduces students to ethics content; the other course is taught later and draws on students' clinical experiences. Other schools teach one course only, often in the early months of the students' senior year.

Many schools do not offer nursing ethics in any formal course because there is no one with expertise to teach it. Other schools integrate ethics throughout the curriculum. Some people who teach ethics are dubious about this method because it assumes that every faculty person has the knowledge base to do this integration. While it is perhaps an ideal solution, this method remains problematic. In the long run, each school will need to work out a solution that fits, given the resources available.

We would like to propose that teachers of nursing ethics not only know ethics content such as presented in this book, but also have some experience with clinical ethics. Experience in applied clinical ethics can be gained in numerous ways, for example, in focused discussions with clinical staff, or through membership on clinical ethics and research ethics committees where they exist. In some healthcare facilities, nurses have organized nursing ethics committees as an arena where nurses can discuss with one another the issues facing them (Gastmans 2002). Not every ethical issue in nursing occurs at the bedside; however, most of what students question is clinical in nature (Lemonidou et al 2004). Clinical ethical issues often have a broader base, which might include questions of justice in the allocation of resources for example. These would certainly include nurses as well as other healthcare resources.

We think it is vital that students have an understanding of clinical ethical problems and learn ways to articulate them to others. Nursing ethics deals with clinical, policy, research and resource allocation issues; students need to think beyond their bedside or community clinical nursing experiences and gain a larger view of the issues.

Another question arises as to whether ethics will be required by faculty or elected by students.

In a recent study conducted in Canada, the authors reported on the role-socialization stresses inherent in new nursing graduates in their transition to professional practice. They found a prevalence among these new graduates of moral distress caused by the inability to live up to their moral convictions (Boychuk Duchscher & Cowin 2004). We seriously doubt that such a situation is limited to Canada. It is just this sort of finding that reinforces the need for ethics in the curriculum and for arenas to discuss ethical issues arising in the clinical setting. It is important for nurse educators to understand fully that ethics should not socialize students into unrealistic ethical positions, but provide them with ways of conceptualizing situations and arriving at some solution that is both ethical and possible. We believe that – ideally – a basic ethics course should be required for every undergraduate student and a more advanced graduate course should be available to help prepare these students for leadership roles.

We also believe that clinical nursing staff need a more systematic understanding of nursing ethics to help them with ethical problems in their work. In addition, the moral development literature indicates that people are often more influenced by their social environment in their ethical decision making than they are by their own values and ethics (Gibbs 2003, Turiel 1998). This finding reinforces the importance of the socio-ethical environment in the workplace.

The moral development literature, usually thought of as a branch of psychology, asks several questions including:

- How do children become moral or ethical?
- What happens when an authority figure tells people to act in such a way that their actions seem to harm another person?
- Do men and women differ in their moral or ethical perspective?
- Does social class status make a difference with regard to how people view ethical questions?

After the faculty decides the who, what, when and how of teaching nursing ethics, the individual or group actually teaching the course needs to refine aspects of these decisions and also think about how to evaluate students enrolled in their ethics course.

EVALUATION OF STUDENTS IN ETHICS COURSES

If the aims of a course are to teach students the language and reasoning processes involved in ethics then this is more akin to the content of other courses and perhaps the students are more easily evaluated. If the aims of the course go beyond this and include students taking ethical positions on various issues, then the evaluation process can become more difficult. Therefore it seems to us that whereas evaluation tends to come at the end of a course, teachers might want to give this some thought when developing a course. For example, the teacher might require graduate students to give an oral presentation in an ethics seminar, with 60% of their grade based on this presentation. One student might take the position that all severely mentally challenged patients in a state-supported institution should be allowed to die by withdrawing their food and fluid. The premise that this student takes is: patients with severe mental challenges do not have humanhood and therefore are not protected by notions of human rights. Such a definition of the people who are severely mentally challenged uses some criteria to establish what constitutes a human being, such as awareness of self and others (Fletcher 1979). This position has several possible consequences that include the ethical justification for helping the patient to die or killing the patient, depending on how one views this. These patients are not terminally ill and cannot indicate their preferences, therefore an interesting procedural question asks:

● Who does make such a decision?

The ethical question is:

● Should such a decision be made?

One argument that might be used to support the student's position is the use of public resources that could be better spent on other groups in society. An argument against this position has to do with the slippery slope problem. If society decides that this group of people is not human and therefore is not to receive public resources, then other vulnerable groups such as elderly senile people, those who are chronically mentally ill or severely physically handicapped might be defined as not having humanhood and therefore be without certain rights.

The larger question is:

● What sort of society do we want to live in?

This question is both fundamental and difficult to answer because all societies, no matter how wealthy they are, have limited resources to meet all the needs of citizens.

Suppose that you as the teacher find this student's position troubling because it makes you think of the mass exterminations in Germany during the 1940s and, more recently, the genocides in parts of Africa.

- What if this student's position seems grossly unethical to you?
- What do you do, if anything, about this and how do you evaluate this student?

The first and perhaps the most important step, in working out such pedagogical problems, is to be aware of them before they happen – preferably as you develop the course – and to decide in advance the means you will use to evaluate students. It seems only fair to the students and perhaps to yourself that the evaluation methods are discussed openly in the seminar.

CASE STUDIES IN TEACHING NURSING ETHICS

Throughout this book, authors have presented case studies because they can anchor ethical problems in the world of patients and nurses. In addition, they provide a specific situation to think about and reason through to some ethically right action. This moves nursing ethics from the general abstract to the more specific concrete. Some situations that are ethical in nature do not have an ethically right answer, therefore people tend to decide on the lesser of the two evils. The son cutting the rope in the mountain climbing incident mentioned earlier is an example of this. From the westerner's perspective it is the lesser of the evils to allow one person to die to save two others. From the Chinese perspective allowing all three to die is less evil than killing the father.

Case studies have traditionally been a major teaching tool in ethics, including nursing ethics. This method has both strengths and weaknesses as a teaching tool. The cases are hypothetical and are therefore safe in that real people are not involved. The strength is that students do not have to cope directly with others in the situation but can think through each case to some ethically justifiable solution. At the same time, this is also a weakness because ethical and unethical actions, as well as ethical quandaries, usually occur in a world with other people. All these people have different roles and statuses, and it is therefore rare that any discussion of ethical problems happens on a level playing field where all involved are equal. Certainly, patients can be extremely vulnerable, given their role and status, and nurses who work in highly stratified organizations, such as is the case in some hospitals, can have similar vulnerabilities. Nevertheless, students can learn from such an exercise and, once they have some experience in thinking through a case study to some ethical solution with the teacher and other students, then they can perhaps deal more readily with similar situations in the clinical arena where relationships are more complex.

Case studies can focus on most clinical situations that are ethically problematic, as well as on policy, resource allocation and research issues. Numerous applied ethics books, including those written for nurses, present case studies (Davis et al 1997, Fry & Johnstone 2002, Fry & Veach 2000, Tschudin 1994, 2003). Journals in the field also provide cases for analysis. In addition, some teachers use case studies found in films. One first task that arises in using these case studies is to collect data by listening and asking questions about the situation such as:

- What do we know?
- What data do we have?
- What should we know and obtain information about?
- What else do we need to know?
- What can we never know?
- How ethically can we think about this case study?
- Can we use ethics theories?

Previous chapters in this book give some examples of case studies and some of the ways to reason through them.

After reading a case study and reasoning it through, students sometimes reach the conclusion that they should take the problem up with the physician and they go no further in their thinking. For example, A is terminally ill and is receiving treatment that the physician believes will help him. One day A says to you, his nurse, 'I am so weary and I know I will die of this disease anyway so I would like to stop treatment and just be kept comfortable.' You reason that the patient is an autonomous person and he is making a choice. Because he is terminally ill, his wish to stop treatment is not doing harm and if he can be kept comfortable, this is doing good. You decide to discuss this with the physician but she says that the patient is responding to the treatment and she thinks it would be harmful to withdraw it now.

- You have taken this problem to the physician but nothing has changed.
- Have you met your obligation to this patient?
- Once you report this information to another person, such as the physician or head nurse, have you met your obligations to the patient?
- Does something have to change for you to meet your obligations?

One important point here is that when you go to another person with an ethical position about a given situation, then you need to be able to articulate this position. The act of bringing a patient's comment for discussion means that you view it in some specific ethical way. This act alone is an ethical act. This type of clinical situation demonstrates the need for ethics courses that teach you the language of ethics and how to reason, using this language, to some conclusion. We suspect that you think that the physician should at least listen to the patient and should possibly withdraw treatment, but it will help the patient if you can articulate your position and the ethical reasons supporting it. Using case studies in teaching ethics is like using the clinical practice laboratory in that it prepares students for when they face a similar situation later.

ETHICS SEMINARS

Undergraduate education does not always lend itself to the seminar teaching format because of the large numbers of students in class. Such a reality is a good argument for teaching ethics in small groupings of students, such as clinical supervision, provided the teacher has the knowledge base to do so. A course that employs small groups discussing case studies can help students to learn the language of ethics and some ways of reasoning through situations. In lectures there is less opportunity for dialogue among students and between students and teacher; however, ethics seminars might be better learning experiences than only lectures. We believe that dialogue is essential to the teaching of nursing ethics (Dierckx de Casterlé et al 2002).

Nursing ethics, as an academic subject, is best undertaken using a seminar format because it requires active participation and learning on the part of students. This is a demanding type of teaching because teachers are not in full control of the flow of ideas and must be able to 'think on their feet'. Teachers must have a good grasp of the concepts in ethics and be able to apply them spontaneously. While demanding, it is also a stimulating teaching method and often gets students deeply involved in the subject. Those who teach in this way must be able to cope with dialogue and disagreement. Students may disagree with teachers, which might show the success of the course. We would suggest that seminar style teaching in ethics is ideal for more experienced nurses and could easily be combined with case studies since the participating nurses bring a wealth of clinical and ethical experience to the class. It can also be used with less experienced nurses and students provided teachers have a knowledge base to guide the dialogue.

THE IMPORTANCE OF REFLECTION

In nursing ethics, as in all other ethics endeavours, there is no cookbook to tell us which ingredients to use and in what amounts to measure them. This is not to say that we have nothing to help us in ethical decision making. Along with values and conceptual ways of thinking about ethically problematic situations, we can also use reflection as an important tool in ethical understanding.

Marian Verkerk and her colleagues (2004) discuss reflection as a way to enhance awareness of the many moral aspects of the daily practice in which professionals function. They developed the reflection enhancement tool, which has three steps:

- Initial reflection: an ethics case situation is presented and individuals write down their reactions. No group interaction occurs.
- Guided reflection: discussion is initiated. The focus is on the agent's core values, social norms, agent's actions, consequences and the social environment. This discussion helps the professionals involved to understand more clearly the values and beliefs that form part of their professional identity. They also see how their beliefs and values may differ from those of other people.
- Mapping responsibilities: after the first two steps, individuals are now ready to reflect on their own positions within the broader moral picture.

Many people reflect on moral/ethical issues when faced with them. This teaching tool structures such an experience and helps teachers to guide students to reflect in a more organized way. The importance of reflection cannot be underestimated in solving ethical problems.

TEACHING NURSING ETHICS IN THE FUTURE

Few people, if any, can predict the future accurately. We tend to extend the past and present into what seems to us a logical future but we do this without knowledge of possible future events. Historians call this the fallacy of uninterrupted trends (Fisher 1970). Scientists might have enough data to give tentative or even more precise predictions about such things as our future natural environment or the impact of ageing populations globally, but sometimes even the scientists disagree. The data on food and healthy eating seem to change from moment to moment so that people become sceptical and do not take comments seriously. Such disagreement is in the nature of knowledge development.

Realizing the dangers of predicting the future, we nevertheless now put forward some comments focused on teaching nursing ethics in the future for you to think about. The surest thing we can say is: as nursing ethics goes, so goes the teaching of nursing ethics. As the healthcare world, including nursing, changes, so will nursing ethics change. New developments in nursing knowledge and in science will have an impact on nursing ethical problems and what content is taught. Already in some nursing ethics courses, genetic counselling is examined and discussed. Nursing ethics content will most likely include a wide range of concerns that include nurse–patient ratios, nurse–patient relationships, nurse–institution accommodations, nursing in the community and such concepts as:

- The role of power
- Emotions
- Relationships
- Moral authority
- Justice issues in resource allocation

Surely the clinical world of nursing will become even more complex and filled with ideas, procedures and technology from the miracles of modern medicine and science. In some parts of the world, the issues will include the infrastructure for clean water and a better waste disposal system.

Many of us have difficulty remembering that it was only three generations ago that surgeons performed amputations without anaesthesia, and that only 60 years ago many of the numerous clinical questions raised routinely today could not have been asked because no knowledge or medical technology existed to make answers possible (Porter 1997). The rapidity of change in the health sciences, particularly in the developed countries, creates an urgency regarding solutions to both age-old problems and newly-created ones.

Ethics courses could be planned around the idea of vulnerable populations such as:

- Women
- Children
- Mentally ill people
- Disabled people
- Refugees
- Elderly people
- Poor people

Some of these issues have a long history and do not seem to go away. Issues of social justice among others frame the content for such a course. A past president of the International Council of Nurses, Nelly Garzón (see Chapter 21), said in her inaugural address that without social justice there is no freedom and no human rights. This remark moves nursing ethics well beyond the bedside in any one country to consider the larger picture. Such a view can help raise questions about the use of the world's resources: who takes what from whom and who gives to whom. This is nursing in the largest, broadest sense.

The focus of any nursing ethics course depends on what teachers want to achieve and this aim may vary both within a specific country and between countries. Whatever the aim of teaching nursing ethics, we believe that teachers need knowledge of ethics and how to apply that knowledge.

As a final word, readers must remember that the four main theories presented in this book were developed in the west. Other parts of the world have values, virtues, ethical principles and notions of caring but they may differ in some fundamental ways from the content of these theories. Exploration of these possible differences is underway and more such investigation is needed (Baker 1998, DeBary 1998, Fan 1999, 2002, Kirkland 1995, Lee 1992, Macklin 1999, Nie 2000, Pang 2003, Pang et al 2004).

Until we know more about possible similarities and differences in nursing ethics globally, we hope this book will assist those who now teach and those who will teach nursing ethics in the future, as well as the students who will enrol in nursing ethics courses or discuss ethical issues during clinical supervision. One thing we know as almost a certainty for the future is that ethical problems will remain in nursing practice, administration, research and education, and that nurses therefore need a knowledge base to understand these problems and the skill to articulate this understanding to others.

References

Arrington RL 1998 Western ethics: an historical introduction. Blackwell, Oxford.

Baker R 1998 A theory of international bioethics: multiculturalism, postmodernism, and the bankruptcy of fundamentalism. Kennedy Institute of Ethics Journal 8:201–231.

DeBary WT 1998 Confucianism and human rights. Columbia University Press, New York.

Boychuk Duchscher JE, Cowin LS 2004 The experience of marginalization in new nursing graduates. Nursing Outlook 52:289–296.

Davis AJ, Aroskar MA, Liaschenko J, Drought TS 1997 Ethical dilemmas and nursing practice. Appleton & Lang, Stanford, CT.

Dierckx de Casterlé B, Meulenbergs T, van de Vijer L et al 2002 Ethics meetings in support of good nursing care: some practice-based thoughts. Nursing Ethics 9:612–622.

Fan R 1999 Confucian bioethics. Kluwer Academic Publishers, Dordrecht.

Fan R 2002 Reconstructionist Confucianism and bioethics: a note on moral difference. In: Engelhardt HT (ed) Bioethics and moral content: national traditions of health care. Morality. Kluwer Academic Publishers, Dordrecht, p 281–287.

Fisher DH 1970 Historians' fallacies: towards a logic of historical thought. Harper and Row, New York.

Fletcher J 1979 Humanhood: essays in biomedical ethics. Prometheus Books, Amherst, NY.

Fry ST, Veach RM 2000 Case studies in nursing ethics. Jones and Barlett, Sudbury, MA.

Fry S, Johnstone M-J 2002 Ethics in nursing practice. A guide to ethical decision making. Blackwell Science, Oxford.

Gaddis JL 2002 The landscape of history: how historians map the past. Oxford University Press, Oxford.

Gastmans C 2002 A fundamental ethical approach to nursing: some proposals for ethics education. Nursing Ethics 9:494–507.

Gibbs JC 2003 Moral development and reality: beyond the theories of Kohlberg and Hoffman. Sage, London.

Kipling R 1889/1982 The portable Kipling. Penguin Books, New York.

Kirkland R 1995 Taoism. In: Reich WT (ed) The encyclopedia of bioethics. Simon & Schuster, New York, vol 5:2463–2469.

Lee SH 1992 Was there a concept of rights in Confucian virtue-based morality? Journal of Chinese Philosophy 19:241–261.

Lemonidou C, Papathanassoglou M, Giannakopoulou M et al 2004 Moral professional personhood: ethical reflections during initial clinical encounters in nursing education. Nursing Ethics 11:122–137.

Macklin R 1999 A defense of fundamental principles and human rights. Kennedy Institute of Ethics Journal 8:389–401.

Nie JB 2000 The plurality of Chinese and American medical moralities: towards an interpretive cross-cultural bioethics. Kennedy Institute of Ethics Journal 10:239–260.

Pang MCS 2003 Nursing ethics in modern China: conflicting values and competing role requirements. Rodopi, New York.

Pang MCS, Wong TSK, Wang CS et al 2004 Towards a Chinese definition of nursing. Journal of Advanced Nursing 46:657–670.

Porter R 1997 The greatest benefits to mankind: A medical history of humanity. Norton, New York.

Tschudin V 1994 Deciding ethically. A practical approach to nursing challenges. Baillière Tindall, Edinburgh.

Tschudin V 2003 Ethics in nursing: the caring relationship. Butterworth-Heinemann, Edinburgh.

Turiel E 1998 The culture of morality: social development, context, and conflict. Cambridge University Press, Cambridge.

Verkerk M, Lindermann H, Maeckelberghe E et al 2004 Enhancing reflection: an interpersonal exercise in ethics education. The Hastings Center Report 34:31–38.

Further reading

Birkelund R 2000 Ethics and education. Nursing Ethics 7:473–480

Cameron ME, Schaffer MA, Park Hyeoun-Ae 2001 Nursing students' experiences of ethical problems and use of ethical decision-making models. Nursing Ethics 8:432–445.

Cassells JM, Redman B 1989 Preparing students to be moral agents in clinical nursing practice. Nursing Clinics of North America 24:463–473.

Fry ST 1989 Teaching ethics in nursing curricula: traditional and contemporary models. Nursing Clinics of North America 24:485–497.

Gaul AL 1989 Ethics content in baccalaureate degree curricula. Nursing Clinics of North America 24:475–483.

Ketefian S 1999 Legal and ethical issues: ethical content in nursing education. Journal of Professional Nursing 15:138–141.

Kikuchi JF 1996 Multicultural ethics in nursing education: a potential threat to responsible practice. Journal of Professional Nursing 12:159–165.

Nylund L, Lindholm L 1999 Ethics in clinical supervision. Nursing Ethics 6:278–286.

Omery A 1989 Values, moral reasoning, and ethics. Nursing Clinics of North America 24:499–508.

Schmitz K 1995 Ethical problems encountered in the teaching of nursing: student and faculty perceptions. Nursing Education 34:42–44.

Silver MC, Sorrel J 1991 Research on ethics in nursing education: an integrative review and critique. National League of Nursing, NY.

Stone JB 1998 Teaching ethics in nursing. Nurse Educator 23:6–10.

van Hooft S 1990 Moral education for nursing decisions. Journal of Advanced Nursing 5:210–215.

Waithe ME 1989 Developing case studies for ethics education in nursing. Journal of Nursing Education 18:175–180.

Glossary

Affective:	in psychology and some other disciplines, affect (affective) refers generally to feelings, emotions, moods. Affective sense of care refers to the various interpersonal emotions associated with this term and the range of feelings that might be invested in a 'caring relationship'.
Agent-centred ethics:	the idea that the most central questions in ethics have to do with the character of the person who is acting: the agent, rather than the character of either the action the agent performs or the outcome of that action. On this view, it is more important to ask about the qualities a person should have than to ask about the nature of (1) good, right or ethical actions or (2) the types of situations that we should try to promote.
AIDS:	acquired immunodeficiency syndrome; a clinical syndrome resulting from diminished immune status as a result of human immunodeficiency virus (HIV) infection.
Anglophone:	a native English speaker.
Anti-theoretical:	against or opposed to theory.
Aphasic:	loss or impairment of power to use or comprehend words, usually resulting from brain damage.
Application:	follows exegesis and interpretation; addresses the question of how believers should live in the light of the critical exegesis and interpretation of a portion of an ancient sacred text.
Aristotelian virtue ethics:	ethics emphasizing the virtue of moderation based on the Greek philosopher, Aristotle.
A-theoretical:	not a theory. A moral position described as a-theoretical might or might not be anti-theoretical. In the case of the a-theoretical virtue perspective, it seems to be anti-theory because for conceptual reasons, it rejects any general statements that claim to capture the nature of morality.
Attitudes:	one's opinion or disposition.

Axiology: a branch of philosophy that studies judgements about values.

Beliefs: the conviction that certain things are true.

Biodiversity: the variability of any living organism from all sources and the ecosystems of which they are part. Diversity is the key to ensuring the continuance of life on earth.

Bioethics: field of study that applies ethical concepts and theories to healthcare issues. Some people view nursing ethics and medical ethics as subsets of bioethics.

Buddhism – Mahayana and Zen: two different sects of Buddhism, a widespread Asian belief and practice system founded in India in the fifth century BCE.

Burn-out: the consequence of unresolved mental tensions and stress. In some countries, nurses experience burn-out due to factors such as work load, low pay.

Caged bed: a device to control mentally ill patients that measures 2.08 m × 0.93 m (7 × 3 ft) and is 1.26 m high. The bed is covered with a strong net and padlocked. Patients cannot stand up, and must eat, sleep and defecate in the bed.

Caliphate: (formerly) a spiritual leader of Islam. The last caliphate in Turkey was held by Ottoman Turkish sultans until it was abolished by Ataturk in 1924.

Canon (n.), canonical (adj.): an established, authoritative list of works or books that are considered to be sacred scripture by a given faith group.

Collectivist: a principle or system of ownership and control of the means of production and distribution by the people collectively, usually under the supervision of the government.

Communism: a classless society and economic system based on Marxist–Leninist ideology. A type of socialism where work is allocated on the basis of abilities and goods are distributed according to necessity.

Compensatory justice: that form of justice that seeks to benefit the least well off in society.

Competence: the demonstration of a range of competencies or abilities with a view to promoting a desired end.

Confidentiality: protection of personal privacy and/or information entrusted to one.

Confucian five cardinal relationships: in Confucianism, human beings are not individuals but interwoven threads of relationships with many people. Relationships are not all equal but are in hierarchy beginning with the most important being: (1) father–son, (2) elder brother–younger brother, (3) husband–wife, (4) friend–friend, (5) ruler–subject. This serves as a major foundation in Asian ethics.

Connections: necessary, contingent and intimate: a necessary condition for something is one without which the thing does not exist or occur. The presence of oxygen is a necessary condition for human life. The contingent is normally what is neither necessary nor impossible. Definitions of contingency are: (1) of entities – the property of not having to exist; (2) of events – the property of not having to occur; (3) of propositions – the property of not having to be true, or of risking the possibility of being false. The phrase 'an intimate connection' is to be understood as lacking the logical requirements of a necessary connection but yet seeming to be stricter than a mere contingent connection. The term 'non-contingent' captures this link in that it is often used for 'logically necessary', but properly it denotes a looser relation: it is possible to say that intention is non-contingently related to action. Any given intentions need not be followed by the relevant action, and therefore the relation is not strictly a necessary one, but the concept of intention could hardly have arisen unless intentions were usually followed by the relevant actions.

Critical scholarship: critical forms of scholarship, e.g. feminism, Marxism, post-colonialism and critical social theory, oppose unequal and oppressive power relations, are committed to social justice and emancipatory politics, give voice to the experiences of the oppressed, and are self-consciously reflective.

Cult: technically, 'cult' refers to formal religious worship or the followers of a religion. It also refers to believers who form a religious group at odds with other religious groups and with society. In this sense, many major religions were initially a cult.

Defensibility: arguments that can support a moral stance and at the same time can refute competing and opposing stances.

Democracy: a political system based on equality before the law, human rights, and fundamental freedoms as well as a multi-political party system where public authority is exercised by elected representatives.

Deontological constraints: refer to negative duties specifying what we cannot justifiably do to others; they do not specify any actions that we should perform for the sake of others.

Deontology: the theory of moral obligation or duty. Holds that some features of actions – other than or in addition to consequences – make actions right or wrong.

Dialectic perspective: pertaining to or of the nature of logical argumentation, a debate or conversation by which the truth of a theory or opinion is arrived at logically.

Discretion: the freedom or authority to make decisions and choices as well as the action or power of discernment and judgement.

Displaced persons: people forced to migrate within the country, abandoning their place of residence and economic activities.

Divinity: the quality of being divine, a deity, God.

Dry sex: a practice commonly described in southern Africa where the woman's vagina is dried to make sexual intercourse 'pleasurable'. Drying agents are herbs, cotton wads, earth/soil and other absorbents.

Eisegesis:	process of reading into a portion of a sacred text a meaning that it does not have.
Empathy:	the ability to perceive accurately the feelings of another person and to communicate this understanding to that person.
Epidictic discourse:	a form of communication that takes place within the group seeking to reaffirm and reinforce the values that the community itself embraces.
Epistemology:	a major branch of philosophy concerned with the nature, source, and validation of knowledge. It answers questions such as: What is knowledge? What knowledge is valid? How do you know?
Equity:	a right founded on the laws of nature; moral justice.
Ethical being:	the demonstration of ethical qualities or character traits.
Ethical competence:	the demonstration of a range of ethical abilities, e.g. knowing, seeing, reflecting, doing and being, directed towards the promotion of ethical ends.
Ethical doing:	the ability to act ethically in relation to others.
Ethical justification:	the set of reasons for providing moral groundings of one's course of action.
Ethical knowing:	the application, understanding of and ability to apply the areas of knowledge applicable to ethics in specific contexts. In health care this includes an appreciation of the nature of professional roles and of their historical and ethical foundations; the ability to distinguish among personal, professional, and theoretical ethics; an understanding of empirical ethics; an appreciation of the complexities and subtleties of everyday ethical issues.
Ethical reflecting:	the ability to scrutinize ethical concepts, ideas, and theories to evaluate practice events or situations and to engage honestly in self-scrutiny, plus learning from and utilizing the ethical insights of colleagues and friends.
Ethical seeing or perception:	the ability to see the ethical components of situations by appreciating the holistic nature of individuals; by understanding common patterns of responses; by demonstrating a commitment to understanding the unique nature of individuals and within health care, a commitment to understanding better the experiences of health, illness, disease and distress.
Ethical justification:	the set of reasons for providing moral groundings of one's course of action.
Ethics of care:	characterized by specific moral considerations: the care and nurturing of self and others, the alleviation of hurt and suffering, the maintenance of relationships, and the emphasis on contextual details of concrete situations. The ethic of care has been contrasted to the ethic of justice characterized by moral considerations such as abstract rules and principles, fairness and reciprocity, and duties and obligations for self and society.
Ethics of maximums:	also called ethics of happiness. Ethics of maximums tries to justify a moral phenomenon in all its complexity, understanding ethics as the

design of a happier way of life. It tries to offer ideals of a good life, models that orient our behaviour, but following it cannot be insisted upon.

Ethics of minimums: civil ethics or justice ethics, which outlines the axiological minimums and norms shared consciously by a pluralistic society. It is those obligations of justice that can be demanded by any rational being and which only imply some minimum demands.

Eudaimonia: happiness or well-being. In Aristotelian philosophy understood as a full and active life governed by reason.

Exegesis: process of critical examination of a passage from an ancient sacred text to uncover how the text's first readers would have understood its meaning.

Feminist ethics: ethical theory that advantages vulnerable populations including women. It differs from feminine ethics.

Fidelity: a faithful devotion to duty or to one's obligations.

Formal justice: treat similar cases in similar ways; equal treatment to equals.

Free will: doctrine that the conduct of human beings expresses personal choice and is not simply determined by physical or divine forces.

Habits: a habitual or characteristic condition of mind or body; a practice or tendency to act in a particular way.

Habituation: to practise and repeat ethical actions and qualities that demonstrate sensitivity to specific contexts and the engagement of judgement and emotions.

Hemiplegic: total or partial paralysis of one side of the body that results from disease or injury to the motor centres of the brain.

Hermeneutics: study of methods of interpretation of ancient sacred texts. The process of critical study involving exegesis and interpretation but not application.

Heterosexual: relationship, including sexual, between members of the opposite gender. In contrast to homosexual.

Hidden curriculum: aspects of student learning that are outside the formal and explicit documented curriculum. Includes role modelling by academics and practitioners, student experiences in health care and support or lack of support for positive (e.g. patient-centred) behaviours.

Intention: a determination to act in a certain way.

Interpretation: follows exegesis; involves discerning how a passage of an ancient sacred text is to be understood today in the light of what it meant to the first readers.

Judeo–Christian dogma: pertaining to the religious writings, beliefs, values, or traditions held in common by Judaism and Christianity.

Kaposi's sarcoma: an endothelial malignant condition commonly diagnosed in AIDS patients. Associated with the human herpes simplex type 8 infection.

	Two types exist: the endemic type, which is indolent and not usually related to HIV; and the aggressive type usually HIV related.
Kurdish:	of or pertaining to the people, language and culture of Kurdistan, a mountainous region of Turkey, Iran and Iraq.
Logical positivism:	philosophy that defines science as the systematic testing of hypotheses.
Logical relationships:	in formal logic, different types of logical relationships are recognized. A one–one relationship is between two items; for example, wife–husband in those cultures that do not permit polygamy. A one–many relationship is between one item and several others; for example, mother–children. A many–many relationship is between any pair of items in a set such as siblings.
Malpractice:	a legal term describing the failure of a professional to exercise a reasonable degree of skill and care. This failure can be due to not acting or acting in a wrong way.
Maternal mortality ratio:	the number of maternal deaths per number of live births, usually expressed per 100 000 live births.
Meiji restoration:	the beginning of Japan's modern history in 1868 and the end of Shogun rule.
Metaethics:	normative ethics (see Normative ethics) concerns itself with ideas and claims about moral standards, what is right and wrong, or what virtues we should have. Metaethics concerns itself with where these standards come from, what their basis is, and what the implications are for the nature of moral thinking and reasoning.
Metaphysics:	it is difficult to say what precisely the distinction between metaphysics and ontology (see Ontology) is. However, metaphysics probably has two broad senses. In the philosophical sense, it is an area of enquiry that concerns itself with concepts such as truth, reality and causation. In a more colloquial sense, it refers, somewhat vaguely, to anything that can be regarded as 'beyond' the normal world of experience.
Modernity:	characteristic of present and recent time; contemporary.
Moral:	pertaining to or concerned with the principles of right conduct or the distinction between right and wrong. Ethics is a system of moral principles; the branch of philosophy dealing with values relating to human conduct. Moral and ethics are sometimes used as synonymously.
Moral agency:	the capacity to recognize, deliberate/reflect on, and act on moral responsibilities.
Moral agent:	one who can act according to his or her own sense of moral integrity.
Moral blindness:	lacking the ability to see the ethical considerations of particular situations, e.g. seeing clinical or research situations with ethical components in purely clinical or research terms.
Moral complacency:	an unwillingness to evaluate or critically scrutinize one's own ethical views or consider that one may be mistaken.

Moral distress:	the conflict that may be experienced when an individual has difficulty in acting in a manner that she or he believes to be ethical due to institutional or other constraints.
Moral justification:	see Ethical justification.
Moral particularism:	argues that the importance of moral considerations is context dependent. Moral particularists, such as feminist ethicists, draw on particular accounts of morality, not on universal accounts. Moral understanding and wisdom are the result of our capacity to discern what features or details of events are of moral significance, not our ability to subsume contextual details under principles or rules.
Moral position:	if one rejects the idea that any of the theories discussed below in moral theory is, in isolation, an adequate account of morality, it is still possible to say that they all provide useful insights into the nature of morality. It is a weaker stance to describe them as positions rather than theories. They remain, however, as useful theoretical accounts but with partial rather than universal significance. The exception to this would be the a-theoretical (see A-theoretical) view of the virtues.
Moral realism:	gets its meaning largely from what it is contrasted with. Any view can be called realist that emphasizes the existence, reality or role of some kind of thing or object such as material objects, propositions, universals. Commitment to moral realism involves subscribing to the idea that there are moral facts and that these pertain, irrespective of cultural differences. Those moral philosophers who consider morality to be underpinned by certain universal facts about human nature are likely to talk about 'moral facts' and would be said to be moral realists.
Moral reflection:	careful consideration or contemplation of what constitutes good or right action.
Moral relativism:	refers to the concern that no objective basis exists to evaluate the merits of particular moral understandings and social practices. At its extreme, moral relativism can take the form of nihilism in which all moral judgements are rejected as unjustifiable, ultimately resulting in the demise of any meaningful moral discourse. Ethical knowledge is not derived from reason alone but requires that it be in collaboration with empirical disciplines. Recognizes the importance of the social environment in determining the content of beliefs about both what is and what ought to be the case, and the possible diversity of such social arrangements. A value relativist maintains that there are no universal standards of good and bad, right and wrong. However, the relativist makes at least one non-relative remark: that there are no universal standards.
Moral theory:	an explanatory account of the nature of morality that says something about what actions are right, and it ought to explain and make intelligible our evaluation of actions, telling us something of what gives actions moral worth and in what way they are made right or wrong. Different moral theories include: consequentialism (e.g. outcome-based utilitarianism), deontology (duty-based), rights-based approaches and virtue

ethics (character/disposition based). These theories compete because their adherents think that their favoured theory presents the best and most comprehensive account of morality.

Morbidity: ill-health.

Muslim: follower of the religion of Islam.

Nasal drip: a tube inserted in the nose to drip fluids into the stomach.

Naturalism: approach to ethics requiring that ethical knowledge, such as ethical concepts and ideals are developed in collaboration with empirical disciplines. Ethical knowledge from this perspective is not derived from reason alone.

Neoliberalism: a political and social philosophy with the following assumptions: (1) markets are the best and most efficient allocators of resources in production and distribution; (2) societies are composed of autonomous individuals (producers and consumers) motivated chiefly or entirely by material or economic considerations; (3) competition is the major market vehicle for innovations.

Nordic: concerning the countries, people and languages of Denmark, Finland, Iceland, Norway, and Sweden.

Normative ethics: concerns itself with general claims about moral standards: what is right and wrong, what virtues a person should have, and so on. It contrasts with applied ethics that examines specific, and usually controversial, issues such as abortion, animal rights, or capital punishment.

Normative evaluation: the process in which justified moral claims are made about the rightness or wrongness of moral practices and understandings. Prescribing ethical norms and standards.

Nursing ethics: the name given to those ethical issues pertinent to nursing and nurses and the body of knowledge used to understand them. Can be viewed as a part of or separate from bioethics.

Nutrition: nourishment.

Obligations: a contract, promise or moral obligation; often a duty imposed legally or socially as a result of a contract, promise, or moral responsibility.

Ontology: it is difficult to say what precisely the distinction between ontology and metaphysics is. However, ontology, in the formal and physical sense is usually taken to be a branch of metaphysics and deals with such questions as: what, ultimately, does the world consist of? What are the most fundamental categories of existence?

Oppression: situations in which people suffer some inhibition of their ability to develop and exercise their capacities and express their needs, thoughts, and feelings. It takes different forms, including exploitation, marginalization, powerlessness, cultural imperialism, and violence.

Ottoman: the Turkish dynasty that ruled the Ottoman Empire from the thirteenth century CE to its dissolution after the First World War.

Particularism:	the view that it is not possible to specify in general terms what is good, right, or ethically correct. Any attempt to do so will by definition generalize over different situations. A particularist believes that moral reasoning makes sense only in the context of a particular set of circumstances, and that each case must therefore be judged entirely on its own merits.
Paternalism:	in bioethics, healthcare professionals act as though they are protective parents caring for children (i.e. patients) even though the patients are adults. Acts or practices that restrict the autonomy or liberty of individuals without their explicit consent.
Patriarchal:	a social system in which the father is the head of the family and men have authority over women and children.
Pneumocystis carinii **pneumonia:**	usually a severe infection affecting individuals with diminished or compromised immune status. The causal organism, *Pneumocystis carinii*, is considered by some to be a protozoon, although others consider it a fungus.
Post-structualism:	In critical theory, this means a widespread skepticism towards metanarratives or grand all-encompassing stories/theories since they dismiss the naturally existing chaos and disorder of the universe and ignore the heterogeneity or variety of human existence. Metanarratives should give way to more modest and localized narratives.
Practice:	any coherent, complex form of socially established cooperative human activity where goods internal to that activity are realized in trying to achieve those standards of excellence appropriate to that form of activity, with the result that human powers to achieve excellence, and human conceptions of the ends and goods involved are systematically extended. Bricklaying is not a practice, but architecture. Nursing is a practice in this sense of the term.
Prima facie:	coming before other considerations. Refers to principles or rules that are always binding unless a competing moral obligation overrides or outweighs it in a particular circumstance. Literally, as it seems first.
Principles:	a fundamental truth or motivating force, especially concerning right conduct.
Proof-texting:	pejorative term that refers to the practice of picking and choosing passages of sacred writings, wresting them from their context without critical analysis or interpretation in order to support a point or justify an assertion.
Redact:	to edit or adapt a written text or oral tradition for public use, often by a specific group such as a faith community.
Relativist:	someone who views ethics as non-universal but as related to individual cultural norms and values.
Rules:	an established regulation or guide for conduct.
Samurai:	a member of the hereditary warrior class in feudal Japan.
Sanctity of life:	human life is to be valued at all costs since it is a gift from God.

Sect:	a dissenting and schismatic religious subgroup that largely embraces but partially diverges from the beliefs or practices of a larger 'parent' religious group.
Secularization:	to draw away from a religious orientation; make worldly.
Shogunate:	the rule of the Shogun or General from the eighth to the twelfth centuries CE in Japan.
Sitz im Leben:	literally 'setting in life' or 'situation in life' meaning the sociological setting.
Social justice:	the virtue that guides people in creating those organized human interactions we call institutions and the responsibility of all continually to perfect institutions as tools of personal and social development.
Solidarity:	unanimity of attitudes or purposes among members of a group or class, as in the slogan: All for one and one for all.
Systematicity:	the use of an organized, orderly, focused and diligent process in framing ethical arguments.
Taoism:	a Chinese philosophy and religion advocating a life of complete simplicity and naturalness and of non-interference with the course of natural events in order to attain a happy, harmonious existence.
Telos:	Greek, meaning end. Teleological moral theories focus on an end view.
Thin and thick descriptions:	Aristotle delineated spheres of human experiences that would figure in any human life such as fear of important damages, especially death or distribution of limited resources. In these spheres, everyone will have to make choices of some kind and there will be ideas of what responding and choosing well would mean. These ideas are the virtues related to the respective spheres. In the above examples, the virtues would be courage and justice respectively. This is the thin or nominal meaning. Work is needed to understand more deeply what problems people encounter in their lives with one another to arrive at a thick definition of what it means to act well in the face of such problems.
Traits:	a distinguishing quality or characteristic, especially of personality.
Transparency testing:	a form of critical reflection at the level of communities to determine who has responsibility for what things and what provisions are available to distribute and evaluate these responsibilities. This type of analysis makes it clear to what the extent differently situated people experience their responsibilities as intelligible and coherent and how the costs and burdens of these responsibilities are distributed. In some circumstances, when some individuals are being exploited, this testing can reveal that equilibriums among people are only apparent.
Ummet (Ummah):	the community of believers or Muslims.
Unani tradition:	a codified system of health traditions in the Indian subcontinent similar to Ayurveda and Siddha.

Universalism: a universal range of knowledge, interests, or activities. The belief that all people hold the same values and use the same ethical ideals.

Utilitarianism: a consequential and a teleological theory with central emphasis on the greatest happiness of the greatest number.

Xenophobia: an unreasonable fear or hatred of foreigners or strangers or of that which is foreign or strange.

Index